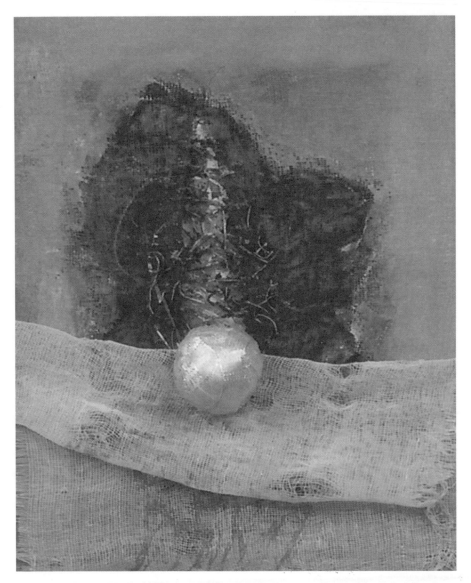

*"Birth"*                    *Danièle M. Marín*

Private Collection

# Mitochondria and the Heart

# Developments in Cardiovascular Medicine

**Previous volumes are still available**

# Mitochondria and the Heart

Edited by

## José Marín-García
The Molecular Cardiology and Neuromuscular Institute,
Highland Park, New Jersey
Department of Physiology & Biophysics,
UMDNJ-Robert Wood Johnson Medical School
Piscataway, New Jersey

With the collaboration of
**Michael J Goldenthal**
The Molecular Cardiology Institute,
Highland Park, New Jersey

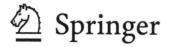 Springer

JosÈ MarÌn-GarcÌa
The Molecular Cardiology and Neuromuscular Institute
Highland Park, New Jersey
Department of Physiology & Biophysics
UMDNJ-Robert Wood Johnson Medical School
Piscataway, New Jersey

Library of Congress Cataloging-in-Publication Data

A C.I.P. Catalogue record for this book is available
from the Library of Congress.

ISBN -10 0-387-25574-5          e-ISBN 0-387-25575-3
ISBN -13 978-0387-25574-3       e-ISBN 978-0387-25575-0
Printed on acid-free paper.

Printed in the United States of America.

9  8  7  6  5  4  3  2  1          SPIN  11055679

springeronline.com

# Dedication

*This book is dedicated to my wife, Danièle, and daughter, Mèlanie, with love*

# Contents

## 1. An Introduction to Mitochondria and the Heart 1

## 2. Mitochondrial Bioenergetics in the Heart    27

# 7. Fatty Acid and Glucose Metabolism in Cardiac Disease                    197

# 8. Mitochondria in Pediatric Cardiology          229

# 9. Mitochondria and the Aging Heart                263

# 10. Heart Mitochondria Signaling
#      Pathways                                        289

## 11. Treatment of Mitochondrial-Based Cardiac Diseases: Targeting the Organelle                                           323

# Preface

Mitochondria have been pivotal in the development of some of the most important ideas in modern biology. Since the discovery that the organelle has its own DNA and specific mutations were found in association with neuromuscular and cardiovascular diseases and with aging, an extraordi-nary number of publications have followed, and the term *mitochondrial medicine* was coined. Furthermore, our understanding of the multiple roles that mitochondria play in cardiac cell homeostasis opened the door for intensive experimentation to understand the pathogenesis and to find new treatments for cardiovascular diseases.

Besides its role in adenosine triphosphate generation, mitochondria regu-late a complex network of cellular interactions, involving (1) generation and detoxification of reactive oxygen species, including superoxide anion, hy-drogen peroxide, and hydroxyl radical; (2) maintenance of the antioxidant glutathione in a reduced state and adequate level of mitochondrial matrix superoxide dismutase; (3) cytoplasmic calcium homeostasis, particularly under conditions of cellular calcium loading; (4) transport of metabolites between cytoplasm and matrix; (5) both programmed (apoptosis) and necrotic cell death; and (6) cell growth and development. It is therefore not surprising that this organelle has come to be the center stage in many current investigations of cardiovascular diseases, aging, and aging-related disease. Concomitant with these advances, an impressive effort is under- way for the development of new tools and methodologies to study mitochondrial structure and function, including powerful ways to visualize, monitor, and alter the organelle function to assess the genetic consequences of these perturbations.

Because the heart is highly dependent for its function on oxidative energy that is generated in mitochondria—primarily by fatty acid $\beta$-oxidation, respiratory electron chain, and oxidative phosphorylation (OXPHOS)—it is understandable that defects in mitochondrial structure and function can be found in association with cardiovascular diseases.

Abnormalities in the organelle structure and function are being increas-ingly reported in association with conditions such as dilated and hypertro-phic cardiomyopathy, cardiac conduction defects and sudden death, ischemic and alcoholic cardiomyopathy, myocarditis, and neuromuscular diseases associated with cardiac disease and aging. Some of the mitochondrial abnormalities may have a genetic basis (e.g., mitochondrial DNA changes might lead to abnormal OXPHOS, and fatty acid oxidation defects might be due to specific nuclear DNA mutations), while other abnormalities may be due to a more sporadic or environmental cardiotoxic insult or may not yet be characterized.

To understand the role that mitochondria play in cardiovascular disease, we discuss the biogenesis and function of cardiac mitochondria during normal growth, development, and aging. Within this context, we then examine the interaction and characterization of mitochondria and mitochondrial abnormalities in cardiac diseases, their diagnosis, therapeutic options currently available, future directions for research, and new frontiers in treatment. While aberrations in the bioenergetic function of the mitochondria are frequently related to cardiac dysfunction, the specific defect causing the bioenergetic abnormalities often resides in a nonbioenergetic pathway (e.g., signaling between the mitochondria and nucleus) or in the overall mitochondrial biogenesis or degradation pathways. Understanding these pathways and the effects that mitochondrial defects have in cardiac pathology is extremely important in establishing the diagnosis and treatment of mitochondrial-based cardiac diseases.

As mitochondria's role in the field of cardiology is strengthened and as research on the multiple functions of this organelle continues its expansion, the time seems appropriate for a book that may integrate known facts, what is developing and what will be known in the near future. In addition to providing a recount of past discoveries, the book deals with areas that are of emerging interest to researchers and clinicians, eyeing potential alternatives that may improve currently available therapies and interventions in the management of cardiovascular diseases in general and the cardiovascular pathology of aging in particular.

It is hoped that this work will further advance the field of mitochondrial medicine.


"New discoveries, fragments of the past, parts of the future."

**José Marín-García**

*Highland Park, New Jersey*

# Chapter 1

# An Introduction to Mitochondria and the Heart

## Overview

This introductory chapter to mitochondria and the heart describes mitochondria and their components, their multiple functions (including their pathology in cardiovascular diseases), and briefly their role in myocardial ischemia/cardioprotection, apoptosis/cell death, and currently available animal models of mitochondrial-based cardiac defects. Most of these subjects merit a more comprehensive discussion and have chapters dedicated to them.

## *What are mitochondria?*

Mitochondria, the powerhouse of the cell, are double-membraned organelles located in the cytoplasm, and their primary cellular role is the generation of bioenergy.

   The components of the mitochondria (Figure 1.1) include a compact mitochondrial genome and their own class of ribosomes. Structural, regulatory, and functional proteins are involved in a variety of tasks that range from enzymatic constituents of bioenergetic pathways —e.g., oxidative phosphorylation (OXPHOS) and respiration, the tricarboxylic acid (TCA) cycle, fatty acid oxidation (FAO); substrate, ion, and nucleotide transport membrane channels; biosynthesis of mitochondrial components e.g., mitochondrial RNA and DNA (mtDNA); the import and assembly of the various protein complexes; and critical elements that are involved in intercellular communication and cell-death pathways (e.g., redox signaling and apoptotic progression).

   While most biological membranes have approximately a 50:50 ratio of protein to lipid, the inner mitochondrial membrane is somewhat exceptional because it exhibits a ratio of 75:25, which is indicative of more densely packed proteins. In cardiac tissue, the anionic phospho-

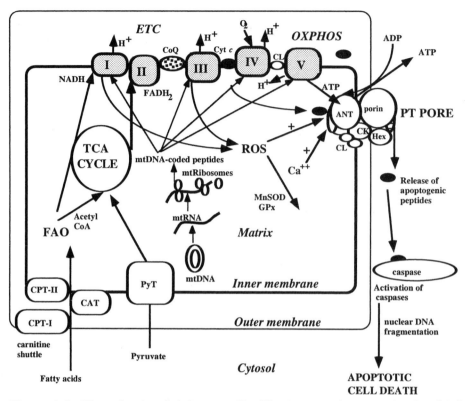

**Figure 1.1. The mitochondrial organelle.** *The inner and outer mitochondrial membranes have numerous points of contact (termed contact sites) and contain a large assortment of integral and peripheral proteins as well as numerous phospholipids. The electron transport chain (ETC) is composed of inner-membrane localized respiratory complexes I–V with associated electron-transfer components, coenzyme Q (CoQ) and cytochrome c (cytc) as shown. Also shown are the matrix associated pyruvate oxidation, fatty acid β-oxidation (FAO), and the TCA cycle pathways. The apoptosis-associated mitochondrial permeability transition (PT) pore is shown including key components such as the adenine nucleotide translocator (ANT), porin, mitochondrial creatine kinase (CK), hexokinase (HEX) and the inner membrane phospholipid, cardiolipin (CL). The release of apoptogenic peptides (e.g., cyt c) from mitochondria precedes caspase activation, leading to apoptotic cell death. Also depicted is the carnitine shuttle pathway for the mitchondrial import of fatty acids including carnitine palmitoyltransferases (CPT-I and CPT-II) and carnitine translocase (CAT), as is the pyruvate transporter (PyT). The generation of ROS from mitochondrial ETC is depicted as are the mitochondrial antioxidants superoxide dismutase (MnSOD) and glutathione peroxidase (GPx). The mtDNA is shown with transcripts( mtRNA) which are translated on mitochondrial ribosomes( mtribosomes) forming peptide subunits of complex I,III, IV, and V.*

lipid, cardiolipin, is particularly prevalent in the mitochondrial inner membrane and at the contact sites. Pores in the outer membrane facilitate the transport of most small molecules (< 5000 kDa) in and out of the mitochondria and are composed primarily of the abundant protein, porin.The inner membrane contains the components of the mitochondrial respiratory electron transport chain (ETC), OXPHOS, and adenine nucleotide transport (ANT). Because the proton and electron flux are located in the inner mitochondrial membrane, the organelle is primarily responsible for the electrochemical potential gradient associated with ATP synthesis and its coupling with electron transport. The inner membrane forms highly folded lamellar structures that are termed *cristae* and that extend the surface area of the inner membrane to within the matrix; the number of cristae sharply increases in highly respiratory-active cardiomyocytes (i.e., threefold more than found in hepatocytes).

The matrix compartment enclosed within the inner membrane contains the mtDNA, ribosomes, transfer, and ribosomal RNAs as well as a multitude of enzymes required for the oxidation of pyruvate, fatty acids, and TCA cycle metabolites.

The number and morphology of mitochondria within the cardiomyocyte can change as a function of diverse physiological stimuli (e.g., exercise, hormones/cytokines, electrical stimulation, etc.), the stage in cardiac development and pathophysiological insult (e.g., cardiac hypertrophy). The population of mitochondria in the cardiomyocytes is controlled by autophagy, a process by which lysosomes regulate the different cellular components.

Under some conditions, more than 1,000 mitochondria can be present in a cardiomyocyte. Typically distributed in a uniform fashion along the entire length of the myofibrillar apparatus (Figure 1.2), they have variable shapes that are likely related to the extent of mitochondrial fusion and division. Mitochondria are involved in cardiac contraction to provide a constant supply of ATP to the sarcomeres. Information concerning the movement of mitochondria within the cardiac cell and its regulation is currently limited; however, it is possible that cardiac mitochondrial movement is mediated by both actin myofilaments and microtubules as has been demonstrated with neural cells [1].

## *How to study mitochondria: New and old*

The *in vitro* growth, culturing, and passaging of cardiomyocytes derived from either neonates or adults have furnished highly informa-

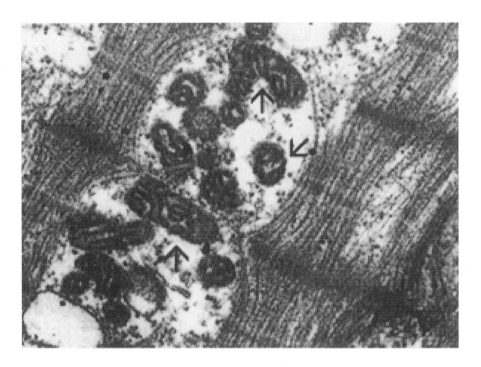

**Figure 1.2. Mitochondria of different shapes (arrows) are distributed along myofibers.**

tive models to study cardiomyocyte phenotype, molecular and biochemical events in response to physiological stresses, the addition and deletion of specific genes, and pharmacological treatments. Moreover, cardiomyocyte culture has proven to be a convenient system for examining rapid signaling changes in membrane channels, mitochondria, transducing kinases, and the receptors associated with myocardial hypertrophy, hypoxia, and apoptosis. In addition, recently developed cardiac myocyte cell lines have provided researchers the opportunity to evaluate the expression of several transcription factors associated with early cardiac development.

Over the last decade, great advances have been made in cytochemical techniques for evaluating mitochondria, both at the ultrastructural and functional levels, including the use of fluorescent dyes. The development of fluorescent imaging technology is improving our ability to measure precisely levels of specific ions and metabolites in the mitochondrial organelle of living cells as well as its subcompartments, such as the mitochondrial matrix. For example, by specifically targeting the $Ca^{++}$ probe aequorin (a $Ca^{++}$ binding photo-protein) to the mitochondrial matrix, free mitochondrial $Ca^{++}$ levels can be determined [2]. A variety of fluorescent probes and potentiometric dyes (listed in Table 1.1) have been used increasingly to evaluate quantitatively overall cardiomyocyte mitochondrial number, membrane potential, oxidative stress and $Ca^{++}$ levels [3–8].

**Table 1.1. Fluorescent dyes**

| Fluorescent Dye | To evaluate | Reference |
|---|---|---|
| Mitotracker green | Mitochondrial number | [8] |
| JC-1 | Membrane potential | [5] |
| CMX-Ros | Membrane potential | [4] |
| Fura-2 | $Ca^{++}$ levels | [7] |
| Dihydrorhodamine 123 | Oxidative stress | [6] |

Other techniques that are available include the fractionation and iso-lation of mitochondria and their membrane-bound subcomparments by differential centrifugation to recover specific membrane fractions; the identification of specific markers of mitochondria and potentially contaminating subcellular organelles (e.g., ER, lysosomes); the devel-opment and availability of a large armamentarium of specific anti-bodies to mitochondrial proteins for use in both immunocytochemical analysis and western immunoblot analysis; easily accessed and updated databases with molecular information to furnish specific probes for molecular genetic and gene expression analysis; a variety of amplification and mutation detection techniques to screen for maternally inherited mtDNA point mutations and Mendelian inherited nuclear DNA mutations; quantitatively accessing large-scale mtDNA deletions; gauging mitochondrial copy number; and improved techniques for the analysis of mtDNA damage. Several excellent books containing updated methods are commercially available.

A recent and critical development in mitochondrial methodology involves the use of cell hybrids (cybrids) to study the effects of specific mutations on mitochondrial function. The development of cultured mammalian cells that lack mtDNA due to growth in low concentrations of ethidium bromide was pivotal in the development of the cybrid technique [9–10] These cells are comparable to yeast petite cells that lack mtDNA and are similarly termed *rho⁰* cells. These cells lack mtDNA, exhibit defective respiration, and adopt an anaerobic phenotype. Cytoplasts containing mitochondria can be prepared from a wide variety of enucleated cells (e.g., platelets and fibroblasts) and fused with *rho*⁰ cells lacking mtDNA to form cybrids, essentially changing the combination of nucleus and mitochondria. Cybrids containing normal mitochondria regain functional respiration, manifest an aerobic phenotype, and can be readily distinguished from cybrids with defective mitochondria. Cybrids can be maintained in culture using the appropriate media supplementation and have been successfully employed to study nuclear-cytoplasmic interactions, as well as the effects of specific mitochondrial mutations in different nuclear backgrounds.

## Mitochondrial bioenergetics

Mitochondria are abundant in energy-demanding cardiac tissue constituting 20% to 40% of cellular volume. Mitochondrial energy production depends on both nuclear and mtDNA-encoded genetic factors that modulate normal mitochondrial function (including enzyme activity and cofactor availability) and on environmental factors (including substrate availability—such as sugars, fats, and proteins— and oxygen). Several interacting bioenergetic pathways contribute to mitochondrial energy metabolism (shown in Figure 1.1), including pyruvate oxidation, the TCA cycle, the β-oxidation of fatty acids, and the common final pathway, OXPHOS, which generates approximately 80% of cellular ATP. OXPHOS is performed by complexes of proteins located at the mitochondrial inner membrane, including the respiratory ETC complexes I–IV, ATP synthase (complex V), and the adenine nucleotide translocator (ANT). Fatty acids are the primary energy substrate for ATP production by OXPHOS in postnatal and adult cardiac muscle. To be fully utilized for bioenergetic production via mitochondrial fatty acid β-oxidation, fatty acids need to be effectively transported into the cardiomyocyte and subsequently into the mitochondria, a process requiring several transport proteins including the carnitine shuttle (carnitine acyltransferase and two carnitine palmitoyltransferases as well as carnitine). Fatty acid β-oxidation and the oxidation of carbohydrates via the TCA cycle generate the majority of intramitochondrial NADH and FADH$_2$, the direct source of electrons for ETC/OXPHOS. The supply of ATP from other sources (e.g., glycolytic metabolism) is limited in normal cardiac tissue. In addition to these bioenergetic pathways and metabolic intermediates, the heart also maintains stored high-energy phosphates (e.g., phosphocreatine) produced by mitochondrial creatine kinase using ATP from closely associated ANT and mitochondrial ATP synthase.

## Mitochondrial biogenesis

Human mitochondria have their own double-stranded circular DNA encoding 13 protein components of 4 of the enzyme complexes (i.e., I, III, IV, and V) involved in electron transport and OXPHOS. These protein-encoding mtDNA genes are transcribed into specific mRNAs that are translated on mitochondrial specific ribosomes. The mtDNA also encodes part of the mitochondrial protein synthesis machinery, including 2 ribosomal RNAs (rRNA) and 22 transfer RNAs (tRNA), as shown in Figure 1.3 [11].

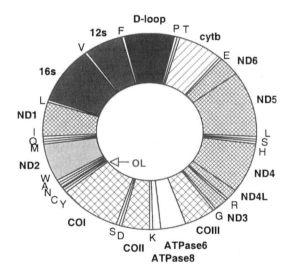

**Figure 1.3. Human mitochondrial double-stranded circular DNA.** *This circular DNA encodes 13 protein components of 4 of the 5 enzyme complexes involved in electron transport and OXPHOS, two rRNAs (12S and 16S), and 22 tRNAs, as shown. The noncoding D-loop region is also shown.*

In general, the cardiomyocyte contains multiple mitochondria (50 to 100 per cell) and each mitochondrion contains multiple copies of mtDNA (1 to 10 copies per mitochondrion).

Pathogenic point mutations and large-scale deletions in mtDNA as well as generalized depletion of mtDNA levels have severe consequences for organs such as the heart, since ATP derived from OXPHOS is needed to maintain myocardial contractility. The nuclear genome encodes the entire complement of proteins involved in mtDNA replication and transcription, protein components of mitochondrial ribosomes, multiple structural and transport proteins of the mitochondrial membranes, and remaining peptide subunits of the respiratory complexes. Synthesized on cytosolic ribosomes, these nuclear-encoded proteins are targeted to mitochondria and imported by a complex but well characterized process involving signal peptide recognition, membrane receptors, proteases, and an array of molecular chaperones. Cardiac-specific regulation of a number of the nuclear genes encoding OXPHOS proteins can be mediated by variable gene expression sensitive to a number of physiological and developmental stimuli and by the presence of tissue-specific isoforms for specific peptides. Therefore, mutations in nuclear genes involved in mitochondrial biogenesis might be expected to contribute to the observed mitochondrial cardiac enzyme and mtDNA defects, including an increased incidence of large-scale mtDNA deletions and mtDNA depletion associated with cardiac disorders. However, thus far only a limited number of mutations have been identified in nuclear genes affecting mitochondrial biogenesis and leading to cardiac disorders. While the nuclear genome controls mitochondrial biosynthesis, mtDNA genes have a much higher mutation rate because of a lack of histones, limited DNA repair, and exposure to reactive oxygen species (ROS) generated by the ETC. Nevertheless, the search for mutations in both nuclear and mitochondrial genomes as well as mutations that affect the cross-talk between the genomes is presently expanding.

Cardiac mitochondrial biogenesis is increased during myocardial hypertrophy, treatment with a variety of agents (e.g., thyroxin and xenobiotics), electrical stimulation, and exercise [12], but the molecular mechanisms that regulate cardiac-specific mtDNA levels and overall mitochondrial number are not known [13].

## Cardiac mitochondrial changes during cardiac growth and development

Variations in mitochondrial substrate utilization, enzyme and membrane activities, growth program, and gene expression occur during the course of cardiac development and in aging, and they reflect changes in cardiac function [14]. Moreover, the role (and demand) for ATP production is clearly modulated during cardiac development as well as during physiological transitions and perturbations.

Among the multiple metabolic changes that occur in cardiac muscle with advancing age are modifications in membrane fatty acid and lipid composition, including increased levels of saturated fatty acids and decreased levels of polyunsaturated fatty acids and cardiolipin [15–16]. Cardiolipin, the most unsaturated cellular phospholipid, is a major component of the mitochondrial inner membrane; plays an intrinsic role in cardiac mitochondrial membrane transport function, fluidity, and stability; and is a facilitator of key mitochondrial inner membrane bioenergetic enzymes. In addition, marked reductions in carnitine and acetylcarnitine levels have also been reported in the aging heart.

A by-product of mitochondrial bioenergetic activity is generation of ROS, including superoxide, hydroxyl radicals, and hydrogen peroxide ($H_2O_2$) [17]. Side reactions of the mitochondrial ETC with molecular oxygen directly generate the superoxide anion radical. Superoxide radicals can be converted to $H_2O_2$ (in the presence of the enzyme superoxide dismutase), which can further react to form the hydroxyl radical. Normally, these toxic by-products, which are powerful cell-damaging oxidants, are neutralized by antioxidant enzymes, some of which are found in the mitochondria (e.g., manganese superoxide dismutase [MnSOD] and glutathione peroxidase) and others of which are found in the cytosol (e.g., CuSOD or catalase) or are scavenged by glutathione. Increased generation of ROS occurs during aging and can also result from myocardial ischemia/reperfusion, inflammation, and impaired antioxidant defenses. This may cause profound effects on cardiac cells, including increased peroxidative damage effecting primarily the membrane phospholipids and proteins. Oxidative damage also targets nucleic acids (particularly mtDNA), causing induction of strand breaks, base modifications and subsequently, point mutations, and deletions [18].

# Mitochondria: The primary site of ROS generation, and also a critical target of its damaging effects

The mitochondrial respiratory chain, located in the inner membrane, is often damaged, resulting in further increase in ROS generation and leading to a vicious cycle of diminished mitochondrial function. In addition to the well characterized cell-damaging effects of ROS, mitochondrial ROS generation and oxidative stress are recognized as having important regulatory functions. Oxidative species (e.g., $H_2O_2$) can function as a potent signal sent from mitochondria to other cellular sites rapidly and reversibly, eliciting an array of intracellular cascades that lead to different physiological end-points for the cardiomyocyte (e.g., apoptosis, necrosis, cardioprotection, and cell proliferation).

## Mitochondrial dysfunction in cardiovascular disease

### *Defects in mtDNA*

Discrete mitochondrial OXPHOS defects or respiratory chain enzyme activity deficiency have been documented in both dilated (DCM) and hypertrophic (HCM) cardiomyopathies [19–20]. In addition, cardiomyopathy can present with specific pathogenic mtDNA point mutations. Pathogenic mtDNA mutations are generally located in nucleotides that are highly conserved in evolution, usually accompanied by reduced levels of myocardial specific respiratory enzyme activity, and frequently present in heteroplasmic fashion (a mixed population of both mutant and wildtype mtDNA genomes) [21–23], albeit recent data suggest that certain pathogenic mtDNA mutations can also be homoplasmic [24].

Mutations in a number of mitochondrial tRNA genes have been detected in association with cardiomyopathy. Specific tRNA genes including Leu, Ile, and Lys appear to be hot spots for mutations in cardiomyopathic patients. In patients with either HCM or DCM, mutations at other mtDNA loci have also been identified (e.g., other tRNAs, rRNA, and in a variety of mtDNA protein-encoding genes). In addition, multisystemic mitochondrial diseases with a wide spectrum of clinical manifestations, which include cardiomyopathy, have been reported with pathogenic mtDNA mutations. These disorders, including Leigh, MELAS (mitochondrial encephalomyopathy with lactic acidosis and strokelike episodes) and MERRF (myoclonic epilepsy with ragged red fibers) syndromes are maternally inherited and often present with a variable cardiac phenotype and a range of neurological symptoms [21]. Specific mtDNA mutations found in association with primary cardiomyopathy can also be present in patients with different combinations of clinical phenotypes. The variability between mitochondrial genotype and phenotype may be related to the involvement of unidentified genetic or environmental cofactor(s) capable of modulating the effect of mtDNA mutations. Similarly, specific phenotype(s) may be caused by a variety of different nuclear and/or mtDNA mutations. For example, Leigh syndrome can be caused by mutations in ATPase-6 subunit [25], point mutation in mitochondrial tRNA$^{Lys}$ gene [26], nuclear DNA mutations in pyruvate dehydrogenase [27], nuclear-encoded complex II subunits [28], or mtDNA depletion [29].

Sporadic large-scale rearrangements of mtDNA can also be associated with cardiac disorders. In Kearns-Sayre syndrome (KSS), cardiac conduction abnormalities typically coexist with somatic large-scale mtDNA deletions [30–31]. The majority of mtDNA deletions in KSS are of a single type; they are not inherited and are mainly detected in skeletal muscle and rarely in blood. In contrast, a multiple mtDNA deletion phenotype associated with DCM may result from genetic defects in unidentified autosomal nuclear loci that can be either dominantly or recessively inherited [32–33]. The mtDNA deletions detected in KSS and in the autosomal disorders tend to be abundant compared to the less abundant, large-scale mtDNA deletions revealed by polymerase chain reaction (PCR) amplification in cardiac tissues of many primary cardiomyopathies [34]. These less abundant deletions reflect specific mtDNA damage (probably as a consequence of ROS) and often occur in an age-dependent manner; however, their role in cardiac pathogenesis is unclear.

Depletion in cardiac mtDNA levels has also been reported in patients with isolated cardiomyopathy, either DCM or HCM [35–36], and also can be induced by drugs such as zidovudine (AZT) and adriamycin (doxorubicin) [37–38].

## *Defects in nuclear DNA-encoded mitochondrial proteins*

Mutations in a wide array of nuclear genes encoding mitochondrial proteins can also cause cardiomyopathy. For example, cardiomyopathy may occur as a consequence of mutations in mitochondrial transport proteins that facilitate the passage of critical metabolites across the inner mitochondrial membrane. Mutations in a mitochondrial transport protein, frataxin, which is involved in mitochondrial iron accumulation, cause Friedreich ataxia (FRDA) with HCM [39]. Moreover, mutations in nuclear genes encoding factors required for the assembly and functioning of the multiple-subunit respiratory complexes have been implicated in some mitochondrial-based diseases such as Leigh syndrome. Mutations in the $SCO_2$ gene encoding a copper chaperone that takes part in complex IV assembly can result in cardiomyopathy [40].

Cardiomyopathy may also be a primary manifestation of several inherited disorders of mitochondrial FAO [41]. Deficiencies in very long-chain acyl-CoA dehydrogenase (VLCAD) [42], long-chain 3-hydroxylacyl-CoA dehydrogenase (LCHAD) [43], short-chain acyl-CoA dehydrogenase (SCAD) [44], and the mitochondrial trifunctional protein (MTP) [45] have been reported to cause cardiomyopathy in young children. Also, defects in carnitine transport into cells and in the carnitine-acylcarnitine shuttle, which is responsible for fatty acid transport into mitochondria, can be associated with cardiomyopathy [46]. The cardiac pathogenesis of these inherited disorders of fatty acid β-oxidation and carnitine metabolism likely includes both a deficient bioenergetic supply to the heart and the accumulation of toxic levels of fatty free acids with subsequent cardiac dysfunction. These disorders primarily occur in early childhood and are usually precipitated by infectious illness or fasting when the heart has increased dependence on FAO for energy. Many of the inherited FAO disorders described above can result in sudden neonatal death [41].

Cardiac conduction defects also occur in patients with specific defects in FAO [47]. Both ventricular and atrial arrhythmias are associated with deficiencies in CPT-II, carnitine translocase, and MTP activities.

Long-chain acylcarnitines possess detergent-like properties and accumulation can extensively modify membrane proteins and lipids with toxic effects on cardiac membrane electrophysiological functions, including ion transport and gap-junction channel activity

[48–49]. Moreover, the accumulation of long-chain fatty acid metabolites plays a pivotal role in the production of ventricular arrhythmias occurring during myocardial ischemia.

Arrhythmias, cardiac failure, and severe DCM with abnormal mitochondria are also common features of Barth syndrome, an X-linked disorder also characterized by cyclic neutropenia and neonatal onset [50–51]. The protein tafazzin responsible for Barth syndrome is encoded by the G4.5 gene and likely belongs to a family of acyltransferases involved in phospholipid synthesis. Its defect results in cardiolipin depletion [52].

## *Myocardial ischemia and ETC*

When the supply of $O_2$ becomes limited (as occurs with myocardial ischemia, OXPHOS and mitochondrial ETC flux decline), creatine phosphate is rapidly depleted, fatty acid and pyruvate oxidation decrease, and ATP production is impaired. The increased hydrolysis of ATP and accumulation of lactate lead to lower intracellular pH and intracellular acidosis, with a direct inhibitory effect on cardiac contractile function. In addition, myocardial ischemia results in reduced activity levels of respiratory complex IV and V and increased levels of mtDNA deletions [53–56]. Sustained ischemia will lead to ATP depletion and finally to necrotic cell death.

Paradoxically, functional mitochondria can exacerbate ischemic damage, especially at the onset of reperfusion. Increased OXPHOS causes increased ROS accumulation with increased lipid peroxidation; this results in lower cardiolipin levels in the inner membrane with consequent effect on complex IV activity [57]. Reperfusion injury mediates an increased opening of the permeability transition (PT) pore, a dynamic megachannel located at contact sites between the mitochondrial inner and outer membranes, which can result in subsequent triggering of apoptotic cell death [58].

As discussed more comprehensively in Chapter 5, a cardioprotective mechanism can be elicited by ischemic preconditioning (IPC) with short bouts of ischemia applied prior to a more prolonged ischemic insult [59–61]. This cardioprotective effect may be mediated by improved ATP production, lowered $Ca^{++}$ overloading in the mitchondrial matrix, and increased ROS generation leading to protein kinase C activation and has been proposed to involve the opening of mitochondrial ATP-sensitive $K_{ATP}$ (mito$K_{ATP}$) and PT pore channels

[62–66]. Several drugs that specifically activate the mitoK$_{ATP}$ channel opening (e.g., diazoxide, nicorandil) mimic ischemic preconditioning [67–68]. Evidence for mitoK$_{ATP}$ channels as effectors of myocardial preconditioning has also been demonstrated in human subjects [69].

## Apoptosis and cell death

Apoptosis (programmed cell death) leading to cardiac cell loss and to extensive left ventricular remodeling has been shown to occur in cardiac failure both in patients with DCM and in animal models. Mitochondria play a pivotal role in the early events of apoptosis. A central outcome in the mitochondrial apoptotic pathway is the release from the intermembrane space into the cytosol of a group of proteins (e.g., cytochrome *c*, Smac, AIF, and endonuclease G) that subsequently triggers a cascade of cytoplasmic changes depicted in Figure 1.1 [70-72]. These apoptogenic mitochondrial proteins form an apoptosome complex on release in the cytosol and are involved in the subsequent activation of downstream cysteine-aspartate proteases (caspases) initiating cell self-digestion and nuclear DNA fragmentation by endonucleases, and leading to apoptotic cell death [73]. The release of the mitochondrial intermembrane peptides occurs primarily as a result of outer membrane permeabilization regulated by the complex interactions of different members of the Bcl-2 family, including Bax, Bid, Bcl-2, and Bcl-X (L) [74]. Proapoptotic membrane-binding proteins (e.g., Bax, Bid, and Bad), translocated from the cytosol to mitochondria, potentiate cytochrome *c* release, whereas antiapoptotic proteins antagonize this event. The release of these proteins is also associated and potentially regulated by the opening of the PT pore, a critical early step of apoptosis preceding the caspase cascade [75]. PT pore opening is promoted by elevated Ca$^{++}$ influx into mitochondria, excessive mitochondrial ROS production, prooxidants, fatty acids, and nitric oxide [73]. PT pore opening is also accompanied by the dissipation of the mitochondrial membrane potential and depolarization. Changes in membrane potential can be either a cause or the result of PT pore opening, since extensive proton influx occurs at this site. There is a continual dynamic in the balance of the proapoptotic proteins (e.g., Bax) and antiapoptotic Bcl-2 factors in modulating the progression of the apoptotic events within the mitochondria.

The PT pore may be a site where mitochondria can integrate multiple cell-signaling stimuli and metabolic responses. Because apoptosis requires energy, the shutdown of OXPHOS either leading or following the PT pore opening is not complete since complete mitochondrial deenergization does not favor apoptosis but rather leads to necrotic cell death [76]. Opening of the PT pore during apoptosis is transient, allowing mitochondria to maintain the ATP levels necessary for fueling the downstream apoptotic responses. It should not be surprising that the early apoptotic events involve the modulation of ATP levels, given the close proximity of the PT pore to the respiratory complexes in the mitochondrial inner membrane as well as its involvement in the mitochondrial loss of cytochrome *c*, a critical molecule in ETC function. Also present at the PT pore site are a number of energy-associated mitochondrial molecules, including ANT, the glycolytic enzyme hexokinase, the outer membrane, voltage-dependent anion channel protein (VDAC or porin), the mitochondrial creatine kinase, and the phospholipid cardiolipin [73, 77].

## Animal models of mitochondrial-associated cardiovascular disease

Gene ablation in mice (i.e., generation of null mutations or gene knockouts) targeting a relatively wide spectrum of nuclear genes encoding mitochondrial proteins results in severe cardiac dysfunction.

Targeted genes include ANT [78], MnSOD [79], factors involved in mitochondrial fatty acid metabolism (e.g., PPAR-α, MTP subunits) [80–81], the mitochondrial transcription factor mtTFA (also termed TFAM) [82], and frataxin [83]. Little information is currently available concerning mtDNA gene ablation since generation of mtDNA gene knockouts presents an especially difficult technical challenge.

The use of cardiac-specific overexpression of specific genes has also been informative in our overall understanding of the role of mitochondria in cardiac dysfunction. Notably, overexpression of a number of nuclear genes that mediate expression and control of cardiac energy metabolism (e.g., PGC-1α, PPAR-α, and TNF-α) can lead to cardiomyopathy with severe cardiac defects and marked changes in mitochondrial structure and function [84–86]. The development of animal models of mitochondrial-based cardiac dysfunction also offers the possibility of direct testing for potential treatments.

## Diagnosis and treatment of mitochondrial-based cardiac diseases

The diagnosis of mitochondrial dysfunction in cardiac disease has emerged largely from clinical studies of endomyocardial biopsies and skeletal muscle using combined histochemical, ultrastructure, OXPHOS, and respiratory enzyme analysis. DNA analysis used to identify specific pathogenic mtDNA mutations, large-scale mtDNA deletions, and evaluation of mtDNA levels can be informative; however, the overall incidence of pathogenic mtDNA mutations is low in patients with cardiac disease, including those with definitive OXPHOS enzymatic defects [87].

Evaluation of fatty acids using a profile of blood-acylcarnitine levels by mass spectroscopy analysis appears to be the most reliable method of assessing a mitochondrial-based FAO metabolic disorder [88–89]. Moreover, biochemical analysis can be used for the determination of levels of other key mitochondrial intermediates, including coenzyme $Q_{10}$, cardiolipin, and carnitine.

Knowledge of the specific molecular and biochemical defect may allow the treatment with metabolic intermediates and vitamins serving as electron donors, transporters, and cofactors for electron transport (e.g., vitamin K, thiamine, ascorbate, and riboflavin), bypassing specific defects in OXPHOS and increasing ATP production [90–91].

Mitochondrial long-chain FAO disorders can be effectively treated with long-term dietary therapy with the replacement of normal dietary fat by medium-chain triglycerides and increased carbohydrates, particularly in the acute cardiomyopathy associated with VLCAD and LCHAD deficiencies [92–93].

## The road ahead

The formation and reintroduction of functioning myocardial cells into damaged myocardium have been achieved with the use of embryonic stem cells derived from blastocyst-stage preembryos [94–95]. More recently, it was demonstrated that a subpopulation of adult cardiac stem cells injected into an ischemic heart was able to fully reconstitute well-differentiated myocardium, differentiating into both cardiomyocytes and new blood vessels [96]. These exciting technologies have numerous potential applications in the treatment of cardiac diseases such as cardiomyopathy by augmentation, regeneration, or replacement of defective cardiomyocytes. They may also be employed in pharmacological testing of cardiotoxic compounds.

The applied use of gene therapy for mtDNA-encoded OXPHOS defects awaits the development of an effective methodology for mitochondrial gene replacement in human cells. Toward this end, various approaches utilizing signal peptide-targeting sequences covalently attached to mitochondrial oligonucleotides have been introduced into the mitochondria of living cells [97–98]. This strategy of mitochondrial transfection can be combined with an antisense approach targeting the expression of defective mitochondrial alleles in the patient's tissue and may prove successful in the treatment of cardiac disorders due to defined mtDNA point mutations.

## References

1.  Morris RL, Hollenbeck PJ (1995) Axonal transport of mitochondria along microtubules and F-actin in living vertebrate neurons. J Cell Biol 131:1315–26

2.  Rizzuto R, Pinton P, Carrington W, Fay FS, Fogarty KE, Lifshitz LM, Tuft RA, Pozzan T (1998) Close contacts with the endoplasmic reticulum as determinants of mitochondrial Ca2+ responses. Science 280:1763–6

3.  Duchen MR, Surin A, Jacobson J (2003) Imaging mitochondrial function in intact cells. Methods Enzymol 361:353–89

4.  Poot M, Zhang YZ, Kramer JA, Wells KS, Jones LJ, Hanzel DK, Lugade AG, Singer VL, Haugland RP (1996) Analysis of mitochondrial morphology and function with novel fixable fluorescent stains. J Histochem Cytochem 44:1363–72

5.  Reers M, Smiley ST, Mottola-Hartshorn C, Chen A, Lin M, Chen LB (1995) Mitochondrial membrane potential monitored by JC-1 dye. Methods Enzymol 260:406–17

6. Mathur A, Hong Y, Kemp BK, Barrientos AA, Erusalimsky JD (2000) Evaluation of fluorescent dyes for the detection of mitochondrial membrane potential changes in cultured cardiomyocytes. Cardiovasc Res 46:126–38

7. Malgaroli A, Milani D, Meldolesi J, Pozzan T (1987) Fura-2 measurement of cytosolic free Ca2+ in monolayers and suspensions of various types of animal cells. J Cell Biol 105: 2145–55

8. Bowser DN, Minamikawa T, Nagley P, Williams DA (1998) Role of mitochondria in calcium regulation of spontaneously contracting cardiac muscle cells. Biophys J 75:2004–14

9. King MP, Attardi G (1989) Human cells lacking mtDNA: Repopulation with exogenous mitochondria by complementation. Science 246:500–3

10. Chomyn A, Meola G, Bresolin N, Lai ST, Scarlato G, Attardi G (1991) In vitro genetic transfer of protein synthesis and respiration defects to mitochondrial DNA-less cells with myopathy-patient mitochondria. Mol Cell Biol 11:2236–44

11. Anderson S, Bankier AT, Barrell BG, De Bruijn MHL, Coulson AR, Drouin J, Eperon IC, Nierlich DP, Roe BA, Sanger F, Schreier PH, Smith AJ, Staden R, Young IG (1981) Sequence and organization of human mitochondrial genome. Nature 290:457–65

12. Attardi G, Schatz G (1988) Biogenesis of mitochondria. Annu Rev Cell Biol 4:289–333

13. Shadel GS, Clayton DA (1997) Mitochondrial DNA maintenance in vertebrates. Annu Rev Biochem 66:409–35

14. Lopaschuk GD, Collins-Nakai RL, Itoi T (1992) Developmental changes in energy substrate use by the heart. Cardiovasc Res 26:1172–80

15. Paradies G, Ruggiero FM (1990) Age-related changes in the activity of the pyruvate carrier and in the lipid composition in rat-heart mitochondria. Biochim Biophys Acta 1016:207–21

16. McMillin JB, Taffet GE, Taegtmeyer H, Hudson EK, Tate CA (1993) Mitochondrial metabolism and substrate competition in the aging Fischer rat heart. Cardiovasc Res 27:2222–8

17. Raha S, Robinson BH (2000) Mitochondria, oxygen free radicals, disease and ageing. Trends Biochem Sci 25:502–8

18. Ames BN, Shigenaga MK, Hagen TM (1995) Mitochondrial decay in aging. Biochim Biophys Acta 1272:165–70

19. Rustin P, Lebidois J, Chretien D, Bourgeron T, Piechaud JF, Rotig A, Munnich A, Sidi D (1994) Endomyocardial biopsies for early detection of mitochondrial disorders in hypertrophic cardiomyopathies. J Pediatr 124:224–8

20. Marín-García J, Goldenthal MJ, Pierpont ME, Ananthakrishnan R. (1995) Impaired mitochondrial function in idiopathic dilated cardiomyopathy: Biochemical and molecular analysis. J Card Fail 1:285–91

21. Schon EA, Bonilla E, DiMauro S (1997) Mitochondrial DNA mutations and pathogenesis. J Bioenerg Biomembr 29:131–49

22. Marín-García J, Goldenthal MJ (2002) Understanding the impact of mitochondrial defects in cardiovascular disease: A review. J Card Fail 8:347–61

23. Shoffner JM, Wallace DC (1992) Heart disease and mitochondrial DNA mutations. Heart Dis Stroke 1:235–41

24. McFarland R, Clark KM, Morris AA, Taylor RW, Macphail S, Lightowlers RN, Turnbull DM (2002) Multiple neonatal deaths due to a homoplasmic mitochondrial DNA mutation. Nat Genet 30: 145–6

25. Pastores GM, Santorelli FM, Shanske S, Gelb BD, Fyfe B, Wolfe D, Willner JP (1994) Leigh syndrome and hypertrophic cardiomyopathy in an infant with a mitochondrial point mutation (T8993G). Am J Med Genet 50:265–71

26. Graf WD, Marín-García J, Gao HG, Pizzo S, Naviaux RK, Markusic D, Barshop BA, Courchesne E, Haas RH (2000) Autism associated with the mitochondrial DNA G8363A transfer RNA(Lys)mutation. J Child Neurol 15:357–61

27. Matthews PM, Marchington DR, Squier M, Land J, Brown R, Brown GK (1993) Molecular genetic characterization of an X-linked form of Leigh's syndrome. Ann Neurol 33:652–5

28. Bourgeron T, Rustin P, Chretien D, Birch-Machin M, Bourgeois M, Viegas-Pequignot E, Munnich A, Rotig A (1995) Mutation of a nuclear succinate dehydrogenase gene results in mitochondrial respiratory chain deficiency. Nat Genet 11:144–9

29. Filiano JJ, Goldenthal MJ, Mamourian AC, Hall CC, Marín-García J (2002) Mitochondrial DNA depletion in Leigh syndrome. Pediatr Neurol 26:239–42

30. Holt IJ, Harding AE, Morgan-Hughes JA (1988) Deletions of mtDNA in patients with mitochondrial myopathies. Nature 331:717–9

31. Zeviani M, Moraes CT, DiMauro S, Nakase H, Bonilla E, Schon EA, Rowland LP (1988) Deletions of mitochondrial DNA in Kearns-Sayre syndrome. Neurology 38:1339–4

32. Bohlega S, Tanji K, Santorelli FM, Hirano M, al-Jishi A, DiMauro S (1996) Multiple mitochondrial DNA deletions associated with autosomal recessive ophthalmoplegia and severe cardiomyopathy severe cardiomyopathy. Neurology 46:1329–34

33. Suomalainen A, Paetau A, Leinonen H, Majander A, Peltonen L, Somer H. (1992) Inherited idiopathic dilated cardiomyopathy with multiple deletions of mitochondrial DNA. Lancet 340:1319–20

34. Marín-García J, Goldenthal MJ, Ananthakrishnan R, Pierpont ME, Fricker FJ, Lipshultz S, Perez-Atayde A (1996) Specific mitochondrial DNA deletions in idiopathic dilated cardiomyopathy. Cardiovasc Res 31:306–14

35. Marín-García J, Ananthakrishnan R, Goldenthal MJ, Pierpont ME (2000) Biochemical and molecular basis for mitochondrial cardiomyopathy in neonates and children. J Inherit Metab Dis 23:625–33

36. Poulton J, Sewry C, Potter CG, Bougeron T, Chretien D, Wijberg FA, Morten KJ, Brown G (1995) Variation in mitochondrial DNA levels in muscle from normal controls. Is depletion of mtDNA in patients with mitochondrial myopathy a distinct clinical syndrome. J Inher Metab Dis 18:4–20

37. Lewis W, Dalakas MC (1995) Mitochondrial toxicity of antiviral drugs. Nature Med 1:417–22

38. Serrano J, Palmeira CM, Kuehl DW, Wallace KB (1999) Cardioselective and cumulative oxidation of mitochondrial DNA following subchronic doxorubicin administration. Biochim Biophys Acta 1411:201–5

39. Monros E, Molto MD, Martinez F, Canizares J, Blanca J, Vilchez JJ, Prieto F, de Frutos R, Palau F (1997) Phenotype correlation and intergenerational dynamics of the Friedreich ataxia GAA trinucleotide repeat. Am J Hum Genet 61:101–10

40. Papadopoulou LC, Sue CM, Davidson MM, Tanji K, Nishino I, Sadlock JE, Krishna S, Walker W, Selby J, Glerum DM, Coster RV, Lyon G, Scalais E, Lebel R, Kaplan P, Shanske S, De Vivo DC, Bonilla E, Hirano M, DiMauro S, Schon EA (1999) Fatal infantile cardioencephalomyopathy with COX deficiency and mutations in $SCO_2$, a COX assembly gene. Nat Genet 23:333–7

41. Kelly DP, Strauss AW (1994) Inherited cardiomyopathies. N Eng J Med 330:913–9

42. Strauss AW, Powell CK, Hale DE, Anderson MM, Ahuja A, Brackett JC, Sims HF (1995) Molecular basis of human mitochondriial very-long-chain acyl-CoA dehydrogenase deficiency causing cardiomyopathy and sudden death in childhood. Proc Natl Acad Sci USA 92:10496–500

43. Rocchiccioli F, Wanders RJ, Aubourg P, Vianey-Liaud C, Ijlst L, Fabre M, Cartier N, Bougneres PF (1990) Deficiency of long-chain 3-hydroxyacyl-CoA dehydrogenase: A cause of lethal myopathy and cardiomyopathy in early childhood. Pediatr Res 28:657–62

44. Tein I, Haslam RH, Rhead WJ, Bennett MJ, Becker LE, Vockley J (1999) Short-chain acyl-CoA dehydrogenase deficiency: A cause of ophthalmoplegia and multicore myopathy. Neurology 52:366–72

45. Brackett JC, Sims HF, Rinaldo P, Shapiro S, Powell CK, Bennett MJ, Strauss AW (1995) Two subunit donor splice site mutations cause human trifunctional protein deficiency. J Clin Invest 95: 2076–82

46. Stanley CA, Treem WR, Hale DE, Coates PM (1990) A genetic defect in carnitine transport causing primary carnitine deficiency. Prog Clin Biol Res 321:457–64

47. Bonnet D, Martin D, de Lonlay P, Villain E, Jouvet P, Rabier D, Brivet M, Saudubray JM (1999) Arrhythmias and conduction defects as presenting symptoms of fatty acid oxidation disorders in children. Circulation 100:2248–53

48. Corr PB, Creer MH, Yamada KA, Saffitz JE, Sobel BE (1989) Prophylaxis of early ventricular fibrillation by inhibition of acyl-carnitine accumulation. J Clin Invest 83:927–36

49. Tripp ME (1989) Developmental cardiac metabolism in health and disease. Pediatr Cardiol 10:150–8

50. D'Adamo P, Fassone L, Gedeon A, Janssen EA, Bione S, Bolhuis PA, Barth PG, Wilson M, Haan E, Orstavik KH, Patton MA, Green AJ, Zammarchi E, Donati MA, Toniolo D (1997) The X-linked gene G4.5 is responsible for different infantile dilated cardiomyopathies. Am J Hum Genet 61:862–7

51. Bissler JJ, Tsoras M, Goring HH, Hug P, Chuck G, Tombragel E, McGraw C, Schlotman J, Ralston MA, Hug G (2002) Infantile dilated X-linked cardiomyopathy, G4.5 mutations, altered lipids, and ultrastructural malformations of mitochondria in heart, liver, and skeletal muscle. Lab Invest 82:335–44

52. Vreken P, Valianpour F, Nijtmans LG, Grivell LA, Plecko B, Wanders RJ, Barth PG (2000) Defective remodeling of cardiolipin and phosphatidylglycerol in Barth syndrome. Biochem Biophys Res Commun 279:378–82

53. Corbucci GG (2000) Adaptive changes in response to acute hypoxia, ischemia and reperfusion in human cardiac cell. Minerva Anestesiol 66:523–30

54. Ylitalo K, Ala-Rami A, Vuorinen K, Peuhkurinen K, Lepojarvi M, Kaukoranta P, Kiviluoma K, Hassinen I (2001) Reversible ischemic inhibition of F(1)F(0)-ATPase in rat and human myocardium. Biochim Biophys Acta 1504:329–39

55. Lesnefsky EJ, Moghaddas S, Tandler B, Kerner J, Hoppel CL (2001) Mitochondrial dysfunction in cardiac disease: Ischemia-reperfusion, aging, and heart failure. J Mol Cell Cardiol 33:1065–89

56. Corral-Debrinski M, Stepien G, Shoffner JM, Lott MT, Kanter K, Wallace DC (1991) Hypoxemia is associated with mitochondrial DNA damage and gene induction. Implications for cardiac disease. JAMA 266:1812–6

57. Paradies G, Petrosillo G, Pistolese M, Di Venosa N, Serena D, Ruggiero FM (1999) Lipid peroxidation and alterations to oxidative metabolism in mitochondria isolated from rat heart subjected to ischemia and reperfusion. Free Radic Biol Med 27:42–50

58. Gottleib RA, Burleson KO, Kloner RA, Babior BM, Engler RL (1994) Reperfusion injury induces apoptosis in rabbit cardiomyocites. J Clin Invest 94:1621–28

59. Murry CE, Jennings RB, Reimer KA (1986) Preconditioning with ischemia: A delay of lethal cell injury in ischemic myocardium. Circulation 74:1124–36

60. Murphy E (2004) Primary and secondary signaling pathways in early preconditioning that converge on the mitochondria to produce cardioprotection. Circ Res 94:7–16

61. Halestrap AP, Clarke SJ, Javadov SA (2004) Mitochondrial permeability transition pore opening during myocardial reperfusion: A target for cardioprotection. Cardiovasc Res 61:372–85

62. O'Rourke B (2004) Evidence for mitochondrial K+ channels and their role in cardioprotection. Circ Res. 94:420–32

63. Oldenburg O, Cohen M, Yellon D, Downey J (2002) Mitochondrial K(ATP) channels: Role in cardioprotection. Cardiovasc Res 55:429-3764.

64. Schulz R, Cohen MV, Behrends M, Downey JM, Heusch G (2001) Signal transduction of ischemic preconditioning. Cardiovasc Res 52:181–98

65. Hausenloy DJ, Maddock HL, Baxter GF, Yellon DM (2002) Inhibiting mitochondrial permeability transition pore opening: A new paradigm for myocardial preconditioning? Cardiovasc Res 55:534–43

66. Pain T , Yang XM, Critz SD, Yue Y, Nakano A, Liu GS, Heusch G, Cohen MV, Downey JM (2000) Opening of mitochondrial K(ATP) channels triggers the preconditioned state by generating free radicals. Circ Res 87:460–466

67. Szewczyk A, Wojtczak L (2002) Mitochondria as a pharmacological target. Pharmacol Rev 54:101–27

68. Garlid KD, Paucek P, Yarov-Yarovoy V, Murray HN, Darbenzio R, D'Alonzo AJ, Lodge NJ, Smith MA, Grover GJ (1997) Cardioprotective effect of diazoxide and its interaction with mitochondrial ATP-sensitive K+ channels: Possible mechanism of cardioprotection. Circ Res 81:1072–82

69. Ghosh S, Standen NB, Galinanes M (2000) Evidence for mitochondrial K ATP channels as effectors of human myocardial preconditioning. Cardiovasc Res 45:934–40

70. Regula KM, Ens K, Kirshenbaum LA (2003) Mitochondria-assisted cell suicide: A license to kill. J Mol Cell Cardiol 35:559–67

71. Danial NN, Korsmeyer SJ (2004) Cell death: Critical control points. Cell 116:205–19

72. Van Gurp M, Festjens N, van Loo G, Saelens X, Vandenabeele P (2003) Mitochondrial intermembrane proteins in cell death. Biochem Biophys Res Commun 304:487–97

73. Kroemer G (2003) Mitochondrial control of apoptosis: An introduction. Biochem Biophys Res Commun 304:433–5

74. Kuwana T, Mackey MR, Perkins G, Ellisman MH, Latterich M,Schneiter R, Green DR, Newmeyer DD (2002) Bid, Bax, and lipids cooperate to form supramolecular openings in the outer mitochondrial membrane. Cell 111:331–42

75. Marzo I, Brenner C, Zamzami N, Susin SA, Beutner G, Brdiczka D, Remy R, Xie ZH, Reed JC, Kroemer G (1998) The permeability transition pore complex: A target for apoptosis regulation by caspases and Bcl-2 related proteins. J Exp Med 187:1261–7

76. Lemasters JJ, Nieminen AL, Qian T, Trost LC, Elmore SP, Nishimura Y, Crowe RA, Cascio WE, Bradham CA, Brenner DA, Herman B (1998) The mitochondrial permeability transition in cell

death: A common mechanism in necrosis, apoptosis and autophagy. Biochim Biophys Acta 1366:177–96

77. Marzo I, Brenner C, Zamzami N, Jurgensmeier JM, Susin SA,Vieira HL, Prevost MC, Xie Z, Matsuyama S, Reed JC, Kroemer G (1998) Bax and adenine nucleotide translocator cooperate in the mitochondrial control of apoptosis. Science 281:2027–31

78. Graham BH, Waymire KG, Cottrell B, Trounce IA, MacGregor GR, Wallace DC (1997) A mouse model for mitochondrial myopathy and cardiomyopathy resulting from a deficiency in the heart/muscle isoform of the adenine nucleotide translocator. Nat Genet 16:226–34

79. Lebovitz RM, Zhang H, Vogel H, Cartwright J Jr, Dionne L, Lu N, Huang S, Matzuk MM (1996) Neurodegeneration, myocardial injury, and perinatal death in mitochondrial superoxide dismutase-deficient mice. Proc Natl Acad Sci USA 93:9782–7

80. Djouadi F, Brandt JM, Weinheimer CJ, Leone TC, González FJ, Kelly DP (1999) The role of the peroxisome proliferator-activated receptor alpha (PPAR alpha) in control of cardiac lipid metabolism. Prostaglandins Leukot Essent Fatty Acids 60:339–43.

81. Ibdah JA, Paul H, Zhao Y, Binford S, Salleng K, Cline M, Matern D, Bennett MJ, Rinaldo P, Strauss AW (2001) Lack of mitochondrial trifunctional protein in mice causes neonatal hypoglycemia and sudden death. J Clin Invest 107:1403–9

82. Wang J, Wilhelmsson H, Graff C, Li H, Oldfors A, Rustin P, Bruning JC, Kahn CR, Clayton DA, Barsh GS, Thoren P, Larsson NG (1999) Dilated cardiomyopathy and atrioventricular conduction blocks induced by heart-specific inactivation of mitochondrial DNA gene expression. Nat Genet 21:133–7

83. Puccio H, Simon D, Cossee M, Criqui-Filipe P, Tiziano F, Melki J, Hindelang C, Matyas R, Rustin P, Koenig M (2001) Mouse models for Friedreich ataxia exhibit cardiomyopathy, sensory nerve defect and Fe-S enzyme deficiency followed by intramitochondrial iron deposits. Nat Genet 27:181–6

84. Finck BN, Lehman JJ, Leone TC, Welch MJ, Bennett MJ, Kovacs A, Han X, Gross RW, Kozak R, Lopaschuk GD, Kelly DP (2002) The cardiac phenotype induced by PPARalpha overexpression mimics that caused by diabetes mellitus. J Clin Invest 109:121–30

85. Lehman JJ, Barger PM, Kovacs A, Saffitz JE, Medeiros DM, Kelly DP (2000) Peroxisome proliferator-activated receptor gamma coactivator-1 promotes cardiac mitochondrial biogenesis. J Clin Invest 106:847–56

86. Kubota T, McTiernan CF, Frye CS, Demetris AJ, Feldman AM (1997) Cardiac-specific overexpression of tumor necrosis factor-alpha causes lethal myocarditis in transgenic mice. J Card Fail 3:117–24

87. Marín-García J, Ananthakrishnan R, Goldenthal MJ, Filiano JJ, Pérez-Atayde A. (1999) Mitochondrial dysfunction in skeletal muscle of children with cardiomyopathy. Pediatrics 103:456–9

88. Pollitt RJ (1995) Disorders of mitochondrial long-chain fatty acid oxidation. J Inherit Metab Dis 18:473–90

89. Saudubray JM, Martin D, de Lonlay P, Touati G, Poggi-Travert F, Bonnet D, Jouvet P, Boutron M, Slama A, Vianey-Saban C, Bonnefont JP, Rabier D, Kamoun P, Brivet M (1999) Recognition and management of fatty acid oxidation defects: A series of 107 patients. J Inherit Metab Dis 22:488–502

90. Shoffner JM, Wallace DC (1994) Oxidative phosphorylation diseases and mitochondrial DNA mutations: Diagnosis and treatment. Annu Rev Nutr 14:535–68

91. Lerman-Sagie T, Rustin P, Lev D, Yanoov M, Leshinsky-Silver E, Sagie A, Ben-Gal T, Munnich A (2001) Dramatic improvement in mitochondrial cardiomyopathy following treatment with idebenone. J Inherit Metab Dis 24:28–34

92. Bonnefont JP, Demaugre F, Prip-Buus C, Saudubray JM, Brivet M, Abadi N, Thuillier L (1999) Carnitine palmitoyltransferase deficiencies. Mol Genet Metab 68:424–40

93. Brown-Harrison MC, Nada MA, Sprecher H, Vianey-Saban C, Farquhar J Jr, Gilladoga AC, Roe CR (1996) Very long chain acyl-CoA dehydrogenase deficiency: Successful treatment of acute cardiomyopathy. Biochem Mol Med 58:59–65

94. Doetschman T, Shull M, Kier A, Coffin JD (1993) Embryonic stem cell model systems for vascular morphogenesis and cardiac disorders. Hypertension 22:618–29

95. Muller M, Fleischmann BK, Selbert S, Ji GJ, Endl E, Middeler G, Muller OJ, Schlenke P, Frese S, Wobus AM, Hescheler J, Katus HA, Franz WM (2000) Selection of ventricular-like cardiomyocytes from ES cells in vitro. FASEB J 14:2540–8

96. Beltrami AP, Barlucchi L, Torella D, Baker M, Limana F, Chimenti S, Kasahara H, Rota M, Musso E, Urbanek K, Leri A, Kajstura J, Nadal-Ginard B, Anversa P (2003) Adult cardiac stem cells are multi-potent and support myocardial regeneration. Cell 114:763–6

97. Geromel V, Cao A, Briane D, Vassy J, Rotig A, Rustin P, Coudert R, Rigaut JP, Munnich A, Taillandier E (2001) Mitochondria transfection by oligonucleotides containing a signal peptide and vectorized by cationic liposomes. Antisense Nucleic Acid Drug Dev 11:175–80

98. Taylor RW, Wardell TM, Lightowlers RN, Turnbull DM (2000) Molecular basis for treatment of mitochondrial myopathies. Neurol Sci 21:S909–12

# Chapter 2

# Mitochondrial Bioenergetics in the Heart

## Overview

Several interacting pathways contribute to the production of bioenergy in the mitochondria, including pyruvate oxidation, the citric acid (TCA) or Krebs cycle, the β-oxidation of fatty acids (FAO), the common final pathway of oxidation phosphorylation (OXPHOS) (which utilizes the energy released from electron transfer) and the generation of a chemiosmotic gradient to drive the conversion of ADP and inorganic phosphate to ATP.

## Introduction

OXPHOS is performed by a series of multiprotein enzymes located at the mitochondrial inner membrane, including the respiratory ETC complexes I–IV and ATP synthase (complex V). These enzyme complexes interact with numerous electron carriers (most of which can be easily dissociated from the membrane complexes) that assist in the transfer of electrons from complex to complex. These carriers as well as the proteins within each complex contain metal groups that bind and transfer the electrons. The directional movement of the electrons between these key carriers is illustrated in Figure 2.1.

NADH→ FMN→ CoQ→ cyt*b*→ cytc1 → cyt*c*→ cyt*aa₃*→ O₂

          ↑

Succinate → FAD

Figure 2.1. Electron transport chain

Reduced NAD (NADH) and FAD (FADH₂) derived mainly from the TCA cycle and FAO are the primary electron donors for the ETC. The electrons derived from the oxidation of NADH are passed to complex I, containing FMN to the lipid ubiquinone (CoQ); electrons from the TCA cycle and from oxidized succinate and FADH₂ enter ETC at complex II, which also transfers them to the ubiquinone acceptor. Complex III containing the noncovalent bound heme cytochrome *b* removes the electrons from ubiquinone and delivers them to the covalent-bound heme containing cytochrome *c*. Electrons are removed by the oxidation of cytochrome *c* at complex IV and transferred to the final acceptor, molecular oxygen. Energy is released from the transfer at specific sites (complexes I, III, and IV) and used to pump protons across the mitochondrial inner membrane from the matrix to the intermembrane space. The generation of this electrochemical proton gradient and the backflow of protons at complex V/ATP synthase (a reverse proton-pump) to synthesize ATP from ADP and inorganic phosphate complete the oxidative phosphorylation.

The production of ATP via anaerobic glycolytic metabolism with its markedly lower yield is limited particularly in normal cardiac tissue. In addition to these bioenergetic pathways and metabolic intermediates, stored high-energy phosphates are generated by mitochondrial creatine kinase, which can serve as bioenergetic reserves for cardiac tissue.

In this chapter, the respiratory ETC and OXPHOS pathways and their regulation are discussed in detail, with particular reference to the heart. Information is provided about interacting pathways such as pyruvate oxidation, the TCA cycle, and the transport of nucleotides and phosphates, which are inextricably linked to OXPHOS.

## Complex I (NADH-ubiquinone oxidoreductase)

The complex I activity combines the transfer of 2 electrons from NADH to ubiquinone coupled with the ejection of 4 protons from the mitochondrial matrix to the intermembrane space contributing to a chemiosmotic gradient to supply the energy necessary for ATP synthesis. The relatively modest function of the enzyme contrasts with the large 900 kD assembly of the beef heart enzyme, containing at least 43 peptide subunits with several cofactors, including FMN and ubiquinone; on the other hand, the enzyme structure in prokaryotic cells contains only 14 peptide subunits. The lower eukaryote yeast *Saccharomyces cerevisiae*, which has a very active electron transport chain, has no complex I at all.

## *Enzyme structure*

Complex I has been characterized as L shaped with a base immersed in the inner membrane forming a "membranous" domain, and a short arm (containing an NADH substrate binding site) extending into matrix [1].

Of its 43 peptide subunits, 7 are encoded by mtDNA (i.e., ND1–6, ND4L). Each of these 7 subunits has bacterial homologues and has been shown to be located in the inner membrane. They are essential for the organization of the enzyme's membranous domain and its ubiquinone hydrogenase activity and are likely responsible for the proton-pump mechanism coupled to NADH oxidation [2]. These subunits interact with lipophilic quinones at 2 binding sites. There are a number of specific complex I inhibitors, the great majority of which interact with the components of the membranous-domain (e.g., rotenone, which interacts with ND1) and target the electron transfer from Fe-S clusters to ubiquinone [3]. Other complex I inhibitors include phenoxan, aureothin, annonin VI, piericidin, and the designer drug methyl-phenyl-tetrahydropyridine (MPTP).

The remaining 36 nuclear encoded subunits are primarily present in the short arm of complex I, which contains the NADH dehydrogenase activity, the FMN cofactor, and a number of Fe-S clusters. Both binding sites for NADH and FMN cofactor are contained within the 51 kD subunit. The exact role of many of these subunit proteins is presently unknown; however, they may participate in the regulation, assembly, and stability of complex I. The majority of the cDNAs for the nuclear complex I genes have been cloned, and their primary structure is available. Chromosomal mapping of more than 12 nuclear genes has revealed a wide pattern of distribution, and single-copy status with 2 pseudogenes identified. Thus far, there is little evidence of tissue-specific isoforms.

Complex I also contains between 22 and 24 atoms of iron and sulfur organized in at least 5 Fe-S clusters (detectable as specific elec-

INTERMEMBRANE SPACE

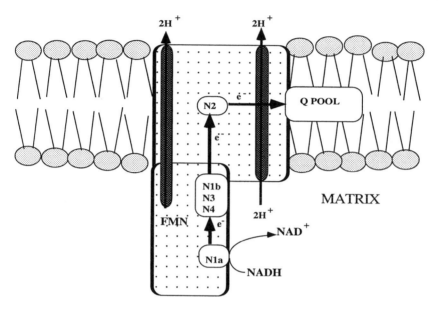

**Figure 2.2. Schematic view of the structure of complex I.** *The two major domains of this L-shaped complex enzyme (containing over 40 polypeptides) are shown and contain the NADH and FMN binding sites and the Fe-S clusters N1a, N1b, N2, N3, and N4, which direct the electron flow to the mobile carrier Q (ubiquinone) pool. Also shown is the proton pump.*

tronic paramagnetic resonance [EPR] structures) [4]. These clusters are denoted N1a, N1b (binuclear clusters), and N2, N3, N4 (tetranuclear clusters), and their relative position within the L-shaped structure of complex I is depicted in Figure 2.2.

## Complex II (Succinate-ubiquinone oxidoreductase)

Complex II consists of 4 nuclear-DNA encoded peptides and is the simplest respiratory complex (Figure 2.3). The 2 largest subunits comprise the succinate dehydrogenase (SDH) activity of the TCA cycle, which catalyzes succinate oxidation to fumarate, thereby reducing covalently attached flavin adenine dinucleotide (FAD). This reaction occurs on the major flavoprotein (Fp) subunit and results in the transfer of 2 electrons from $FADH_2$ to the inner membrane, for-

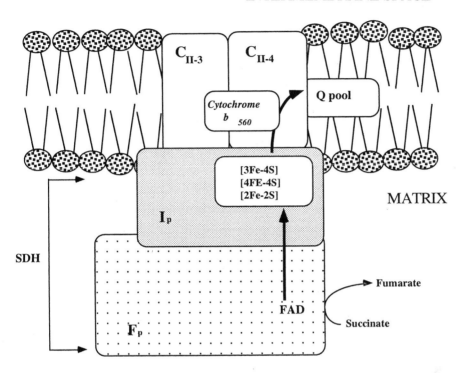

**Figure 2.3. Schematic representation of complex II succinate-ubiquinone oxidoreductase.** *Depicted are the two anchoring membrane protein subunits (C$_{II-3}$ and C$_{II-4}$) with cytochrome b$_{560}$, the Ip (iron protein) subunit with its 3 Fe-S clusters, and the Fp (flavoprotein) subunit containing the FAD cofactor and nearby-substrate binding site (e.g., succinate); SDH comprises the Fp and Ip subunits.*

ming ubiquinone. Hence it represents a pivotal link between the TCA cycle and the ETC. These peripheral proteins are linked to the inner membrane through 2 integral membrane (anchor) proteins of 11 and 9 kD [5], encoded by SDHC and SDHD, respectively.

The 70 kD subunit is covalently linked to FAD at a histidine residue, and the substrate analogue malonate binds as competitive inhibitor at the active site. The Fp gene (SDHA) has been sequenced from the human heart [6]. The second subunit is an iron-protein (Ip) subunit of 27 kD containing 3 nonheme Fe-S centers involved in electron transport function. Ip contains 3 highly conserved cysteine clusters that are involved in the structure of the 3 Fe-S clusters. The Ip gene (SDHB) has been sequenced in human [7]. Ip, like other Fe proteins, has primarily a posttranscriptional mode of regulation. Iron regulatory elements (IRE) are present in the Ip mRNA transcript, which can form a stem-loop structure at the 5' untranslated region on binding iron regulatory proteins (IRP). In the absence of IRP, Ip mRNA is normally translated, whereas if IRP is present, there is decreased translation of Ip [8].

The Fp-Ip complex (SDH) can be easily dissociated by treatment with chaotropic agents, and the dissociated SDH can oxidize succinate to fumarate by using artificial electron acceptors such as ferricyanide, PMS, or tetrazolium but cannot interact directly with the more lipophilic ubiquinone. Therefore, the interaction with ubiquinone can occur only on the association of Fp-Ip with both anchor proteins ($C_{II-3}$ and $C_{II-4}$) within the membrane.

The overall structure of complex II is similar to complex I. It comprises a matrix-localized peripheral subcomplex (SDH) with a substrate binding site, hydrogen acceptor (FAD), and 3 Fe-S centers conducting electron transfer linked to the membrane-bound subcomplex containing a cytochrome $b_{560}$ that is distinct from the cytochrome $b$ associated with complex III and also features a ubiquinone binding site.

## Complex III (Ubiquinol-cytochrome $c$ oxidoreductase)

Complex III catalyzes the oxidation of ubiquinol and the transfer of electrons to the mobile carrier cytochrome $c$ coupled to the transfer of protons across the inner membrane. Complex III is also termed $bc1$ complex after its 2 cytochrome components.

The mitochondrial $bc1$ complex in most species contain up to 11 subunits per monomer, whose central feature is 3 redox centers, cytochrome $b$ (with 2 heme groups), cytochrome $c1$ (one heme), and an iron-sulfur protein, Rieske protein, which are all highly conserved in evolution [9]. The other subunit proteins (including the core 1 and core 2 proteins and subunits VI to XI) are less conserved but manifest secondary structure similarities. All the $bc1$ proteins are encoded by the nuclear genome except the mtDNA-encoded cytochrome $b$. The importance of the 3 redox proteins cytochrome $b$, $c1$, and Rieske iron-sulfur protein to complex III function is underscored by their primary role in both electron transfer and accompanying proton translocation, as well as by the fact that the corresponding $bc1$ complex in bacteria contains only these 3 proteins.

Structural studies demonstrated that the functional $bc1$ complex is present as a dimer [10]. Each monomer contains 13 transmembrane helices, 8 contributed by cytochrome $b$, 1 from cytochrome $c1$ and 1 from the iron-sulfur protein. Cytochrome $b$ contains 1 heme ($b_L$) oriented closely to the positive side of the membrane and 1 heme ($b_H$) attached to 2 histidines positioned proximal to the negative side of the membrane. The core I and II proteins, constituting roughly 50% of the molecular mass of the $bc1$ complex, are located on the matrix side of the inner membrane and serve primarily a structural rather than functional role.

The Rieske iron-sulfur protein and the domain of cytochrome $c1$ containing heme are located on the outside of the membrane (P side) facing the intermembrane space. The Rieske protein contains a Fe-S cluster that is coordinated by two histidine and two cysteine residues. In cytochrome $c1$, the heme is covalently bound to 2 cysteines contained within the hydrophilic N-terminus extending into the intermembrane space; its C terminus contains a transmembrane anchoring sequence.

A recently identified ancillary protein (BCs1L) contributes to the assembly of complex III by assisting in the maturation of the Rieske protein.

## *The Q cycle and bc1 function*

Complex III like complex I contains two reaction centers for ubiquinone, $Q_N$ and $Q_P$ [11]. $Q_N$ is located on the matrix (negative) side of the membrane, while $Q_P$ is located on the intermembrane space (positive) side of the membrane (see Figure 2.4). At $Q_P$, the oxidation of the 2 electron donor ubiquinol ($QH_2$) into ubiquinone occurs; electrons are accepted and divided into two pathways, half to be recycled and half to be transferred via the Fe-S center and cytochrome $c1$ to cytochrome $c$. At $Q_N$, the ubiquinone molecule is reduced into ubiquinol, recycling electrons back into the quinone pool with an associated uptake of protons from the matrix.

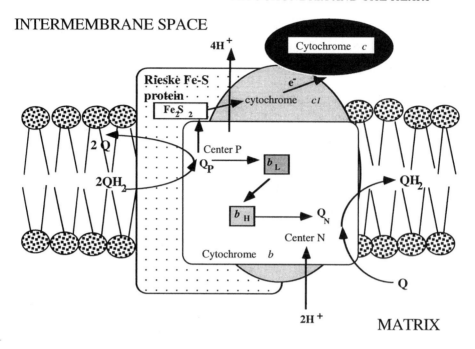

**Figure 2.4. The Q cycle and electron flow through complex III.** *The 3 catalytic subunits of the mitochondrial bc1 complex (the Rieske Fe-S protein and cytochromes c1 and b) are shown highlighting the major sites of electron transfer as detailed in the text. The flow of electrons resulting from the oxidation of QH₂ to the mobile carrier cytochrome c is shown as is the proton pump at this site.*

The Q cycle is initiated with the oxidation of ubiquinol ($QH_2$) supplied by complex I or complex II at the $Q_P$ site. One electron is transferred to the Fe-S center of the Rieske protein, which is subsequently oxidized by cytochrome $c1$, which in turn is oxidized by the mobile carrier cytochrome $c$ (with a single electron transferred) and 2 protons are released into the intermembrane space. The semiquinone intermediate, resulting from the oxidation of ubiquinol, donates a second electron to the heme $b_L$ and becomes oxidized to ubiquinone (Q). Heme $b_L$ is then reoxidized by heme $b_H$, which reduces a quinone into a semiquinone at $Q_N$. This constitutes the first half of the Q cycle with a net oxidation of $QH_2$ to semiquinone, reduction of cytochrome $c$, and transfer of two protons to the intermembrane space.

The second half of the Q cycle is started by a second round of ubiquinol oxidation at $Q_P$ resulting in reduced cytochrome *c*, the release of 2 more protons into the intermembrane space, and the successive reduction of cytochrome hemes $b_L$ and $b_H$ culminating with the complete reduction at $Q_N$ of the semiquinone (formed in the first half of the cycle) to ubiquinone. This reaction sequence results in the uptake of 2 protons from the matrix. A net result of the Q cycle is that for every pair of electrons transferred from ubiquinol to cytochrome, 4 protons are translocated to the intermembrane space, and 2 protons are removed from the matrix.

Specific inhibitors of electron transport have proved to be extremely valuable in arresting electron flux at specific sites allowing the isolation of portions of the electron chain for detailed evaluation [12]. A number of complex III inhibitors can block ubiquinol oxidiation at $Q_P$ (e.g., myxothiazol, mucidin). Myxothiazol binds to cytochrome *b* midway between heme $b_L$ and the Fe-S center of the Rieske protein. Other inhibitors (e.g., antimycin and diuron) prevent the oxidation by ubiquinone at $Q_N$. The antimycin binding site is located within a transmembrane region of cytochrome *b* near $b_H$.

## Complex IV (Cytochrome *c* oxidase)

Complex IV (COX) accepts 4 electrons from cytochrome *c* and transfers them to molecular oxygen, which is reduced to water, consuming 4 protons; simultaneously, 4 protons are translocated from the matrix to the intermembrane space creating the proton electrochemical gradient to be used to generate ATP.

The mammalian COX enzyme contains 13 subunits with 2 hemes, cytochrome $aa_3$, and 2 copper centers; Fe is the ligand bound to the hemes. In total, there are actually 3 redox centers, denoted CuA, heme *a*, and heme $a_3$-CuB (Figure 2.5).

The mtDNA-encoded subunits COX I, II, and III have extensive homology to subunits present in the bacterial enzyme and form the enzyme's catalytic core, containing the metallic centers, the binding sites for $O_2$ and cytochrome *c*, and the bulk of the proton and electron pathways. Subunit I binds the heme *a* and $a_3$ prosthetic groups and forms the CuB redox center. Subunit II binds the CuA center, whereas subunit III is involved in proton pumping and in electron transport through its metal centers.

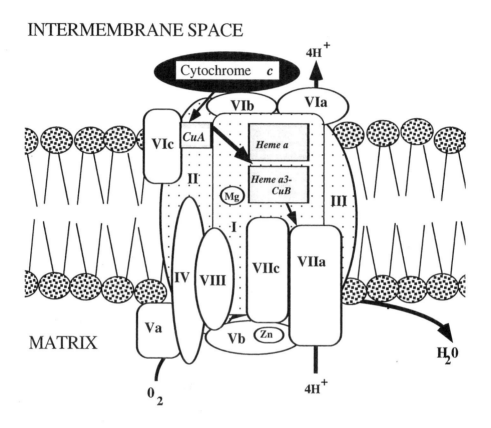

**Figure 2.5. Structure of the heart COX (complex IV) monomer**. *The relative orientation of the COX subunits containing the heme Cu centers, Zn and Mg site. The cytochrome c binding site, and the proton pump are shown.*

The nuclear encoded subunits IV, Va, Vb, VIa, VIb, VIc, VIIa, VIIb, VIIc, and VIII are considered to contribute to the biogenesis, stability, assembly, and regulation of the mammalian COX enzyme. However, their precise function has not yet been completely determined. Many use the designation CO rather than COX in designating the complex IV genes (e.g., COI encodes COXI).

## COX enzyme structure

The elucidation of COX enzyme structure, with its 13 subunits at the 2.8 A° resolution from beef heart [13], as well as in soil bacteria (*P.*

*denitrificans*) [14], has been critical to our understanding of the role of COX in the ETC. These enzymes were found to have striking homology at the level of redox center organization and structure.

Subunit I of COX contains 12 transmembrane $\alpha$ helices organized in 3 groups of 4 helices; each group has a pore in the center; 1 contains heme $a$, another, heme $a_3$-CuB center, and the third is empty.

Histidine residues play a key role as ligands; heme $a_3$ is linked by His$^{376}$, CuB is bound to His$^{240}$ and His$^{290}$, and heme $a$ binds His$^{61}$ and His$^{378}$. Heme $a$ and $a_3$-CuB center are located near the cytochrome $c$ binding site, 13 A° from the membrane surface. Subunit II carries the CuA atoms coordinated with 2 cysteines—a methionine and a glutamate residue. Subunit III contains 7 transmembrane helices and is bound to subunit I on the opposite side of subunit II.

Most of the nuclear-encoded COX subunits have a transmembrane $\alpha$ helix interacting with other nuclear and mitochondrial subunits. Three subunits are peripherally located; subunits Va and Vb are present on the matrix side, and VIb is located on the intermembrane space side (Figure 2.5).

Subunit Vb is bound to I and III; it contains a Zn atom linked to 4 Cys and to a zinc finger motif; the function of the relatively isolated Zn site is unknown. A Mg site is located on the cytoplasmic side at the junction of subunit II (Glu$^{298}$) and subunit I (His$^{368}$, Asp $^{369}$), between heme $a_3$ and CuA. Beef-heart COX enzyme is a dimer whose monomers are linked by subunits VIa and VIb.

## *COX subunit gene structure and expression*

The nucleotide primary sequence is available for all the cDNAs of human COX, and the chromosome location of the majority of these genes has been determined. The specific features of the human nuclear COX genes—including chromosomal location, isoform, cDNA and mature protein size—are presented in Table 2.1.

There are tissue-specific isoforms of subunits IV, VIa, VIb, VIIa, VIII. Isoforms H (present in heart and skeletal muscle) and L (mainly in liver) have been identified for subunits VIa, VIIa, and VIII in beef but only for VIa and VIIa in humans. A lung-specific isoform for subunit IV (COXIV-2) has been recently reported in human, rat, and mice [15], and a testes-specific isoform for subunit VIb [16]. An important regulatory function involving ATP-binding has been assigned

**Table 2.1. Human nuclear COX subunits**

| Subunit | cDNA | Mature Protein Size | Chromosomal Location |
|---------|------|---------------------|----------------------|
| IV | 668 bp | 147 aa | 16 q22–q24 |
| Va | 647 bp | 109 aa | 15 q25 |
| Vb | 494 bp | 98 aa | 2 cen–113 |
| VIa | VIa-L: 543 bp | VIa-L: 86 aa | 12 q24.2 |
|     | VIa-H: 371 bp | VIa-H: 86 aa | 16p |
| VIb | 439 bp | 86 aa | 19 q13.1 |
| VIc | 421 bp | 75 aa | 8 q22–q23 |
| VIIa | VIIa-L: 408 bp | VIIa-L: 60 aa | 4 q31–qter |
|      | VIIa-H: 341 bp | VIIa-H: 58 aa | 19q13.1 |
| VIIb | 468 bp | 56 aa | N.A. |
| VIIc | 334 bp | 47 aa | 5 q14 |
| VIII | 472 bp | 44 aa | 11 q12–13 |

*Note*: N.A. = not available.

to the subunit isoform VIa-H, which is not found with its isoform VIa-L. ATP binding to the heart enzyme uncouples proton flux from electron transfer [17].

The sequences of most of the COX subunit genes, including the complete promoter sequence for many of the nuclear genes, are available. Subunits Vb, VIa-L, VIa-H [18], VIIa-L [19] and VIIa-H [20] have been fully analyzed.

The transcriptional regulation of the H isoforms is largely attributed to the presence of muscle-specific promoter elements (e.g., Myo D) in VIa-H and VIIa-H, whereas L isoform expression is primarily regulated at the posttranscriptional level. During the transition from fetal to adult rat, the expression of VIa-H and VIII-H subunits increases, while their isoforms (liver-specific forms) decrease [21]. Various hormones (e.g., thyroid hormone and adrenal steroid hormone) have been reported to induce specific isoform expression.

As noted in the following chapter on mitochondrial biogenesis, many of the COX genes contain within their promoters binding sites for the SP1, NRF-1, and NRF-2 regulatory proteins. These multiple *cis*-acting sites and *trans*-acting regulatory factors that govern trans-criptional expression of the COX subunit genes allow for diverse stimuli to modulate enzyme biosynthesis and can also be integrated for coordinated biosynthesis.

Several ancillary nuclear proteins that do not belong to the COX enzyme complex have been reported as essential in its assembly. Phylogenetically conserved proteins with roles in COX enzyme assembly and function, originally identified in yeast, have been found in humans, including COX10, OXA1, SCO1, $SCO_2$, and SURF1. Specific defects in the genes encoding these proteins may result in COX deficiency with a variety of clinical phenotypes, including Leigh syndrome and other neuropathies. Defects in $SCO_2$ and in COX15 (the latter involved in the biosynthesis of heme required for COX enzyme assembly) result in fatal infantile HCM [22–23].

## *COX activity regulation*

The mechanistic pathway of electron transfer is better understood than the mechanism of proton pumping. The binding site for cytochrome *c* occurs on the intermembrane space side of the enzyme and involves residues from subunits II, VIa, and VIb. The highly conserved residues $Glu^{109}$ and $Asp^{139}$ of subunit II are essential to cytochrome *c* binding. Electrons from reduced cytochrome *c* are first transferred to the CuA center then to heme *a* and finally to the heme $a_3$-CuB center where the oxygen reduction site is located, with the hydrogen-bond networking playing a pivotal role in electron transfer.

With respect to electron transfer and oxygen-reduction activity, the monomeric form of COX is as active as the dimeric form; however, only the dimeric form can perform proton pump function. A nucleotide binding site (for adenine nucleotides) is located between $Arg^{14}$ and $Arg^{17}$ of the VIa-H subunit isoform and $Trp^{275}$ of subunit I of the other monomer. This interaction is thought to contribute to dimer stability. Also ATP can modulate COX activity through subunits IV and VIA by allosteric interactions [17].

## Complex V (F$_0$-F$_1$ ATPase; ATP synthase)

### *Subunit composition, structure, and function*

ATP synthase is the primary enzyme of oxidative phosphorylation responsible for ATP synthesis from ADP and inorganic phosphate. In the bovine heart, there are 16 subunits for complex V, including two subunits denoted ATPase6 and ATP6L (also termed ATPase8) encoded by mtDNA genes, while the remaining 14 subunits are encoded by the nuclear DNA. The overall complex V structure is shown in Figure 2.6. Early studies employing biochemical, ultrastructural, and electron microscopy analysis depicted the enzyme as a lollipop-like structure with a spherical headpiece projected into the mitochondrial matrix attached by a central stalk to an inner membrane basepiece [24]. Further studies have modified the original model of mammalian ATP synthase structure to include a second stalk extending from the basepiece to the top of the headpiece, as well as a ringlike disc or "collar" surrounding the central stalk [25]. Biochemical studies have demonstrated that complex V can be dissociated into a soluble F1-ATPase (contained within the spherical headpiece) and an insoluble membrane complex called F$_0$. In all species studied, including bacteria, the spherical head contains the catalytic F$_1$-ATPase subcomplex comprised of 5 different peptide subunits — α, β, γ, δ, and ε in the ratio 3:3:1:1:1. The mammalian enzyme also contains an ancillary protein that binds the β subunit (IF1) and functions as an inhibitor of ATP synthesis or hydrolysis.

The central stalk combined with the membrane portion of the F$_0$ subcomplex has the ability to translocate protons across the membrane and on coupling with the F$_1$ subcomplex can synthesize ATP. The central stalk and membrane segments of the F$_0$ subcomplex contain the OSCP (oligomycin sensitivity conferring protein), b, d, F6, e, f, g, and A6L subunits, and the hydrophobic transmembrane proteins subunits a and c (the latter referred to as the DCCD binding protein). The stoichiometry of the F$_0$ subunits in the mammalian enzyme may be variable; the ratio of a, b, and c subunits is usually 1:2:n, where n is between 9 and 12.

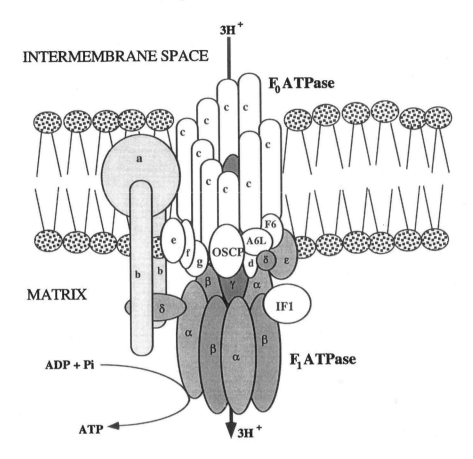

**Figure 2.6. Schematic representation of complex V.** *The peripherally located $F_1ATPase$ containing subunits $\alpha$, $\beta$, $\gamma$, $\delta$, and $\varepsilon$ and associated inhibitor protein IF1 are shown, as is the membrane-embedded $F_0ATPase$ containing the integral subunits c and a along with their associated subunits A6L, b, d, e, f, F6, g, and OSCP comprising the major and minor stalks located at the juncture of the $F_0$-$F_1ATPase$ subcomplexes. ATP synthesis is driven by proton flow from the intermembrane space into the matrix as indicated.*

In the $F_1$ subcomplex, 3 $\alpha$ and 3 $\beta$ subunits are alternately arranged around the central $\gamma$ subunit. Nucleotide binding sites are situated at the interfaces of each $\alpha$ and $\beta$ junction. Each $\alpha$ subunit and one $\beta$ subunit ($\beta_{TP}$) contains AMP-PP; another $\beta$ subunit ($\beta_{DP}$) contains ADP; while the third $\beta$ subunit ($\beta_E$) is empty. These include the 3 catalytic active sites at which nucleotide turnover occurs.

The binding of ADP and inorganic phosphate at one of the active sites provides the energy needed for combining the substrates to make ATP, since ATP formation is spontaneous and does not require additional energy input. However, the release of the newly formed ATP is energetically unfavorable in the face of the strong nucleotide binding and requires energy provided by proton translocation. The release is triggered by changes in affinity for ATP driven by conformational variations in the enzyme. A model of a rotary molecular motor has been used to describe the $F_1$-ATPase stucture [26–30]. The movement of the motor and changes in conformation of the protein are accomplished by the transient and cyclical occupancy of the catalytic sites, driven by energy coming from $F_0$ transduced through the $\gamma$ subunit, the motor's shaft. The rotation of the $\gamma$ subunit inside the 3 $\alpha$–$\beta$ couples has been directly observed. The input energy from $F_0$ to $F_1$ functions not to phosphorylate ADP but to change the conformation of the $\alpha$–$\beta$ couples effecting nucleotide binding and their release.

Inhibition of complex V activity can be affected at either the $F_1$ or $F_0$ levels. $F_1$ specific inhibitors such as aurovertin, efrapeptin, and the natural protein inhibitor (IF1) interfere either with nucleotide binding to $F_1$ or with the conformational changes essential to enzyme catalysis. Aurovertin binds to $\beta_{TP}$ and $\beta_E$, whereas efrapeptin interacts with $\gamma$ and prevents the conformational changes occurring by nucleotide binding at $\beta_E$. Uncouplers such as carbonylcyanide p-trifluoromethoxyphenylhydrazone (FCCP) or 2-4 dinitrophenol (DNP) dissipate the proton gradient, thereby eliminating the energy source. Inhibitors such as oligomycin or carbodiimide prevent proton translocation through $F_0$. Oligomycin binds to the stalk OSCP subunit blocking proton flow. Dicyclohexylcarbodiimide (DCCD) binds to Glu residues contained within the hydrophobic $\alpha$ helices of the c subunit. Despite the fact that there are between 9 and 12 c subunits per $F_0$ subcomplex, the binding of a single DCCD molecule is sufficient to block proton transfer and entirely abolish the activity of the enzyme. This finding has suggested a model of complex V function in which the single integral a subunit and 9 to 12 c subunits, embedded in the inner membrane $F_0$, form a path for proton flux across the membrane with the proton movement passing through all of the c subunits before the transfer to $F_1$. Movement of the c subunits in $F_0$, within the lipid bilayer, may rotate coupled with the rotation of the central shaft ($\gamma$ subunit) of $F_1$ [26–27].

As in other complicated biological systems, supercomplexes involved in bioenergetic metabolism (i.e., metabolons) exist in the mitochondria [31]. One or more have been identified with the ETC complexes (e.g., complexes II and IV) [32], and there is biochemical evidence for a supercomplex composed of ATP synthase, ANT, and the phosphate carrier [33]. These supercomplexes provide increased efficiency by eliminating the diffusion of substrates and other products and as a means of channeling intermediates to individual complexes, leading to catalytic enhancement. In the case of ATP synthase, the advantages of having the key membrane carriers for ADP, phosphate, and ATP proximal to the enzyme responsible for synthesis and hydrolysis may be particularly critical given the large number of avidly competitive binding molecules (Table 2.2.).

**Table 2.2. Subunits of human ATP synthase: Mature proteins, presequence size, and the mapped locale of genes**

| Subunit | Mature Protein Size | Gene Location | Presequence |
|---|---|---|---|
| **F$_1$-subcomplex** | | | |
| α | 55.1 kD (510 aa) | 18q12–q21 | 43 aa |
| β | 51.6 kD (480 aa) | 12p13–qter | 49 aa |
| γ | 30.2 kD (272 aa) | 10q22–q23 | 25 aa |
| δ | 15.1 kD (146 aa) | 19p13.3 | 22 aa |
| ε | 5.7 kD (51aa) | 20q13.2→q13.3 | N.A. |
| **F$_0$-subcomplex** | | | |
| c (ATPase9) | 14.7 kD (75 aa) | 3 functional genes | |
| | | P1 chromosome 17 | 61 aa |
| | | P2 chromosome 12 | 66 aa |
| | | P3 chromosome 2 | 66 aa |
| OSCP | 23.2 kD (190 aa) | 21q22.1–22.2 | 23 aa |
| b | 24.6 kd (214 aa) | N.A. | 42 aa |
| d | 18.4 kD (161 aa) | 12q13 | N.A. |
| e | 7 kD (66 aa) | 4p | N.A. |
| f | 10.7 kD (88 aa) | N.A. | 5 aa |
| g | 11.4 kD (100 aa) | 3Q27 | N.A. |
| F6 | 12.6 kD (76 aa) | Chromosome 10 | 32 aa |
| IF1 | 12.2 kD (106 aa) | N.A. | 25 aa |
| Factor B | 20.3 kD (175 aa) | 14q21.3 | 40 aa |
| a (ATPase6) | 24.8 kD (226 aa) | mtDNA | None |
| A6L | 7.9 kD (68 aa) | mtDNA | None |

*Note:* N.A. = not available; aa = amino acid residues.

There are two tissue-specific isoforms identified for the $\gamma$ gene, and these are derived from a single gene by alternative splicing of exon 9 [34]. The H isoform is prevalent in cardiac and skeletal muscle, whereas the L isoform that contains additional sequences at its C-terminus is found in other tissues. The gene for the $\delta$ subunit also uses alternative splicing to generate two transcripts whose differential function and expression are unknown [35]. The c subunit is encoded by 3 different functional genes, P1, P2, and P3, resulting in 3 isoforms with different signal sequences but identically sized mature proteins. The c isoforms have different expression patterns in regard to tissue-specificity, physiological regulation, hormone treatment, and development [36]. Besides the functional nuclear genes encoding ATP synthase subunits, several pseudogenes have also been identified.

As noted in our analysis of the COX genes, several of the ATP synthase genes (e.g., ATP $\alpha$ and $\beta$) contain *cis* binding sites for the SP1, OXBOX, and NRF-2 regulatory proteins. However, little information is currently available concerning the promoter elements of the majority of human ATP synthase genes.

## *ATP synthase defects and related pathologies*

Although this subject is treated in depth in later chapters, it is relevant to briefly mention here that defects in ATP synthase have significant clinical consequences. The best characterized mtDNA mutation in ATPase6 at nt 8993 causes Leigh syndrome with HCM. This mutation modifies the $F_0$ subunit a conformation, blocking proton transfer and reducing complex V stability [37]. In Batten disease (or neuronal ceroid lipofuscinosis), a hereditary neurodegenerative disease, an aberrant accumulation of the $F_0$ subunit c is found in several tissues, including brain and heart [38]. The targeting of specific tissues, with electrical excitability in the Batten neurodegenerative disorder, has prompted the suggestion that the $F_0$ subunit c has a role in membrane electrical response, ion pore formation, and calcium signaling [39]. In Batten patients, none of the 3 nuclear genes encoding the c protein contain mutations; the genetic defect lies in the CLN3 gene implicated in mitochondrial and lysosomal proteolytic processing of the c subunit.

Myocardial ,ATP synthase regulation may be abnormal in alcoholic cardiomyopathy [40]. Decreased ATP synthase activity has been found in several patients with primary cardiomyopathy with no defects in the mtDNA genes encoding the ATP synthase subunits. The enzyme abnormalities have been attributed to mutations in nuclear genes involved in the structure of the enzyme or its biosynthesis [41].

## Other enzymes of bioenergetics

### *Adenine nucleotide translocator (ANT)*

ANT's primary physiological role is to control the flux of ADP and ATP. In the mitochondria, it is responsible for maintaining an adequate supply of ADP for the ATP synthase generation of ATP and the transfer of ATP from its site of synthesis out of the mitochondria for utilization when and where needed (e.g., myofibril and membrane pumps). A strict exchange stoichiometry is maintained by ANT with 1 ADP entering the matrix for 1 ATP released outside the mitochondria, keeping the mitochondrial adenine nucleotide level relatively constant. ANT can function as a critical factor in modulating the OXPHOS rate through respiratory control, dependent on the developmental and metabolic conditions of supply and demand and on the tissue. From studies in several animal models, there is evidence that ANT exerts greater effects on the respiratory control of the newborn heart than in the adult heart. However, in the adult heart under conditions of high workload and hypertrophy, the involvement of myocardial ANT in controlling respiration appears to increase [42–43]. In addition, ANT actively participates in channeling and directing adenine nucleotides to specific microcompartment-containing enzymes (e.g., creatine kinase) [44], and it has been identified as an intrinsic component of the PT pore implicated in the early events of apoptosis (a role that is examined in more detail in Chapter 4). The interaction with the outer membrane VDAC/porin is also critical to the overall ANT function. Besides regulating the entry of cytosolic ADP through the outer membrane pores to reach the ANT carrier, porin transfers ATP to the cytosol. In some cases, this passage through the outer membrane serves as a limiting factor for ADP entry.

Moreover, ANT interacts with the proximal ATP synthase and the mitochondrial creatine kinase isoforms, which play a pivotal role in the ADP/ATP flux  (Figure 2.7). ANT function is also electrogenic and sensitive to the mitochondrial membrane potential.  Significantly, ADP influx involves the translocation of a proton into the matrix resulting in lower pH.

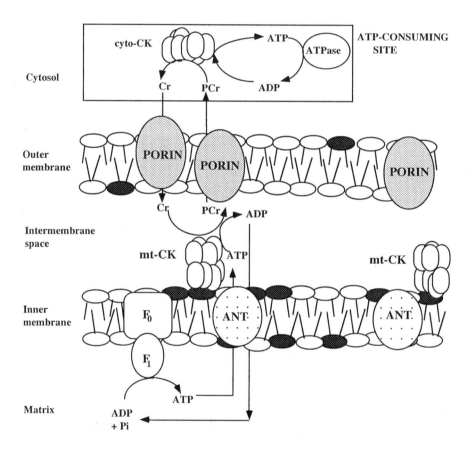

**Figure 2.7. View of the interaction of ATP synthase, ANT, VDAC/ porin, and CK at a contact site and in the transfer of ATP and ADP to and from the mitochondria.** *The relative orientation of the ATP synthase, the ANT, the octomeric mitochondrial creatine kinase (mt-CK) within the intermembrane space, and  the outer membrane located VDAC/porin are shown as are cytosolic sites (e.g., myofibrils) where ATP is delivered and utilized. Also depicted in the lipid bilayer are cardiolipin residues (dark circles) to which mt-CK molecules attach. The metabolites phosphocreatine (PCr) and creatine(Cr) are also shown.*

## ANT structure

ANT is an integral mitochondrial inner-membrane protein with a molecular weight of approximately 32 kD with 3 large sequence repeats encompassing approximately 100 aa; each repeat contains 2 motifs of transmembrane helices. Overall, the ANT protein has 6 transmembrane domains with both its N- and C-termini present on the same side of the inner membrane, facing the intermembrane space.

Three highly specific inhibitors (atractyloside, carboxyatractyloside, and bongkrekic acid) have been useful in the analysis and purification of the ANT protein. These inhibitors bind to opposite sides of the carrier; atractyloside binds from the outside and binds to the cytoplasmic side; bongkrekic acid enters the mitochondria and binds only to the matrix side.

## ANT regulation in the heart

Mitochondrial ATP synthesis is tightly coupled to cytosolic ATP utilization, in both the developing heart and the mature heart. Mitochondrial OXPHOS *in vitro* responds to increases in cytosolic ADP with respiration displaying first-order Michaelis-Menten kinetics, a pattern found *in vivo* in the newborn myocardium. In contrast, *in vivo* studies in mature adult myocardium have shown that a substantial increase in oxygen consumption is accompanied by minimal ADP changes indicating less respiratory control [45]. In the mature heart, during high work states, increased level of ANT carrier sites are found that likely modulate a greater sensitivity of OXPHOS to ADP levels [46]. Levels of myocardial ANT isoforms are modulated during cardiac development, with thyroid hormone treatment, and also in cardiac hypertrophy [42]. It is not known if alteration in human myocardial ANT level occurs during aging and senescence.

## ANT genes and their expression

Data concerning the human 3 ANT gene isoforms and their chromosomal locations are presented in Table 2.3. It includes other nomenclatures used in several studies (e.g., ANC1, ANC2, and ANC3), which can be confusing since ANT2 corresponds to ANC3 and ANT3 corresponds to ANC2.

**Table 2.3. Human adenine-nucleotide translocator genes**

| Isoform | Alternative Designation | Chromosome Location | Isoform Expression/ Regulation |
|---------|-------------------------|---------------------|-------------------------------|
| ANT1 | ANC1 | 4q35–qter | High-level expression in heart and skeletal muscle; low-level expression in proliferating myoblasts; promoter contains TATA, CCAAT, and OXBOX sites |
| ANT2 | ANC3 | Xp22.2 | Low-level expression in heart; Increased level of expression in proliferating cells; promoter contains SP1 and TATA but no CCAAT or OXBOX sites |
| ANT3 | ANC2 | Xq13→ Xq25–q26 | Ubiquitously present in most tissues; "housekeeping" type expression; no TATA, CCAAT, or OXBOX sequences in promoter |

While both ANT2 and ANT3 are located on the X chromosome, only ANT2 is subjected to X-inactivation (i.e., one transcribed copy in males compared to two copies in females). All 3 ANT genes have similar genomic structures but contain numerous differences in their promoter regions, likely responsible for the differences found in tissue-specific expression [47] as depicted in Table 2.3.

## *ANT dysfunction plays a key role in cardiac pathology*

In transgenic mice, a knockout mutation of ANT1 gene leads to severe cardiac hypertrophy and dramatic proliferation of mitochondria in both skeletal and cardiac muscle. ANT1 deficient mice display the histological, metabolic, and physiological characteristics of mitochondrial cardiomyopathy [48]. In addition, significant changes in the level of ANT1 expression in patients with MERRF, MELAS, and KSS [49] have been reported. Antibodies against ANT1 isoform are rather prevalent in the sera of patients with DCM and myocarditis [50–51] and considerable decline in transport of adenine nucleotides, accompanied by a significant elevation in ANT1 protein, have been found in the myocardium of these patients. On the other hand, no changes in ANT protein or carrier activity have been detected in patients with ischemic or valvular heart disease.

Similar to the newborn heart, the hypertrophic heart displays lower ANT protein levels and ADP-dependent respiratory kinetics, which may contribute to myocardial remodeling and heart failure [42].

## Creatine kinase

Mitochondrial creatine kinase (mt-CK) is responsible for the transfer of high-energy phosphates from mitochondria to the cytosolic carrier, creatine, and exists in mammals as two isoenzymes, sarcomeric mt-CK and ubiquitous mt-CK (Table 2.4). As shown in Figure 2.7, at the inner membrane site, the mitochondrial enzyme forms phosphocreatine and ADP from ATP generated by ATP synthase and translocated out of the mitochondria by ANT. The phosphocreatine is shuttled to cytosolic sites, where it can be utilized and hydrolyzed by cytosolic CK isozymes to provide ATP for utilization in muscle contraction and ion transport. Creatine kinase has been described as a major phosphotransfer system in cells with high-energy demand such as the cardiomyocyte, facilitating intracellular energetic communication by its integration with other enzymatic systems [52]. The expression and functional coupling of mt-CK is highly tissue and species specific, is subject to short-term and long-term adaptations, and shows developmental regulation. The mode of action of mt-CK is related to its precise localization within the mitochondrial intermembrane space, and its amount can control the quantitative aspects of the coupling to ATP-generating pathways [53].

The close interaction of mt-CK and ANT in mitochondria allows for the direct translocation of ATP from the active site of ANT into the active site of mt-CK. As a result, the ATP concentration increases and the concentration of ADP decreases in the active site of mt-CK, providing a high rate of unidirectional synthesis of phosphocreatine

**Table 2.4. Mitochondrial creatine kinase genes and proteins**

| Isoform | Genetic Locus | Mature Protein Size (aa) | Pre-sequence Size (aa) | Expression Pattern |
|---------|---------------|--------------------------|------------------------|--------------------|
| Sarcomeric mt-CK | 5q13.3 | 419 aa (47.5 kD) | 39 aa | Highly and exclusively expressed in heart and skeletal muscle |
| Ubiquitous mt-CK | 15q15 | 417 aa (47 kD) | 39 aa | Low-level of expression in tissues, including heart and skeletal muscle |

and ADP. No stable pool of creatine or phosphocreatine is present in the mitochondrial matrix in contrast to a large creatine pool localized in the cytoplasm; therefore, creatine must be continually brought into the mitochondria through the outer membrane.

While the mitochondrial creatine kinase is found in either dimeric and octameric forms, both *in vitro* and *in vivo* [54], the mt-CK octamer is the predominant form *in vivo*. Impairment of heart function and mitochondrial energy metabolism have been found to be associated with a significant decrease of mt-CK octamer/dimer ratios and reduced mt-CK activities. A significant decrease of the octamer/dimer ratio is found in heart with induced ischemia, and a decrease of octamer stability occurs *in vitro*, on induction by peroxynitrite radicals. The loss of mt-CK octamers impairs the channeling of high-energy phosphates from the mitochondria and compromises heart function in general.

## *Structure*

The two mitochondrial isoforms of creatine kinase are similar in size and quaternary structure (i.e., all form dimeric and octameric structures) to the 3 cytoplasmic CK isoforms (e.g., MM, BB, and MB). Nevertheless, all CK isoforms exhibit substantial differences in primary structure, and there is more sequence divergence between the different cellular CK isoforms in the same organism than there is in the same CK isoform of different species [55–56]. All of the CK isoforms represent distinct gene products of related but separate genes, and the mitochondrial isoforms are physically distinguishable from their cytosolic counterparts not only by their mitochondrial location but also by their higher isoelectric point. They contain a N-terminal presequence of 39 aa for targeting the mt-CK proteins to the intermembrane space. Mt-CK gene expression is tissue-specific and developmentally regulated, undetectable in the early fetal heart and increasing in a concerted fashion with their cytosolic counterparts during cardiac growth and development [57]. The elevated expression of the mitochondrial isozymes, and the development of the phosphocreatine shuttle is also coordinated with the development of the myocardial contractile apparatus [58] and with the transition in bioenergetic substrates from glycolytic to oxidative pathways [59].

## *Creatine kinase and the heart*

It is well established that both acute ischemia-reperfusion and chronic ischemia result in the loss of the stimulatory effect of creatine for mt-CK and affect the outer mitochondrial permeability to cytochrome $c$ and ADP. This can be explained by an ischemia-induced alteration of the intermembrane space leading to the loss of intracellular adenine nucleotide compartmentation and functional coupling of mt-CK and ANT. Such effects can be prevented by ischemic preconditioning or pharmacological preconditioning using mitochondrial ATP-sensitive potassium channel openers. The protective effect of preconditioning is associated with the preservation of mitochondrial function, as evidenced by maintenance of affinity constants and $V_{max}$ for ADP in mitochondrial respiration and the preservation of functional coupling between mt-CK and ANT [60].

Opening of the mitoK$_{ATP}$ channel during ischemic preconditioning has been suggested as critical in maintaining the intermembrane space environment needed to ensure low outer membrane permeability to ADP and ATP [61].

In transgenic mice with CK deficiency, energy delivery for muscular contraction is compromised as are intracellular cardiac handling and signal communication to membrane sensors such as the K$_{ATP}$ channel [62–63]. Studies with mice containing null mutations in either the ubiquitous or sarcomeric mt-CK genes have shown little bioenergetic abnormalities and unchanged phosphocreatine levels relative to controls [64–66]. However, deletion of both the ubiquitous mt-CK and sarcomeric mt-CK genes leads to significant alterations in myocardial high-energy phosphate metabolites. [66]. Alternative high-energy phosphotransfer routes can rescue cellular bioenergetic dysfunction in cells with defective CK [62]; these alternative routes include adaptive increases in other CK isoforms as well as increased levels of adenylate kinase and glycolytic pathway function [62, 67].

Finally, studies in both clinical and experimental models of cardio-myopathy (the latter of either hereditary or of diabetic etiology) have found significant reductions in mt-CK activity levels [68–69].

## *PDH and the TCA (Krebs) cycle*

The TCA cycle is preceded by the production of acetyl-CoA and NADH from the oxidation and decarboxylation of pyruvate transport-ed into the mitochondria by pyruvate dehydrogenase (PDH). Pyruvate oxidation has an essential role in aerobic energy metabolism and is catalyzed by the multimeric pyruvate dehydrogenase complex (PDHC) located in the mitochondrial matrix. This large assembly includes 132 subunits (30 E1 dimers, 60 E2 monomers, and 6 E3 di-mers) with a variety of coenzymes including thiamine pyrophosphate, lipoamide, CoA, FAD, and NAD and also contains 3 catalytic subunits responsible for different enzymatic reactions. PDHC is regu-lated by end-product inhibition, as well as by the activation/inactiva-tion of its catalytic components (i.e., E1, E2, and E3) by their dephosphorylation/ phosphorylation. Activation of the E1 component is catalyzed by a PDH-phosphatase (PDHP) requiring $Mg^{++}$ and $Ca^{++}$; inactivation of E1 activity is accomplished by an ATP-dependent pyruvate kinase that is subject to inhibition by pyruvate or dichloro-acetate and activation by increased ratios of NADH/NAD, acetyl-CoA/CoA, and ATP/ADP. Both the activating phosphatase and deac-tivating PDH kinase have several cardiac-specific isoforms subject to regulation by diverse developmental, dietary, and hormonal stimuli [70–71]. The PDH kinase (PDHK) 1 isoform is up-regulated in the adult compared to the neonatal heart and is primarily involved in regulating glucose oxidation through the inhibitory phosphorylation of PDHC. Expression of the cardiac PDH kinase 4 isoform is responsive to changes in the myocardial lipid supply; its early up-regulation in the postnatal heart contributes to the perinatal developmental switch to fatty acids as the primary myocardial energy source. This myocardial kinase isoform is also up-regulated in response to thyroid hormone and high-fat diet. Starvation and diabetes decrease the level of PDHC in the heart by both activating PDHK gene expression and by the inactivation of myocardial PDH phosphatase activity, effected largely by promoting reduced expression of the PDHP2 gene [72].

All but 1 enzyme of the TCA cycle are soluble enzymes situated within the mitochondrial matrix, with SDH (the peripheral part of the membrane-bound complex II) being the exception. The TCA enzymes are highly organized as a supercomplex or metabolon within the matrix, providing a kinetic advantage in concentrating intermediates and channeling substrates within the supercomplex [73]. Substrate and product concentration are the immediate controlling factors determining the flux through the cycle, and ATP, ADP, and $Ca^{++}$ are significant allosteric effectors of TCA cycle enzymes. Several of the TCA enzymes (i.e., isocitrate dehydrogenase, $\alpha$-ketoglutarate dehydrogenase, and malate dehydrogenase) also require $NAD^+$ as a cofactor to produce NADH. While a major contribution of the TCA cycle is as a direct source of intramitochondrial reducing equivalents NADH and $FADH_2$ for the ETC, the supply of NAD is critical (supplied by complex I oxidation) and indicates the necessity of coupling the TCA and ETC pathways to regulate oxygen consumption, NADH oxidation and ATP synthesis. Although the majority of the primary sequences of the cDNAs for the human TCA cycle enzymes have been reported, information regarding either the genomic structure or regulatory sequences for these genes, their expression and overall regulation is rather limited at this time.

## Overall regulation of mitochondrial bioenergetics in the heart

### *Supply and demand: substrates, oxygen and ATP-ADP levels*

If adequate substrates are supplied, the rate of oxygen consumption (a direct measure of OXPHOS) depends largely on the ADP and phosphate levels. In the absence of ADP (i.e., state 4 respiration), oxygen consumption is an order of magnitude lower. With lower levels of ADP available as substrate, ATP synthesis by complex V declines, the membrane potential is not dissipated, and subsequent proton translocation and electron transport are adversely affected. Under these circumstances (i.e., absence of ADP), increased proton leakage can increase the rate of respiration by abolishing the proton gradient (causing less coupling). This proton leakage can occur either with damaged (or frozen) mitochondria, with naturally occurring proteins that promote proton leaks (termed uncoupling proteins), or by treatment with uncouplers (e.g., dinitrophenol) that provide a path for protons across the bilayer membrane, collapsing the electrochemical gradient.

ATP consumption (the majority of which occurs in the cytosol) also plays a critical role in regulating respiration. Since the ratio of ATP/ADP *in vivo* is generally very high, changes in ATP level are smaller compared to ADP. It has been argued that respiratory control is exerted by the ATP/ADP ratio, but the consensus view supports the concept that ADP levels in mitochondria are more often critical. Analysis of whole hearts by NMR has failed to demonstrate sufficient changes in adenine nucleotide levels to account for the increases in oxygen consumption that occur with an increased workload.

Another way that adenine nucleotides can impact on respiration is by direct effects on the bioenergetic enzymes involved. Both ADP and ATP can exert allosteric effects on enzymes involved in bioenergetic production (e.g., both cytosolic glycolytic enzymes and mitochondrial dehydrogenases) and on ATP utilization. In addition, a role for ATP and ADP in the allosteric control of COX activity is well established. This is particularly relevant to the heart enzyme in which the tissue-specific COX enzyme interacts and is stimulated by ADP, an effect not seen with the liver COX. This regulation is pertinent to COX since it is the only respiratory enzyme with tissue-specific isoform subunits (VIa, VIIa, and VIII). The interaction with ADP is likely to involve the N-terminus of the VIa-H subunit. Recently, it has been found that myocardial cytochrome *c* oxidase activity is also profoundly regulated by NO levels [74] and by cAMP-dependent phosphorylation of specific COX subunits [75], which may modulate the ATP-COX interaction.

Other substrates such as NADH and NAD are also important in metabolic control, but they are rarely limiting since NADH can be resupplied by many diverse reactions with individual regulation. The NADH level is controlled and elevated with increased ADP. Levels of oxygen are also rarely rate-limiting in mammalian tissues except under hypoxic conditions.

Cytoplasmic and mitochondrial calcium levels are controlled by diverse stimuli including hormones and growth factors and by electrical signals. Specific transporters including a $Ca^{++}$ uniporter and a $Na^+/Ca^{++}$ exchanger have been implicated in the influx and efflux, respectively, of mitochondrial $Ca^{++}$. Increases in mitochondrial $Ca^{++}$ stimulate several TCA cycle dehydrogenases (e.g., isocitrate and α-ketoglutarate dehydrogenase), phosphatase-activated PDH, and ATP synthase activities. This $Ca^{++}$-mediated enzyme activation results in increased intramitochondrial NADH, elevated membrane potential, and increased ATP synthesis [76]. It is noteworthy that an increase in cardiac work is often associated with increased cytosolic $Ca^{++}$. Studies with isolated cardiomyocytes support this model; however, it is technically difficult to measure mitochondrial matrix $Ca^{++}$ levels in the *in vivo* heart. Elevated levels of mitochondrial NADH/NAD, expected with calcium stimulation of the dehydrogenases, accompanying increased myocardial $O_2$ consumption *in vivo* have been reported under conditions of increased heart rate [77]. However, other studies have found a decreased mitochondrial NADH level with increased cardiac workload [78].

Another key modulator of enzyme activity, which can influence the overall respiration rate, are lipids, which contribute to the mitochondrial membrane milieu. Cardiolipin, an exclusive mitochondrial membrane component, has been found to be necessary for COX stability and activity. In addition, it plays a key role in binding mt-CK to the inner membrane.

The construction of integrated models of cardiac mitochondrial energy metabolism has been made to predict the results of various effectors (e.g., hormones, metabolic inhibitors, and substrates) on OXPHOS rates [79–80]. These models reveal that there is no single rate-limiting step and support the importance of ADP, ATP, proton leak, and calcium levels in regulating respiration. Control over bioenergetic flux may occur at multiple sites (e.g., ATP synthase, ANT, and ETC) to minimize levels needed for any one regulatory factor.

# References

1.  Walker JE (1992) The NADH: ubiquinone oxidoreductase (complex I) of respiratory chains. Q Rev Biophys 25:253–324

2.  Brandt U (1997) Proton-translocation by membrane-bound ligand NADH: ubiquinone-oxidoreductase (complex I) through redox-gated ligand conduction. Biochim Biophys Acta 1318:79–91

3.  Albracht SP, Mariette A, de Jong P (1997) Bovine-heart NADA: ubiquinone oxidoreductase is a monomer with 8 Fe-S clusters and 2 FMN groups. Biochim Biophys Acta 1997 1318:92–106

4.  Degli Esposti M (1998) Inhibitors of NADH- ubiquinone reductase: An overview. Biochim Biophys Acta 1364:222–35

5.  Cochran B, Capaldi RA, Ackrell BA (1994) The cDNA sequence of beef heart CII-3, a membrane-intrinsic subunit of succinate-ubiquinone oxidoreductase. Biochim Biophys Acta 1188:162–6

6.  Morris AA, Farnsworth L, Ackrell BA, Turnbull DM, Birch-Machin MA (1994) The cDNA sequence of the flavoprotein subunit of human heart succinate dehydrogenase. Biochim Biophys Acta 1185:125–8

7.  Au HC, Ream-Robinson D, Bellew LA, Broomfield PL, Saghbini M, Scheffler IE (1995) Structural organization of the gene encoding the human iron-sulfur subunit of succinate dehydrogenase. Gene 159:249–53

8.  Melefors O (1996) Translational regulation in vivo of the Drosophila melanogaster mRNA encoding succinate dehydrogenase iron protein via iron responsive elements. Biochem Biophys Res Commun 221:437–41

9.  Gonzalez-Halphen D, Lindorfer MA, Capaldi RA (1988) Subunit arrangement in beef heart complex III. Biochemistry 27:7021–31

10. Xia D, Yu CA, Kim H, Xia JZ, Kachurin AM, Zhang L, Yu L, Deisenhofer J (1997) Crystal structure of the cytochrome bc1 complex from bovine heart mitochondria. Science 277:60–6

11. Brandt U, Trumpower B (1994) The protonmotive Q cycle in mitochondria and bacteria. Crit Rev Biochem Mol Biol 29:165–97

12. Link TA, Haase U, Brandt U, von Jagow G (1993) What information do inhibitors provide about the structure of the hydroquinone oxidation site of ubihydroquinone: cytochrome c oxidoreductase? J Bioenerg Biomembr 25:221–32

13. Tsukihara T, Aoyama H, Yamashita E, Tomizaki T, Yamaguchi H, Shinzawa-Itoh K, Nakashima R, Yaono R, Yoshikawa S (1996)

The whole structure of the 13-subunit oxidized cytochrome c oxidase at 2.8 A. Science 272:1136–44

14. Iwata S, Ostermeier C, Ludwig B, Michel H (1995) Structure at 2.8 A resolution of cytochrome c oxidase from Paracoccus denitrificans. Nature 376:660–9

15. Huttemann M, Kadenbach B, Grossman LI (2001) Mammalian subunit IV isoforms of cytochrome c oxidase. Gene 267:111–23

16. Huttemann M, Jaradat S, Grossman LI (2003) Cytochrome c oxidase of mammals contains a testes-specific isoform of subunit VIb-the counterpart to testes-specific cytochrome c. Mol Reprod Dev 66:8–16

17. Anthony G, Reimann A, Kadenbach B (1993) Tissue-specific regulation of bovine heart cytochrome-c oxidase activity by ADP via interaction with subunit VIa. Proc Natl Acad Sci USA 90:1652–6

18. Bachman NJ, Riggs PK, Siddiqui N, Makris GJ, Womack JE, Lomax MI (1997) Structure of the human gene (COX6A2) for the heart/muscle isoform of cytochrome c oxidase subunit VIa and its chromosomal location in humans, mice, and cattle. Genomics 42:146–51

19. Wolz W, Kress W, Mueller CR (1997) Genomic sequence and organization of the human gene for cytochrome c oxidase subunit (COX7A1) VIIa-M. Genomics 45:438–42

20. Yu M, Jaradat SA, Grossman LI (2002) Genomic organization and promoter regulation of human cytochrome c oxidase subunit VII heart/muscle isoform (COX7AH). Biochim Biophys Acta 1574:345–53

21. Schagger H, Noack H, Halangk W, Brandt U, von Jagow G (1995) Cytochrome c oxidase in developing rat heart: Enzymic properties and amino-terminal sequences suggest identity of the fetal heart and the adult liver isoform. Eur J Biochem 230:235–41

22. Papadopoulou LC, Sue CM, Davidson MM, Tanji K, Nishino I, Sadlock JE, Krishna S, Walker W, Selby J, Glerum DM, Coster RV, Lyon G, Scalais E, Lebel R, Kaplan P, Shanske S, De Vivo DC, Bonilla E, Hirano M, DiMauro S, Schon EA (1999) Fatal infantile cardioencephalomyopathy with COX deficiency and mutations in $SCO_2$, a COX assembly gene. Nat Genet 23:333–7

23. Antonicka H, Mattman A, Carlson CG, Glerum DM, Hoffbuhr KC, Leary SC, Kennaway NG, Shoubridge EA (2003) Mutations in COX15 produce a defect in the mitochondrial heme biosynthetic

pathway, causing early-onset fatal hypertrophic cardiomyopathy. Am J Hum Genet 72:101–14

24. Walker JE (1995) Determination of the structures of respiratory enzyme complexes from mammalian mitochondria. Biochim Biophys Acta 1271:221–7

25. Ko YH, Hullihen J, Hong S, Pedersen PL (2000) Mitochondrial F(0)F(1) ATP synthase. Subunit regions on the F1 motor shielded by F(0), Functional significance, and evidence for an involvement of the unique F(0) subunit F(6). J Biol Chem 275:32931–9

26. Junge W, Lill H, Engelbrecht S (1997) ATP synthase: An electrochemical transducer with rotatory mechanics. Trends Biochem Sci 22:420–3

27. Kaim G, Matthey U, Dimroth P (1998) Mode of interaction of the single a subunit with the multimeric c subunits during the translocation of the coupling ions by F1F0 ATPases. EMBO J 17: 688–95

28. Hong S, Pedersen PL (2003) ATP synthases: Insights into their motor functions from sequence and structural analyses. J Bioenerg Biomembr 35:95–120

29. Capaldi RA, Aggeler R (2002) Mechanism of the F1F0-type ATP synthase, a biological rotary motor. Trends Biochem Sci 27:154-60

30. Boyer PD (1997) The ATP synthase: A splendid molecular machine. Annu Rev Biochem 66:717–49

31. Robinson JB Jr, Inman L, Sumegi B, Srere PA (1987) Further characterization of the Krebs tricarboxylic acid cycle metabolon. J Biol Chem 262:1786–90

32. Schagger H (2001) Respiratory chain supercomplexes. IUBMB Life 52:119–28

33. Ko YH, Delannoy M, Hullihen J, Chiu W, Pedersen PL (2003) Mitochondrial ATP synthasome: Cristae-enriched membranes and a multiwell detergent screening assay yield dispersed single complexes containing the ATP synthase and carriers for Pi and ADP/ATP. J Biol Chem 278:12305–9

34. Matsuda C, Endo H, Hirata H, Morosawa H, Nakanishi M, Kagawa Y (1993) Tissue-specific isoforms of the bovine mitochondrial ATP synthase gamma-subunit. FEBS Lett 325:281–4

35. Shoffner JM, Kaufman A, Koontz D, Krawiecki N, Smith E, Topp M, Wallace DC (1995) Oxidative phosphorylation diseases and cerebellar ataxia. Clin Neurosci 3:43–53

36. Andersson U, Houstek J, Cannon B (1997) ATP synthase subunit c expression: Physiological regulation of the P1 and P2 genes. Biochem J 323:379–85

37. Tatuch Y, Robinson BH (1993) The mitochondrial DNA mutation at 8993 associated with NARP slows the rate of ATP synthesis in isolated lymphoblast mitochondria. Biochem Biophys Res Commun 192:124–8

38. Rowan SA, Lake BD (1995) Tissue and cellular distribution of subunit c of ATP synthase in Batten disease (neuronal ceroid-lipofuscinosis). Am J Med Genet 57:172–6

39. McGeoch JE, Guidotti G (2001) Batten disease and the control of the Fo subunit c pore by cGMP and calcium. Eur J Paediatr Neurol 5:147–50

40. Das AM, Harris DA (1993) Regulation of the mitochondrial ATP synthase is defective in rat heart during alcohol-induced cardiomyopathy. Biochim Biophys Acta 1181:295–9

41. Houstek J, Klement P, Floryk D, Antonicka H, Hermanska J, Kalous M, Hansikova H, Hout'kova H, Chowdhury SK, Rosipal T, Kmoch S, Stratilova L, Zeman J (1999) A novel deficiency of mitochondrial ATPase of nuclear origin. Hum Mol Genet 8:1967–74

42. Portman MA (2002) The adenine nucleotide translocator: regulation and function during myocardial development and hyper-trophy. Clin Exp Pharmacol Physiol 29:334–8

43. Portman MA, Xiao Y, Song Y, Ning XH (1997) Expression of adenine nucleotide translocator parallels maturation of respiratory control in vivo. Am J Physiol Heart Circ Physiol 27:H1977–83

44. Saks VA, Khuchua ZA, Vasilyeva EV, Belikova OYu, Kuznetsov AV (1994) Metabolic compartmentation and substrate channelling in muscle cells: Role of coupled creatine kinases in in vivo regulation of cellular respiration—A synthesis. Mol Cell Biochem 133-134:155–92

45. Doussiere J, Ligeti E, Brandolin G, Vignais PV (1984) Control of oxidative phosphorylation in rat heart mitochondria: The role of the adenine nucleotide carrier. Biochim Biophys Acta 766:492–500

46. Schonfeld P. Schild L, Bohnensack R (1996) Expression of the ADP/ATP carrier and expansion of the mitochondria (ATP + ADP) pool contribute to postnatal maturation of the rat heart. Eur J Biochem 241:895–900

47. Stepien G, Torroni A, Chung AB, Hodge JA, Wallace DC (1992) Differential expression of adenine nucleotide translocator isoforms in

mammalian tissues and during muscle cell differentiation. J Biol Chem 267:14592–7

48. Graham BH, Waymire KG, Cottrell B, Trounce IA, MacGregor GR, Wallace DC (1997) A mouse model for mitochondrial myopathy and cardiomyopathy resulting from a deficiency in the heart/muscle isoform of the adenine nucleotide translocator. Nat Genet 16:226–34

49. Heddi A, Stepien G, Benke PJ, Wallace DC (1999) Coordinate induction of energy gene expression in tissues of mitochondrial disease patients. J Biol Chem 274:22968–76

50. Dorner A, Schulze K, Rauch U, Schultheiss HP (1997) Adenine nucleotide translocator in dilated cardiomyopathy: Pathophysiological alterations in expression and function. Mol Cell Biochem 174:261–9

51. Schultheiss HP, Bolte HD (1985) Immunological analysis of auto-antibodies against the adenine nucleotide translocator in dilated cardiomyopathy. J Mol Cell Cardiol 17:603–17

52. Dzeja PP, Terzic A (2003) Phosphotransfer networks and cellular energetics. J Exp Biol 206:2039–47

53. Jacobus WE (1985) Respiratory control and the integration of heart high-energy phosphate metabolism by mitochondrial creatine kinase. Annu Rev Physiol 47:707–25

54. Schlegel J, Zurbriggen B, Wegmann G, Wyss M, Eppenberger HM, Wallimann T (1988) Native mitochondrial creatine kinase forms octameric structures. I. Isolation of two interconvertible mitochondrial creatine kinase forms, dimeric and octameric mitochondrial creatine kinase: Characterization, localization, and structure-function relationships. J Biol Chem 263:16942–53

55. Payne RM, Haas RC, Strauss AW (1991) Structural characterization and tissue-specific expression of the mRNAs encoding isoenzymes from two rat mitochondrial creatine kinase genes. Biochim Biophys Acta 1089:352–61

56. Haas RC, Strauss AW (1990) Separate nuclear genes encode sarcomere-specific and ubiquitous human mitochondrial creatine kinase isoenzymes. J Biol Chem 265:6921–7

57. Tiivel T, Kadaya L, Kuznetsov A, Kaambre T, Peet N, Sikk P, Braun U, Ventura-Clapier R, Saks V, Seppet EK (2000) Developmental changes in regulation of mitochondrial respiration by ADP and creatine in rat heart in vivo. Mol Cell Biochem 208:119–28

58. Hoerter JA, Kuznetsov A, Ventura-Clapier R (1991) Functional development of the creatine kinase system in perinatal rabbit heart. Circ Res 69:665–76

59. Payne RM, Strauss AW (1994) Expression of the mitochondrial creatine kinase genes. Mol Cell Biochem 133-134:235–43

60. Laclau MN, Boudina S, Thambo JB, Tariosse L, Gouverneur G, Bonoron-Adele S, Saks VA, Garlid KD, Dos Santos P (2001) Cardioprotection by ischemic preconditioning preserves mitochondrial function and functional coupling between adenine nucleotide translocase and creatine kinase. J Mol Cell Cardiol 33:947–56

61. Dos Santos P, Laclau MN, Boudina S, Garlid KD (2004) Alterations of the bioenergetics systems of the cell in acute and chronic myocardial ischemia. Mol Cell Biochem 256-257:157–66

62. Dzeja PP, Bortolon R, Perez-Terzic C, Holmuhamedov EL,Terzic A (2002) Energetic communication between mitochondria and nucleus directed by catalyzed phosphotransfer. Proc Natl Acad Sci USA 99:10156–61

63. Abraham MR, Selivanov VA, Hodgson DM, Pucar D, Zingman LV, Wieringa B, Dzeja PP, Alekseev AE, Terzic A (2002) Coupling of cell energetics with membrane metabolic sensing: Integrative signaling through creatine kinase phosphotransfer disrupted by M-CK gene knock-out. J Biol Chem 277:24427–34

64. Steeghs K, Oerlemans F, Wieringa B (1995) Mice deficient in ubiquitous mitochondrial creatine kinase are viable and fertile. Biochim Biophys Acta 1230:130–8

65. Steeghs K, Heerschap A, de Haan A, Ruitenbeek W, Oerlemans F, van Deursen J, Perryman B, Pette D, Bruckwilder M, Koudijs J, Jap P, Wieringa B (1997) Use of gene targeting for compromising energy homeostasis in neuromuscular tissues: The role of sarcomeric mitochondrial creatine kinase. J Neurosci Methods 71:29–41

66. Spindler M, Niebler R, Remkes H, Horn M, Lanz T, Neubauer S (2002) Mitochondrial creatine kinase is critically necessary for normal myocardial high-energy phosphate metabolism. Am J Physiol Heart Circ Physiol 283:H680–7

67. Boehm E, Ventura-Clapier R, Mateo P, Lechene P, Veksler V (2000) Glycolysis supports calcium uptake by the sarcoplasmic reticulum in skinned ventricular fibres of mice deficient in mitochondrial and cytosolic creatine kinase. J Mol Cell Cardiol 32:891–902

68. Veksler V, Ventura-Clapier R (1994) In situ study of myofibrils, mitochondria and bound creatine kinases in experimental cardiomyopathies. Mol Cell Biochem 133-134:287–98

69. Ingwall JS, Atkinson DE, Clarke K, Fetters JK (1990) Energetic correlates of cardiac failure: Changes in the creatine kinase system in the failing myocardium. Eur Heart J 11:108–15

70. Sugden MC, Langdown ML, Harris RA, Holness MJ (2000) Expression and regulation of pyruvate dehydrogenase kinase isoforms in the developing rat heart and in adulthood: Role of thyroid hormone status and lipid supply. Biochem J 352:731–8

71. Denton RM, McCormack JG, Rutter GA, Burnett P, Edgell NJ, Moule SK, Diggle TA (1996) The hormonal regulation of pyruvate dehydrogenase complex. Adv Enzyme Regul 36:183–98

72. Huang B, Wu P, Popov KM, Harris RA (2003) Starvation and diabetes reduce the amount of pyruvate dehydrogenase phosphatase in rat heart and kidney. Diabetes 52:1371–6

73. Srere PA, Sumegi B, Sherry AD (1987) Organizational aspects of the citric acid cycle. Biochem Soc Symp 54:173–8

74. Brookes PS, Zhang J, Dai L, Zhou F, Parks DA, Darley-Usmar VM, Anderson PG (2001) Increased sensitivity of mitochondrial respiration to inhibition by nitric oxide in cardiac hypertrophy. J Mol Cell Cardiol 33:69–82

75. Bender E, Kadenbach B (2000) The allosteric ATP-inhibition of cytochrome c oxidase activity is reversibly switched on by cAMP-dependent phosphorylation. FEBS Lett 466:130–4

76. Territo PR, Mootha VK, French SA, Balaban RS (2000) Ca(2+) activation of heart mitochondrial oxidative phosphorylation: Role of the F(0)/F(1)-ATPase. Am J Physiol Cell Physiol 278:C423–35

77. Scholz TD, Laughlin MR, Balaban RS, Kupriyanov VV, Heineman FW (1995) Effect of substrate on mitochondrial NADH, cytosolic redox state, and phosphorylated compounds in isolated hearts. Am J Physiol 268:H82–91

78. Ashruf JF, Coremans JM, Bruining HA, Ince C (1995) Increase of cardiac work is associated with decrease of mitochondrial NADH. Am J Physiol 269:H856–62

79. Jafri MS, Dudycha SJ, O'Rourke B (2001) Cardiac energy metabolism: Models of cellular respiration. Annu Rev Biomed Eng 3: 57–81

80. Cortassa S, Aon MA, Marban E, Winslow RL, O'Rourke B (2003) An integrated model of cardiac mitochondrial energy metabolism and calcium dynamics. Biophys J 84:2734–55

# Chapter 3

# Heart Mitochondrial Biogenesis

## Overview

Mitochondrial DNA (mtDNA) defects including point mutations, large-scale deletions and depletion may be associated with cardiac disorders. Most of the proteins participating in mitochondrial biogenesis—including mtDNA maintenance, transcription, and replication—are encoded by the nuclear genome and may be implicated in cardiac mtDNA defects. How mitochondrial biogenesis normally proceeds and how it can be affected by physiological stresses and disease are discussed in this chapter, keeping in mind that a coordinated expression of both nuclear and mitochondrial genomes must be maintained. Understanding the stimuli, signals, and transducers that govern the mitochondrial biogenesis pathways may have critical significance in the management of certain cardiac disorders.

## Introduction

Pathogenic point mutations and large-scale deletions in the mitochondrial genome as well as generalized depletion of mtDNA levels have severe consequences for organs such as the heart, since ATP derived from OXPHOS is steadily needed to maintain normal myocardial function. The nuclear genome encodes the entire complement of proteins involved in mtDNA replication and transcription, protein components of mitochondrial ribosomes, multiple structural and transport proteins of the mitochondrial membranes, and the remaining peptide subunits of the respiratory complexes (other than the 13 mtDNA-encoded peptide subunits).

These nuclear-encoded proteins are synthesized on the cytosolic ribosomes, targeted to mitochondria, and imported by a complex process.

The mtDNA genes exhibit a much higher mutation rate than the nuclear genes since they lack histones, have a rather limited DNA repair machinery, and are exposed to ROS generated by the ETC. A comprehensive analysis of the mitochondria and nuclear genome interactions and the overall regulation of biogenesis is presented in this chapter, with particular emphasis on heart mitochondria.

## Structure of mtDNA

Mammalian cardiac mitochondria have their own double-strand DNA circular molecule encompassing slightly over 16,000 bp and encoding 13 proteins that constitute a portion of the 5 enzyme complexes involved in the OXPHOS-respiratory chain [1]. The protein-encoding mtDNA genes are transcribed into mRNAs that are translated on a mitochondrial ribosome/protein synthesis apparatus. The mtDNA also encodes 2 ribosomal RNAs (e.g., 12S and 16S rRNA) and 22 tRNAs that contribute to the mitochondrial protein synthesis apparatus. The organization of the mitochondrial genome (Figure 3.1) and the sequence of its genes are highly conserved in evolution. This genome is highly compact and organized with structural genes generally separated by tRNA genes. Some of the proteins genes are overlapping.

Two mRNAs are translated in two different reading frames generating 4 proteins (ATPase 6 and 8, ND4 and ND4L). The structural genes of cardiac mtDNA (unlike either nuclear genes or plant and yeast mtDNA genes) contain no introns. A control region of approximately 1,100 nucleotides in size contains nearly all the mtDNA noncoding sequences, including the majority of sequence elements for the regulation of mitochondrial transcription and DNA replication. This region located between the $tRNA^{Pro}$ and $tRNA^{Phe}$ contains a short triple-stranded structure called the displacement loop or D-loop (Figure 3.1) in which a nascent H-strand DNA is annealed to the complementary parental L-strand DNA, displacing the parental H-strand. The D-loop region contains 3 blocks of sequences denoted CSB I-III with evolutionary conservation and also contains sequences that show an extremely high degree of variation ("hypervariable region"), including base substitutions.

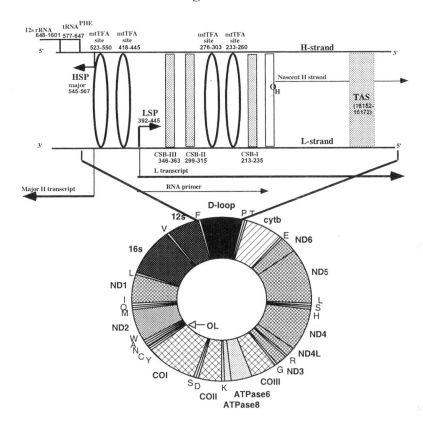

**Figure 3.1. Diagram of the human mitochondrial genome and its D-loop region.** *The circular human mtDNA molecule depicts the location of the 22 tRNAs identified by their cognate amino acid using single-letter code (F,V,L,I,Q,M,W,A,N, C,Y,S,D,K,G,R,H,S,L,E,T,P), 2 ribosomal RNA genes (12S and 16S), all 13 protein-encoding genes (ND1-ND6, COI-COIII, cytb, ATPase6, and ATPase8), the noncoding D-loop region including the origin of replication for the heavy strand ($O_H$), and promoters for transcription of the light (LSP) and heavy strand (HSP). Also shown are the binding sites for mitochondrial transcription factor (mtTFA), the highly conserved sequence blocks (CSB I-III), the start sites of the nascent DNA strand, the L and H transcripts produced by mtDNA replication, and transcription and TAS (termination association sequence). Also shown is the origin of replication for the L strand ($O_L$).*

In mammalian mitochondria, the mitochondrial genetic code differs from the "universal" genetic code found in bacteria, animal and plant nuclear DNA. The "universal" termination codon UGA is translated as Trp, while AGA and AGG (which normally encode Arg) are recognized as termination codons. In addition, AUA is recognized as Met instead of Ile. Moreover, there is a higher flexibility in the pairing of the third base of mitochondrial anticodons compared with their cytosolic counterparts. This allows the limited set of 22 tRNA species encoded by human mtDNA to be sufficient to translate all mitochondrial proteins.

MtDNA undergoes a higher mutation rate than nuclear DNA [2]. This has been attributed to the proximity of the mtDNA to oxidative free radicals generated by the mitochondrial bioenergetic machinery present in the inner membrane, as well as to a rather limited mtDNA repair system. An increased incidence of heart mtDNA mutations has been found in association with aging and cardiac disease [3].

While the maps of animal mtDNA are often presented in linear form, it is important to emphasize its circular nature as well as its topological structure, which is most often supercoiled. The covalently closed circular mtDNAs are molecules with each duplex composed of a heavy (H) and a light (L) strand, distinguishable on the basis of their base composition. Both the circularity and the supercoiled nature of mtDNA impose constraints on its replication and transcriptional functions as well as on the maintenance of the mtDNA genome.

Mitochondrial DNA has often been characterized as essentially naked, compared to the histone-enveloped nuclear DNA and its complex chromatin structure. Although mtDNA is localized within the mitochondrial matrix, it binds to the inner-membrane proteins [4–5]. In lower eukaryotes such as yeast and the slime mold, *Physarum*, a mitochondrial nucleoid-like structure, is present. The mtDNA from higher eukaryotes, including human, has also been found to be packaged in a nucleoid structure [6–8].

## MtDNA Function

### Replication

The replication cycle of the mtDNA begins with the initiation of the leading H-strand synthesis at the replication origin ($O_H$) with an RNA primer transcribed from the light strand promoter (LSP) [9–10]. The synthesis of this primer requires both a mtRNA polymerase and the mitochondrial transcription factor (mtTFA). The RNA primer exists as a stable and persistent RNA:DNA hybrid (also known as an R-loop), which is formed during transcription at human $O_H$ [11].

Therefore, the replication of mammalian mtDNA is intimately linked with mitochondrial transcription. H-strand DNA replication is initiated within the D-loop at 4 major and 3 minor sites. Three of these sites correspond to the L-strand transcription stop sequences, containing the conserved sequence blocks (CSB I-III) shown in Figure 3.1.

The mtTFA binds throughout the D-loop with a 40 to 50 base pair periodicity, with the CSBI most strongly bound. The mtTFA sites, downstream from CSBI, correspond to the DNA synthesis initiation sites, suggesting that mtTFA exerts a role in defining the transition from RNA to DNA synthesis. Evidence that mtTFA is a limiting factor for mtDNA replication has been demonstrated *in vivo* in mice [12]. The essential role of mtTFA in maintaining the overall mitochondrial structure and function in the heart has been well documented in mtTFA-null transgenic mice, which exhibit DCM and severe abnormalities in the structure and function of heart mitochondria [13].

The initial L strand primer transcript is enzymatically processed to yield the mature RNA 3' termini, most likely by a mitochondrial RNA processing endonuclease (MRP RNase), a ribonucleoprotein [9]. The MRP RNase requires a nuclear-encoded RNA of 265 nucleotides to guide the precise cleavage events. The processed-primer is then further elongated by mitochondrial DNA polymerase $\gamma$ to generate a short piece of H strand DNA (7S DNA), at which DNA replication apparently pauses. Arrested nascent H-strands remain annealed to their template L strand and form triplex D-loop structures. While the role of these triplex D-loop structures is presently unclear, they are particularly abundant in the heart and probably correlate with the capacity of the tissue to perform oxidative metabolism [14]. All 7S DNA molecules end at a site located about 50 nucleotides beyond a short conserved sequence element termed the termination-associated sequence (TAS), which interacts with a sequence-specific termination protein of 48kD [15]. Further elongation and completion of synthesis of the H-strand daughter DNA may be mediated by either antitermination or reinitiation events at the TAS site. These events and their regulation may be key determinants in the mtDNA copy number [16].

Eventually, the leading H-strand synthesis proceeds beyond the 7S DNA and around the L-strand template. After traversing approximately two-thirds of the genome, a second site, the L-strand replication origin ($O_L$), is exposed. The $O_L$ origin delimits a region of 30 bp within a cluster of tRNA genes. Displacement of the parental H-strand, which adopts a stem and loop structure, is recognized by a different enzyme, mtDNA primase, which provides a short RNA primer for L-strand DNA synthesis [17]. Following the synthesis of these primers, subsequent L strand elongation proceeds by mtDNA polymerase γ. Following the RNA primer removal and ATP-dependent DNA ligation events, the ensuing replication of covalent mtDNA circles is completed (estimated to occur within 2 hours).

Mammalian mtDNA polymerase γ, the only DNA polymerase present in mitochondria, is composed of a 140-kD catalytic subunit and a smaller accessory protein of 43-54 kD [18]. The major catalytic subunit of human mtDNA polymerase γ has been cloned and sequenced, and its content and activity do not significantly change during development or aging [19–20]. The DNA polymerase γ is stably expressed in cell cultures devoid of mtDNA, in contrast to mtTFA, whose amount and stability depend on mtDNA [21]. These findings have also suggested that the binding of mtTFA to mtDNA protects it from proteolytic degradation, since in the absence of mtDNA, the mtTFA is more easily degraded.

Other protein factors are involved in mtDNA replication. These include a mitochondrial single-strand binding protein (mtSSB), which maintains the integrity of exposed single-stranded regions of mtDNA found in the replication intermediates and which also has been reported to stimulate mtDNA polymerase activity. The levels of mtSSB protein correlate with mtDNA content and are up-regulated during early postnatal development of the heart [20]. DNA topoisomerases (enzymes that change the supercoiling of DNA) have been identified in mitochondria of leukemia cells and human platelets [22]. Specific genes involved in the synthesis of mtDNA topoisomerase have not yet been identified; they may represent modified isoforms of the nuclear DNA topoisomerase genes derived by differential expression or splicing [23]. In addition, a human ligase III gene has been shown to encode both a nuclear and a mitochondrial isoform [24]. While a role for the ligase III activity in mtDNA repair has been recently demonstrated, its precise role in mtDNA replication has not been determined (although likely required in the formation of covalently closed mtDNA circles). Other proteins, considered to play a role in mtDNA replication, include the ATP-dependent helicases (enzymes that separate the strands of DNA), which have been identified and partially purified from mitochondria. The protein encoded by the gene Twinkle has striking homology to bacteriophage helicases, exhibits a DNA helicase activity with 5' to 3' directionality, and is involved with events at the mitochondrial replication fork [25]. *In vitro* reconstitution experiments have shown that in combination with purified DNA polymerase $\gamma$ and mtSSB, Twinkle forms a functional mtDNA replisome capable of replicating the full-length mtDNA molecule at a rate not significantly different than that found *in vivo* [26]. Mutations in either DNA polymerase $\gamma$ or Twinkle can cause autosomal dominant progressive external ophthalmoplegia (adPEO), a disorder associated with deletions in mtDNA [27].

## *Regulation of mitochondrial DNA replication:*

Mitochondrial DNA replication can be regulated by the following:
1. Synthesis or modulation of RNA polymerase, mtTFA activity, and binding controlling LSP transcription;
2. Synthesis and cleavage activity by MRP RNAse, regulation of elongation, and termination, or antitermination of D-loop;
3. Modulating mtDNA polymerase $\gamma$ and mtDNA primase synthesis and activity;
4. Regulation of nucleotide levels (defects in nucleotide metabolism can severely impact mtDNA levels and cause mitochondrial cytopathy [28]);
5. Regulation of import of these nuclear proteins to mitochondria.

Mitochondrial proliferation is frequently accompanied by a high rate of mtDNA replication [29]. Nuclear-encoded transcription factors (e.g., NRF-1 and NRF-2) are responsive to a number of the stimuli that increase mitochondrial biogenesis [30]. These factors modulate the transcriptional expression of several genes implicated in mtDNA replication, including mtTFA, the RNA component of the MRP RNase, mtSSB, and mtDNA polymerase $\gamma$ subunits, reinforcing the notion that many of the regulatory steps for mtDNA replication are likely exerted at the nuclear level as discussed later.

In general, multiple copies of mtDNA are present in each cardiac cell (estimated at 1 to 10 genomes/mitochondria) [29]. The molecular mechanism(s) that regulate cardiac-specific mtDNA levels remains unknown. However, it has been reported that mtTFA is critical in the regulation of mtDNA levels; knockouts of mtTFA function decrease mtDNA copy number, while mtTFA overexpression elevates mtDNA levels [31–32]. The turnover of mtDNA is relatively short; the half-life for rat heart mtDNA is estimated at approximately 1 week compared to 1 month in brain [33]. The number of mtDNA molecules may change during cell differentiation and in response to different physiological conditions in contrast to the 2 copies of the nuclear genome found in somatic cells. The occurrence of a high copy number for mtDNA molecules, genes, and alleles has important ramifications for the effect of mutant mtDNA alleles on phenotype, cellular distribution, transmission at mitosis, and inheritance of mitochondrial genes, as well as in the regulation of cardiac mitochondrial gene expression.

## *Mitochondrial transcription and RNA processing*

The characterization of *trans*-acting factors involved in mtDNA replication, transcription and translation has generally been hampered by their low concentration, as well as by problems with nuclear/cytosolic contamination. However, several key genes have recently been identified during the screening of human gene data bases with sequences of genes derived from yeast and lower eukaryotes involved in mitochondrial replication, transcription, and translation. This has allowed rapid progress in carrying out functional studies.

In vertebrates, mtDNA is transcribed by mtRNA polymerase with at least 1 transcription factor (mtTFA) conferring transcriptional specificity (i.e., promoter selectivity) [34–35]. The human mtRNA polymerase is a single-subunit enzyme of 145 kD whose gene has recently been identified and whose protein residues (particularly within the C-terminal half of the polypeptide) share significant sequence homology with yeast mitochondrial and bacteriophage T3, SP6, and T7 RNA polymerases [36]. The mitochondrial transcription factor mtTFA (also known as TFAM) possesses 2 high-mobility group (HMG) domains involved in DNA-binding as well as a C-terminal transcriptional activating domain [37–38]. It is noteworthy that related HMG proteins have been implicated in both transcriptional activation and packaging of nuclear DNA in chromatin. Moreover, mtTFA binds to mtDNA at a variety of sites in addition to the promoter sites raising the possibility that mtTFA may have additional functions in mitochondrial maintenance or distribution. This is supported by new reports that mtTFA is present in human cells at a concentration well in excess of that required for transcriptional function, and by mtTFA's ability to wrap around the mtDNA in a histone-type fashion [39–41].

Critical to its transcriptional function, the mtTFA protein acts bidirectionally by binding to 2 sites within the D-loop that are located immediately upstream (between 10 to 40 bp) of each transcriptional start site of the light- and heavy-strand promoters (i.e., LSP and HSP). Each promoter element contains a 15 bp consensus sequence 5'-CANACC(G)CC(A)AAAGAYA surrounding the transcription initiation sites. Despite the close proximity of these 2 promoters (approximately 150 bp apart), these elements do not overlap and are functionally independent. A second initiation site for H-strand transcription (HSP2) is located at position 638 in the tRNA$^{Phe}$ gene, adjacent to the 12S rRNA. It has limited homology with the 15 bp consensus sequence, is used less frequently, and is considered a minor promoter. The mtTFA has the ability to wrap and unwind DNA *in vitro,* and can bend mtDNA at the promoters [39]. At low concentrations of mtTFA, the L-strand is transcribed from LSP, presumably due to its higher affinity for its binding site near LSP. In contrast, at higher concentrations of mtTFA, the H-strand is transcribed from both major and minor promoter regions, albeit the extent of mtTFA-stimulation of H-strand transcription is moderate and likely requires accessory factors. In lower eukaryotes, such as yeast and *Xenopus laevis*, a second transcription factor (mtTFB) with extensive sequence homology with the dissociable sigma subunit of bacterial RNA polymerase is required for mtDNA transcription [9]. Recently, 2 related homologues of mtTFB were identified (e.g., TFB1M and TFB2M) in human and mouse. They have been shown to participate in the activation of mtDNA transcriptional initiation [42–43].

The transcription of each mtDNA strand is polycistronic [44]. L-strand transcription produces a large genome-size precursor transcript, which is rapidly processed to yield mature transcripts for 1 polypeptide (ND6) and 8 tRNAs (P, S$^{UCN}$, Q, A, C, N, Y, E). Similarly, H-strand transcription generates large, full-genome-length precursor transcripts which are rapidly processed to produce discrete mature transcripts for 12S and 16S rRNAs, the remaining 12 polypeptides, and 14 tRNAs (F, V, L$^{UUR}$, M, I, W, D, K, G, T, R, H, S$^{AGY}$, L$^{CUN}$). The previously described transcriptional attenuation sequence located at nt 3237–3249 (near the end of the 16S rRNA gene within tRNA$^{Leu}$)

is a highly conserved motif in mtDNA and functions to regulate the rRNA/mRNA transcript ratio. Binding of a protein complex (including a 34 kD multileucine zipper-containing protein termed mTERF) to this sequence (and perhaps to mtRNA polymerase) terminates mtDNA transcription, resulting in a 15 to 100-fold higher synthesis of rRNA (16S and 12S rRNAs) relative to genes located downstream [45]. The mTERF termination activity but not its DNA-binding function is regulated by phosphorylation, and mTERF is active as a monomer but not as a dimer [46–47]. The functional significance of the mTERF regulatory site is underscored by the demonstration that point mutations within TAS are associated with MELAS, which may be a consequence of mitochondrial trans-criptional dysfunction [48].

## Regulation of mitochondrial transcription and processing

There is no evidence for differential activity of the two major mitochondrial transcription promoters [29]. The presence of mtRNA polymerase in combination with 1 major accessory factor is thought to determine a steady state rate of transcription from both promoters. Modulation of the overall level of mitochondrial transcription is primarily regulated by levels of the mtRNA polymerase and mtTFA, controlled by nuclear factors. However, recent data have shown that mitochondria transcription can be more directly regulated without invoking changes in nuclear transcription factors and nuclear gene expression. Studies with isolated mitochondria (also termed *in organello*) show that mtDNA transcription can be maintained for several hours in the absence of nuclear and cytoplasmic interactions; however, processing of rRNA precursors and the stability of the mature rRNAs, but not transcription itself, is severely impaired after short periods of incubation [49–50]. This supports the view that rRNA processing is dependent on the mitochondrial interaction with the nucleo-cytoplasmic compartment, whereas events leading to the synthesis of mitochondrial mRNAs do not require the continuous supply of nucleocytoplasmic factors (likely accumulated in excess by mitochondria). In addition, the relative transcription rates of rRNA and mRNA are modulated by ATP levels [51]. It appears that ATP levels directly impact mtRNA polymerase activity, both *in organello* and *in vitro*, suggesting that mtRNA synthesis is regulated in response to changes in intramitochondrial ATP levels [49]. Footprinting analysis of protein-DNA interactions suggests that ATP affects transcription primarily by acting at the level of transcriptional initiation at specific promoter sites and not on transcription termination sites [52]. In addition, *in organello* mitochondrial transcription studies have demonstrated that thyroid hormone directly modulates mtRNA levels and transcription rate, affecting the mRNA/rRNA ratio. This is achieved by selective modification of the specific H-strand initiation sites and does not require previous activation of nuclear gene expression [50].

There is also evidence that posttranscriptional control plays a contributory role in regulating mitochondrial gene expression [29]. Differential RNA stability accounts for 20 to 150-fold higher levels of tRNA compared to individual mRNAs derived from the same transcriptional event [53] and likely contributes to the different steady-state levels of individual mature RNA species derived from the same transcript [54]. Changes in mtRNA stability can also occur as a function of developmental or physiological transition, resulting in marked changes in the steady-state levels of specific mitochondrial transcripts. In the developing liver, high transcript levels of mtDNA-encoded subunits of ATP synthase (i.e., ATPase 6 and 8) result from altered stability of the specific mitochondrial transcripts [55]. Similar findings have been found with the mRNAs of the nuclear-encoded ATP synthase subunit β [56]. These findings indicate that the developmental regulation of nuclear and mitochondrial genes during biogenesis of mammalian mitochondria can be concertedly controlled by a posttranscriptional mechanism involving regulation of degradation of mRNA derived from both genomes.

## Mitochondrial translation

### *Mitochondrial ribosomes*

Translation of mitochondrial mRNAs occurs exclusively on mitochondrial ribosomes. The rRNA of mitochondrial ribosomes are encoded by mtDNA, while the ribosomal proteins are entirely encoded by nuclear DNA [57]. The ribosomes present in mammalian mitochondria have a lower sedimentation coefficient (i.e., 55S) than cytoplasmic ribosomes and are composed of small (28S) and large (39S) subunits. They are characterized by a significantly lower percentage of rRNA, compared to bacterial or cytoplasmic ribosomes, and a compensatory increase in the number and mass of ribosomal proteins [58]. The small subunit of the mitochondrial ribosome contains a 12S rRNA and about 30 proteins, whereas the large subunit consists of a 16S rRNA and approximately 48 proteins [59]. This total of nearly 80 proteins is significantly higher than that observed in bacterial ribosomes and eukaryotic cytoplasmic ribosomes. At present, the available data are limited in regard to the content and number of ribosomes/ mitochondria in human cells as a function of development, cell-type, or physiological condition.

Although the importance of the mitochondrial translation products is well known, the information available in mammalian mitochondria concerning the identity of the protein components of the translational machinery is limited. A comprehensive effort to identify and characterize mammalian and human genes involved in the mitochondrial ribosome is currently underway. Recently, proteins from both the large and small subunits of the mammalian mitochondrial ribosome have been primarily characterized by peptide sequencing coupled to extensive use of the expressed sequence tag (EST) databases to deduce the full-length cDNAs and the corresponding amino acid sequences [60–65]. Of the 48 proteins present in mammalian mitochondrial large ribosomal subunit, 28 shared extensive homology with *E. coli* ribosomal proteins; the remaining 20 proteins had no homology with either bacterial, chloroplast, or cytosolic ribosomal proteins, indicating that they were novel [65]. The majority of the identified genes encoding the mitochondrial ribosomal proteins have been mapped and show a pattern of wide dispersion throughout the nuclear genome [66].

Although all of the polypeptides synthesized by the mitochondrial translational system are localized in the inner membrane, it has not yet been determined whether they are actually synthesized on membrane-bound ribosomes or if the insertion of these polypeptides is a cotranslational or posttranslational process. Unlike yeast mitochondrial and nuclear mRNAs, animal mitochondrial mRNAs lack significant 5'- and 3'-untranslated nucleotides. The start codon is generally located within 3 nucleotides of the 5' end of the mRNA. In addition, there is no 5' 7-methylguanylate cap structure (found in nuclear mRNAs), nor is there a Shine-Delgarno sequence for appropriately positioning the ribosome for efficient translation such as found in bacteria [29]. In general, the stop codon of mitochondrial mRNA is immediately followed by a poly (A) tail added posttranscriptionally. A significant fraction of bovine mitochondrial ribosomes are associated with the inner membrane and most ribosomes can be released from the inner membrane by high salt (indicating electrostatic interactions) or detergent. In addition, there is evidence that the nascent peptide insertion is not involved in ribosome-membrane attachment [67].

Protein synthesis from mammalian mitochondrial ribosomes like their prokaryotic counterparts is sensitive to chloramphenicol but insensitive to cycloheximide. The binding site for chloramphenicol can be modified by a mutation in the rRNA gene resulting in chloramphenicol-resistant ($CAP_R$) mutants, the first mitochondrial mutation to be investigated in mammalian cell culture studies [68].

Chloramphenicol has been widely used to selectively inhibit mitochondrial protein synthesis without effecting the cytoplasmic protein synthesis machinery. Conversely, cycloheximide is used to inhibit cytoplasmic protein synthesis with little immediate effect on mitochondrial protein synthesis.

Mutations or polymorphisms in mtRNA molecules involved in processing and translation may be a primary cause of some OXPHOS disorders and may modulate the severity and tissue specificity of pathogenic mitochondrial DNA mutations [69]. A cardiac-specific splice variant of a mitochondrial ribosomal protein (L5) has been recently identified as a potential candidate in the cardiac specificity of mitochondrial-based disease [70]. In addition, compared to their cytosolic counterparts, the mitochondrial ribosomes have also been shown to be extremely sensitive to toxic agents such as alcohol. Chronic ethanol feeding in rats can produce a marked decrease in the number of intact 55S mitochondrial ribosomes, as well as decreased levels of a selected number of ribosomal subunit proteins, suggesting impaired mitochondrial assembly [71]. However, no such defects were observed with cytoplasmic ribosomes. These changes in ribosomes may be the cause for the decreased hepatic mitochondrial protein synthesis and impaired OXPHOS observed with increased alcohol consumption [72].

## Initiation and elongation of translation

Identifying and reconstituting the *in vitro* factors, enzymes and substrates comprise the classical molecular approach toward understanding complex molecular phenomena such as replication, transcription, and translation. Over the last 2 decades, while *in vitro* systems have been successfully developed and employed with both human mitochondrial DNA replication and transcription, no *in vitro* system has yet been developed for the study of mitochondrial translation. Hence, there has been a lag in identifying elongation and initiation factors for mitochondrial translation.

The following has been revealed thus far in mammalian protein synthesis:

1. Small ribosomal subunits bind mRNA tightly in the absence of initiating factors or tRNA (unlike prokaryotic or eukaryotic cytosolic systems). At least 400 nucleotides of the messenger template are minimally required for efficient binding to the ribosomal subunit, which may explain why genes for ATPase8 and ND4L (which encode < 300 nt transcripts) may have to be part of a larger message [73].

2. Two initiating factor (IF-2 and IF-3) have been identified and cloned. IF2 belongs to a family of GTPases and exhibits strong structural and functional homology with *E. coli* IF-2, promoting fMET-tRNA binding to the small ribosomal subunit in the presence of GTP and mRNA template [74–75].

3. Three mitochondrial elongation factors (EF-TU, EF-TS and EF-G) have been purified and cloned from mammalian sources and show structural and functional homology with the corresponding prokaryotic factors [76–78].

## Mitochondrial DNA repair

It has been assumed for some time that mtDNA repair was not present, poorly developed, or inefficient. More recently, the presence of mtDNA repair in mammalian cells has been unequivocally demonstrated, and a number of defects are removed from mtDNA in cells exposed to various chemicals [79–80]. The activity of several proteins that process damaged mtDNA has been detected in mitochondria. Specific evidence has been found for mitochondrial base excision repair (BER), mismatch repair, and recombinational repair mechanisms, while mitochondrial nucleotide excision repair (NER) has not been demonstrated.

In aerobic cells, the most frequent type of injury encountered by nuclear DNA and even more by mtDNA is DNA damage arising from ROS. This damage includes single-strand breaks and oxidative base damage. Mitochondria are proficient at removing oxidized and alkylated lesions by the monofunctional alkylating agent alloxan and acridine orange damage, which are typically repaired by base excision repair. These agents enter the cell, undergo redox cycling, and produce ROS similar to that normally generated in mitochondria. Addition of 5 mM alloxan to cultured rat cells increased the rate of oxidative base damage and by several fold the frequency of mtDNA defects. After alloxan removal, the frequency of oxidized bases decreased rapidly, returning to levels found in mitochondria from untreated cells, indicating that mitochondrial repair of these defects is extremely efficient [81].

A number of enzymatic activities involved in DNA repair have been found in mitochondria. Three uracil glycosylases have been identified and characterized [82–84]. A mitochondrial apurinic (AP) endonuclease activity that is UV-inducible has also been found [85]. Examination of CHO cells exposed to acridine orange plus light for the purpose of introducing 8-oxoG and other oxidative DNA damage lesions showed that these lesions were rapidly removed from mtDNA (with more than 60% of the defects repaired within 4 hours), suggesting that mammalian cells possess mitochondrial enzymes that recognize and remove 8-oxoG. A mitochondrial endonuclease, reactive to oxidative damage, is responsible for the recognition and incision of 8-oxoG and abasic sites [86]. Another mitochondrial endonuclease (endonuclease G) has been proposed to play a contributory role in both mtDNA replication and in repair of both single-strand breaks and intrastrand cross-links [87–89]. However, endonuclease G's role in mtDNA repair and replication has been recently challenged because this nuclease appears to be exclusively located within the mitochondrial intermembrane space and not in the matrix compartment, in which mtDNA resides [90–91]. The release from the mitochondrial intermembrane space into the cytoplasm (and eventual delivery to the nucleus) of endonuclease G, along with cytochrome *c*, AIF, and Smac/diablo proteins, represents a pivotal event in apoptotic progression [92]. It is also noteworthy that endonuclease G activity is markedly elevated in both fetal and adult heart mitochondria, compared to other tissues, and displays significant decline in the senescent heart [93].

Other DNA repair enzymes identified in mammalian mitochondria include a DNA ligase III activity [24] involved in repairing single-strand nicks [89] and a poly (ADP-ribose) polymerase (PARP) implicated in repairing alkylation damage to mtDNA by facilitating the removal of N-methylpurines induced by methylnitrosourea treatment [94]. In addition, mtDNA polymerase $\gamma$ can be recruited to fill single-nucleotide gaps during base excision repair, in contrast to the "patch" repair found in nuclear DNA [95].

Distinct mtDNA repair systems are utilized for repairing missing and mismatched bases (e.g., BER), and also in the repair of cytosine and guanosine deamination in human fibroblasts (e.g., repair of NO-induced mtDNA damage) [96]. Thus far, there has been only limited investigation of mtDNA repair at the regulatory level, although there is indication of the existence of both tissue-specific and developmental-specific regulation of mtDNA repair. For instance, there are striking variations in glial cell responses to mtDNA damage with astrocytes being more effective at removing some types of alkylating damage compared to oligodendrocytes [97]. This variability appears to correlate with the ability to withstand oxidative stress. Moreover, recombinational repair of mtDNA in mammalian cells has also been demonstrated [98]. This is consistent with the observed mitochondrial repair of cisplatin-induced interstrand lesions in mtDNA [99]. Such interstrand DNA abnormalities are repaired in bacteria and in yeast nuclear DNA by homologous recombination, suggesting that mammalian mitochondria may utilize a homologous recombination-based process to repair damaged DNA. Recombination intermediates involving all regions of the mitochondrial genome are particularly prevalent in human heart muscle and are considered products of mtDNA repair [100]. Studies of mtDNA repair of inter- and intrastrand defects, double-strand scissions, or bulky adducts that likely involve NER have been rather equivocal. While repair of UV-induced mtDNA photolesions was not detected in cultured mouse or human cells [101–102], the repair of UV-induced photolesions and of some bulky adducts and interstrand lesions in mtDNA has been reported in murine leukemia [103] and yeast [104].

# Nuclear participation in mitochondrial biogenesis

## *Nuclear regulatory proteins and coordination of transcriptional events*

Mitochondria have been estimated to contain more than 1,000 polypeptides, and most of them are nuclear-DNA-encoded. With a limited (but essential) contribution of 13 proteins, 2 ribosomal rRNAs, and 22 tRNAs, mitochondria are obviously not self-supporting organelles. The entire complement of enzymes and regulatory factors required for mtDNA replication and repair, transcription, RNA processing, and translation is encoded by nuclear DNA. In addition, the large network of enzymes involved in generating bioenergy, via the TCA cycle and FAO pathways, are encoded by nuclear genes, and the respiratory enzyme complexes of OXPHOS and ETC are of hybrid origin with the majority of enzyme subunits (over 70) being encoded by nuclear DNA, as shown in Table 3.1.

**Table 3.1. MtDNA-and nuclear-DNA-encoded subunits of ETC/OXPHOS complexes**

|  | MtDNA-Encoded Subunits | Nuclear-DNA Encoded Subunits |
|---|---|---|
| Complex I | 7 | 35 |
| Complex II | 0 | 4 |
| Complex III | 1 | 10 |
| Complex IV | 3 | 10 |
| Complex V | 2 | 14 |

These nuclear-encoded proteins are synthesized on cytosolic ribosomes, targeted to mitochondria, and imported by a complex process.

In this section, we address the major nuclear regulatory circuits in mitochondrial protein biosynthesis and examine the pathway from the nucleus to the mitochondria.

The transcriptional signals governing the nuclear gene synthesis of mitochondrial proteins are of 2 major classes, *cis* elements and *trans* regulatory factors (primarily activators). Regulatory *cis* elements are located within the promoter sequences of the structural genes to be transcribed. These are responsive to diverse tissue and developmental specific signals, as well as to an array of physiological stimuli that are gradually being revealed. Specific *cis* elements involved in the regulation of specific nuclear transcripts of mitochondrial proteins have been identified within the promoter regions of genes encoding selected subunits of ATP synthase, cytochrome *c* oxidase, ANT, cytochrome *c*, and several FAO and TCA cycle enzymes. While some of these *cis* sequences respond to general transcriptional activators (e.g., SP1, CCAAT, cAMP response element binding or CREB), others respond to specific mitochondrial *trans* activators (e.g., OXBOX activators).

The OXBOX enhancer element has been located in 5' regions and promoters of ANT, ATP $\beta$, and ATP $\alpha$ genes [105] and is bound by transcription factors, present only in muscle cells [106]. The OXBOX sequence element is also present in a highly conserved sequence block within the mtDNA D-loop [107]. Mitochondrial element-binding proteins (MtEBPs) are present in the mitochondria of human, bovine, and rat cells. MtEBPs purified from human mitochondria, using mitochondrial element-specific DNA affinity chromatography, recognize specific *cis* acting sequences in the cytochrome *c* gene, COXVb, mitochondrial creatine kinase, and a mitochondrial element-like sequence within the mtTFA binding site for the heavy-strand promoter [108]. These findings suggest a role for OXBOX and MtEBP in coordinating nuclear and mitochondrial gene expression.

Nuclear respiratory factors (e.g., NRF-1 and NRF-2) are presently the best characterized of the *trans* activators involved in mitochondrial biogenesis [30, 109–110]. These factors bind sites within the promoters of genes for complex IV subunits, including COXIV, COXVIIa, COXVb, several complex I, III, and V subunits, cytochrome *c*, mtTFA, and $\delta$-aminolevulinate (ALA) synthase, the rate-limiting enzyme in heme biosynthesis and expression regulation as shown in Table 3.2. The NRF-2 factor also known as the GA-binding protein (GABP) binds to a *cis* sequence element containing a GGAA/T motif [111], present in many of the same genes as the NRF-1 *cis* element. The transcription factor NRF-1 has a central role in augmenting mitochondrial biogenesis during states of increased respiratory uncoupling (which increases oxygen consumption and lowers energy reserves). Moreover, by translating physiological signals into an increased capacity for generating energy, it plays a pivotal role in cellular adaptation to energy demands [112].

Interestingly, the expression of the NRF family is itself regulated by the master transcriptional regulator, PGC-1α [113].

**Table 3.2.  Regulatory sites in nuclear genes specifying mitochondrial proteins**

| | OXPHOS Genes | MtDNA Biogenesis | Other Mitochondrial Functions |
|---|---|---|---|
| NRF-1 | Cytochrome *c* | MRP RNA | 5-ALA synthase |
| | Complex I  (subunit 8) | mtTFA | TOM20 |
| | Complex II  (subunits SDHB, SDHC,SDHD) | rp S12 | VDAC |
| | Complex III (core and ubiquinone binding proteins) | | |
| | Complex IV (subunits Vb, VIc, VIa, and VIIa) | | |
| | Complex V (subunits β and γ) | | |
| NRF-2 | Complex II (subunits SDHB, SDHC,SDHD) | mtTFA | TOM20 |
| | Complex V (subunit β) | TFB1M | SURF1 |
| | Complex IV (subunits IV, Vb VIa, VIIa, and Vb) | TFB2M | VDAC |
| | | rp S12 | |
| | | mtSSB | |
| OXBOX | ANT | N.D. | N.D. |
| | ComplexV (subunits α and β) | | |

*Note:* ND = not determined; rp S12 = ribosomal protein S12.

A number of nuclear genes encoding mitochondrial proteins respond to thyroid hormone by virtue of the *cis* element, TRE (thyroid hormone responsive element) within their promoter sequences. In addition, the global regulator PPAR-α regulates several of the FAO enzymes [114]. In Table 3.2, a list of several *cis* elements and their *trans* activators identified in the gene activation of specific nuclear-encoded mitochondrial proteins is presented, including nuclear OXPHOS and targeted biogenesis genes. Several of the *cis* sequences are present not only in nuclear gene promoter regions but also are found within the mtDNA D-loop region as well (e.g., TRE and OXBOX elements), suggesting a mechanism of coordinated regulation of both nuclear and mtDNA gene expression. While a number of important OXPHOS genes have several *cis* regulatory sites, recognized by these *trans*-acting factors, many of the genes involved in OXPHOS and ETC do not contain any of the forementioned *cis* elements as a recognizable consensus sequence.

## *Hormones affecting both mitochondrial transcription and nuclear transcription*

It has been reported that a number of nuclear and mitochondrial-encoded genes exhibit a similar pattern of transcriptional regulation in cardiac tissue [115]. However, the analysis of transcript and peptide levels, of both nuclear and mtDNA-encoded enzyme subunits, assessed in response to physiological transition (e.g., thyroid hormone treatment and cell-growth activation), have revealed a more complex pattern of transcriptional regulation of nuclear genes encoding mito-chondrial proteins, indicating multiple regulatory circuits [116–117].

In mitochondria, hormone receptors serve as transcription factors, previously thought to be solely located in the nucleus. For example,a protein (denoted c-ErbAα1) displaying affinity for triiodothyronine (T3), similar to that of the T3 nuclear receptor, was found in the mitochondrial matrix of rat liver [118]. The c-ErbAα1 protein, a truncated version of the T3 nuclear receptor, specifically binds to 4 sites with sequence homology to nuclear T3 response elements; 2 of the sites are located within the mtDNA D-loop. The binding of the c-ErbAα1 protein to its response element causes an increase in levels of both precursor and mature mitochondrial transcripts and in the ratio of mRNA to rRNA in a T3-dependent manner, leading to the stimulation of mitochondrial protein synthesis [119]. Experiments using immuno-fluorescence labeling and confocal laser-scanning microscopy have similarly localized a glucocorticoid receptor in the mitochondrial matrix [120]. Evidence of mtDNA sequence similarity to nuclear glucocorticoid-responsive elements has also been demonstrated [121]. However, unlike the thyroid hormone receptor, direct evidence of a glucocorticod receptor-mediated action of steroid hormones on mitochondrial gene transcription has not yet been reported.

The presence of hormone receptors in mitochondria, which bind both nuclear and mitochondrial hormone-response elements, further assists the coordination of the bi-genomic response to hormone stimulation and regulation. At least in the case of the T3 receptor, such pathways appear to be operative in both short-term physiological responses, providing a direct and rapid mitochondrial response to hormone stimulation and in overall myocyte development and differentiation [122].

## *Mitochondria import and assembly of proteins*

The translocation of proteins into mitochondria (as with other organelles such as the chloroplast and peroxisome) is post-translational (after protein is completely synthesized). Therefore, it is unlikely that cytoplasmic ribosomes, either free or associated with endoplasmic reticulum (ER), are bound to the mitochondrial organelle [123].

Protein translocation occurs at mitochondrial "contact" sites joining outer and inner membranes. Signal sequences (signal peptides 20 to 80 residues long) on the imported proteins are a prerequisite for their efficient translocation into the mitochondrial matrix; a second signal (normally composed of hydrophobic residues) is required for insertion into the inner membrane. Specific receptors are present on the mitochondrial outer membrane and bind signal peptides. These receptors are part of the translocase outer-membrane complex (TOM 20) [124–126]. Translocation requires both mitochondrial membrane potential and ATP hydrolysis, and mitochondrial protein import is mediated by the action of chaperone proteins e.g., heat-shock proteins (HSPs) located in both the cytoplasm and mitochondria. These chaperones sequentially fold the proteins before entering mitochondria and unfold them once inside the matrix (e.g., mitochondrial HSP70). Within the matrix, a signal-peptidase rapidly cleaves off the signal peptide as shown in Figure 3.2.

Tissue-specific mitochondrial protein import can be affected by hormones. Thyroid hormone can modify the cardiac mitochondrial phenotype by increasing the rate of mitochondrial protein import [127]. The import of matrix-localized precursor proteins malate dehydrogenase (MDH), and ornithine carbamoyl transferase was increased coinciding with thyroid hormone-induced changes in the expression of protein import machinery components (i.e., elevated levels of the outer-membrane receptor TOM20 and the mtHSP70.

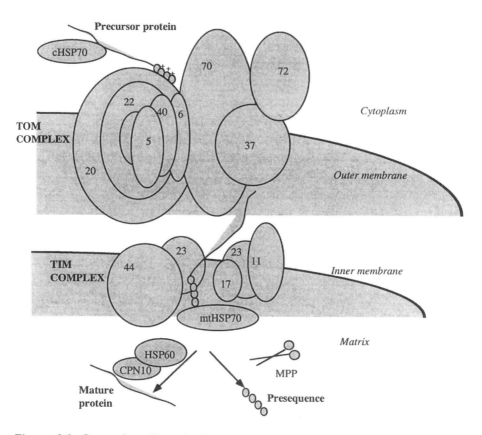

**Figure 3.2. General outline of mitochondrial protein import.** *A typical matrix-destined precursor preprotein, containing a mitochondrial-targeting presequence, is unfolded and directed to the import machinery by a cytosolic chaperone (e.g., cytosolic HSP protein of 70 kd, cHSP70). The denatured form of the precursor protein is recognized by receptors on the outer membrane (TOM 20/22 and 37/70). The preprotein is translocated through the outer membrane (TOM complex) and transferred to the translocase on the inner membrane (TIM complex). The matrix chaperone mtHSP70 pulls in the precursor, and the signal sequence is cleaved by the mitochondrial processing peptidase (MPP). Subsequently, the mature protein is refolded by matrix chaperones HSP60 and CPN 10.*

## Relevance of mitochondrial biogenesis

While the issue of mitochondrial nonautonomy is an open and shut case, the interactions between nucleus and mitochondria for a coordinated regulation of gene expression are recognized as having a large, subtle, and rich interrelationship that is gradually being deciphered. This relationship is considered to be a two-way dialogue or cross-talk between the two genomes, allowing an integration of responses to a variety of extracellular and intracellular stimuli and signals. In addition to physiological stimulation of mitochondrial biogenesis in skeletal and cardiac muscle in response to increased contractile activity (e.g., exercise), electrical stimuli, and thyroid hormone [128], there is evidence that the mitochondrial biogenesis pathways may be implicated in mitochondrial-based diseases. Coordinated increases in both mitochondrial and nuclear gene expression have also been reported in patients with mitochondrial diseases with OXPHOS defects, including mitochondrial cardiomyopathy [129,3]. Understanding the stimuli, signals, and transducers that govern the mitochondrial biogenesis pathways may have critical significance in the effective treatment of cardiovascular disorders.

## References

1. Anderson S, Bankier AT, Barrell BG, de Bruijn MH, Coulson AR, AR, Drouin J, Eperon IC, Nierlich DP, Roe BA, Sanger F, Schreier PH, Smith AJ, Staden R, Young IG (1981) Sequence and organization of human mitochondrial genome. Nature 290:457–65
2. Neckelmann N, Li K, Wade RP, Shuster R, Wallace DC (1987) cDNA sequence of a human skeletal muscle ADP/ATP translocator: Lack of a leader peptide, divergence from a fibroblast translocator cDNA, and coevolution with mitochondrial DNA genes. Proc Natl Acad Sci USA 84:7580–4
3. Marín-García J, Goldenthal MJ (2002) Understanding the impact of mitochondrial defects in cardiovascular disease: A review. J Card Fail 8:347–61
4. Albring M, Griffith J, Attardi G (1977) Association of a protein structure of probable membrane derivation with HeLa cell

mitochondrial DNA near its origin of replication. Proc Natl Acad Sci USA 74:1348–52

5. Hillar M, Rangayya V, Jafar BB, Chambers D, Vitzu M, Wyborny LE (1979) Membrane-bound mitochondrial DNA: Isolation, transcription and protein composition. Arch Int Physiol Biochim 87:29–49

6. Kanki T, Nakayama H, Sasaki N, Takio K, Alam TI, Hamasaki N, Kang D (2004) Mitochondrial nucleoid and transcription factor A. Ann NY Acad Sci 1011:61–8

7. Legros F, Malka F, Frachon P, Lombes A, Rojo M (2004) Organization and dynamics of human mitochondrial DNA. J Cell Sci 117:2653–62

8. Bogenhagen DF, Wang Y, Shen EL, Kobayashi R (2003) Protein components of mitochondrial DNA nucleoids in higher eukaryotes. Mol Cell Proteomics 2:1205–16

9. Shadel GS, Clayton DA (1997) Mitochondrial DNA maintenance in vertebrates. Annu Rev Biochem 66:409-35

10. Taanman JW (1999) The mitochondrial genome: Structure, transcription, translation and replication. Biochim Biophys Acta 1410: 103–23

11. Xu B, Clayton DA (1996) RNA-DNA hybrid formation at the human mitochondrial heavy-strand origin ceases at replication start sites: An implication for RNA-DNA hybrids serving as primers. EMBO J 15:3135–43

12. Larsson NG, Wang J, Wilhelmsson H, Oldfors A, Rustin P, Lewandoski M, Barsh GS, Clayton DA (1998) Mitochondrial transcription factor A is necessary for mtDNA maintenance and embryogenesis in mice. Nat Genet 18:231–6

13. Wang J, Wilhelmsson, Graff C, Li H, Oldfors A, Rustin P, Bruning JC, Kahn CR, Clayton DA, Barsh GS, Thoreen P, Larsson N G (1999) Dilated cardiomyopathy and atrioventricular conduction blocks induced by heart-specific inactivation of mitochondrial gene expression. Nature Genet 21:133–7

14. Annex BH, Williams RS (1990) Mitochondrial DNA structure and expression in specialized subtypes of mammalian striated muscle. Mol Cell Biol 10:5671–8

15. Madsen CS, Ghivizzani SC, Hauswirth WW (1993) Protein binding to a single termination-associated sequence in the mitochondrial DNA D-loop region. Mol Cell Biol 13:2162–71

16. Moraes CT (2001) What regulates mitochondrial DNA copy number in animal cells? Trends Genet 17:199–205

17. Wong TW, Clayton DA (1985) Isolation and characterization of a DNA primase from human mitochondria. J Biol Chem 260:11530–5

18. Kaguni LS (2004) DNA polymerase gamma, the mitochondrial replicase. Annu Rev Biochem 73:293–320

19. Ropp PA, Copeland WC (1996) Cloning and characterization of the human mitochondrial DNA polymerase, DNA polymerase gamma. Genomics 36:449–58

20. Schultz RA, Swoap SJ, McDaniel LD, Zhang B, Koon EC, Garry DJ, Li K, Williams RS (1998) Differential expression of mitochondrial DNA replication factors in mammalian tissues. J Biol Chem 273:3447–51

21. Davis AF, Ropp PA, Clayton DA, Copeland WC (1996) Mitochondrial DNA polymerase gamma is expressed and translated in the absence of mitochondrial DNA maintenance and replication. Nucleic Acids Res 24:2753–9

22. Castora FJ, Lazarus GM, Kunes D (1985) The presence of two mitochondrial DNA topoisomerases in human acute leukemia cells. Biochem Biophys Res Commun 130:854–66

23. Wang Y, Lyu YL, Wang JC (2002) Dual localization of human DNA topoisomerase III alpha to mitochondria and nucleus. Proc Natl Acad Sci USA 99:12114–9

24. Lakshmipathy U, Campbell C (2001) Antisense-mediated decrease in DNA ligase III expression results in reduced mitochondrial DNA integrity. Nucleic Acids Res 29:668–76

25. Korhonen JA, Gaspari M, Falkenberg M (2003) TWINKLE has 5'→3' DNA helicase activity and is specifically stimulated by mitochondrial single-stranded DNA-binding protein. J Biol Chem 278:48627–32

26. Korhonen JA, Pham XH, Pellegrini M, Falkenberg M (2004) Reconstitution of a minimal mtDNA replisome in vitro. EMBO J 2004 23:2423–9

27. Spelbrink JN, Li FY, Tiranti V, Nikali K, Yuan QP, Tariq M, Wanrooij S, Garrido N, Comi G, Morandi L, Santoro L, Toscano A, Fabrizi GM, Somer H, Croxen R, Beeson D, Poulton J, Suomalainen A, Jacobs HT, Zeviani M, Larsson C (2001) Human mitochondrial DNA deletions associated with mutations in the gene encoding Twinkle, a phage T7 gene 4-like protein localized in mitochondria. Nat Genet 28:223–3

28. Marti R, Nishigaki Y, Vila MR, Hirano M (2003) Alteration of nucleotide metabolism: A new mechanism for mitochondrial disorders. Clin Chem Lab Med 41:845–51

29. Attardi G, Schatz G (1988) Biogenesis of mitochondria. Annu Rev Cell Biol 4:289–333

30. Scarpulla RC (1997) Nuclear control of respiratory chain expression in mammalian cells. J Bioenerg Biomembr 29:109–19

31. Matsushima Y, Garesse R, Kaguni LS (2004) Drosophila mitochondrial transcription factor B2 regulates mitochondrial DNA copy number and transcription in Schneider cells. J Biol Chem 279:26900–5

32. Ekstrand MI, Falkenberg M, Rantanen A, Park CB, Gaspari M, Hultenby K, Rustin P, Gustafsson CM, Larsson NG (2004) Mitochondrial transcription factor A regulates mtDNA copy number in mammals. Hum Mol Genet 13:935–44

33. Gross NJ, Getz GS, Rabinowitz M (1969) Apparent turnover of mitochondrial deoxyribonucleic acid and mitochondrial phospholipids in the tissues of the rat. J Biol Chem 244:1552–62

34. Clayton DA (1992) Transcription and replication of animal mitochondrial DNAs. Int Rev Cytol 141:217–32

35. Fernandez-Silva P, Enriquez JA, Montoya J (2003) Replication and transcription of mammalian mitochondrial DNA. Exp Physiol 88:41–56

36. Tiranti V, Savoia A, Forti F, D'Apolito MF, Centra M, Rochi M, Zeviani M (1997) Identification of the gene encoding the human mitochondrial RNA polymerase (h-mtRPOL) by cyberscreening of the Expressed Sequence Tags database. Hum Mol Genet 6:615–25

37. Fisher RP, Parisi MA, Clayton DA (1989) Flexible recognition of rapidly evolving promoter sequences by mitochondrial trans-cription factor 1. Genes Dev 3:2202–17

38. Parisi MA, Clayton DA (1991) Similarity of human mitochondrial transcription factor 1 to high mobility group proteins. Science 252:965–9

39. Fisher RP, Lisowsky T, Parisi MA, Clayton DA (1992) DNA wrapping and bending by a mitochondrial high mobility group-like transcriptional activator protein. J Biol Chem 267:3358–67

40. Takamatsu C, Umeda S, Ohsato T, Ohno T, Abe Y, Fukuoh A, Shinagawa H, Hamasaki N, Kang D (2002) Regulation of mitochondrial D-loops by transcription factor A and single-stranded DNA-binding protein. EMBO Rep 3:451–6

41. Ghivizzani SC, Madsen CS, Nelen MR, Ammini CV, Hauswirth WW (1994) In organello footprint analysis of human mitochondrial DNA: Human mitochondrial transcription factor A interactions at the origin of replication. Mol Cell Biol 14:7717–30

42. Falkenberg M, Gaspari M, Rantanen A, Trifunovic A, Larsson NG, Gustafsson CM (2002) Mitochondrial transcription factors B1 and B2 activate transcription of human mtDNA. Nat Genet 31:289–94

43. McCulloch V, Seidel-Rogol BL, Shadel GS (2002) A human mitochondrial transcription factor is related to RNA adenine methyltransferases and binds S-adenosylmethionine. Mol Cell Biol 22:1116–25

44. Montoya J, Ojala D, Attardi G (1981) Distinctive features of the 5'-terminal sequences of the human mitochondrial mRNAs. Nature 290:465–70

45. Daga A, Micol V, Hess D, Aebersold R, Attardi G (1993) Molecular characterization of the transcription termination factor from human mitochondria. J Biol Chem 268:8123–30

46. Prieto-Martin A, Montoya J, Martinez-Azorin F (2004) Phosphorylation of rat mitochondrial transcription termination factor (mTERF) is required for transcription termination but not for binding to DNA. Nucleic Acids Res 32:2059–68

47. Fernandez-Silva P, Martinez-Azorin F, Micol V, Attardi G (1997) The human mitochondrial transcription termination factor (mTERF) is a multizipper protein but binds to DNA as a monomer, with evidence pointing to intramolecular leucine zipper interactions. EMBO J 16:1066–79

48. Hess JF, Parisi MA, Bennett JL, Clayton DA (1991) Impairment of mitochondrial transcription termination by a point mutation associated with the MELAS subgroup of mitochondrial encephalomyopathies. Nature 351:236–9

49. Enriquez JA, Fernandez-Silva P, Perez-Martos A, Lopez-Perez MJ, Montoya J (1996) The synthesis of mRNA in isolated mitochondria can be maintained for several hours and is inhibited by high levels of ATP. Eur J Biochem 237:601–10

50. Enriquez JA, Fernandez-Silva P, Montoya J (1999) Autonomous regulation in mammalian mitochondrial DNA transcription. Biol Chem 380:737–47

51. Gaines G, Rossi C, Attardi G (1987) Markedly different ATP requirements for rRNA synthesis and mtDNA light strand transcription

versus mRNA synthesis in isolated human mitochondria. J Biol Chem 262:1907–15

52. Micol V, Fernandez-Silva P, Attardi G (1997) Functional analysis of in vivo and in organello footprinting of HeLa cell mitochondrial DNA in relationship to ATP and ethidium bromide effects on transcription. J Biol Chem 272:18896–904

53. King MP, Attardi G (1993) Post-transcriptional regulation of the steady-state levels of mitochondrial tRNAs in HeLa cells. J Biol Chem 268:10228–37

54. Gelfand R, Attardi G (1981) Synthesis and turnover of mitochondrial ribonucleic acid in HeLa cells: the mature ribosomal and messenger ribonucleic acid species are metabolically unstable. Mol Cell Biol 1:497–511

55. Ostronoff LK, Izquierdo J, Cuezva JM (1995) mt-mRNA stability regulates the expression of the mitochondrial genome during liver development. Biochem Biophys Res Commun 217:1094–8

56. Izquierdo J, Ricart J, Ostronoff LK, Egea G, Cuezva JM (1995) Changing patterns of transcriptional and post-transcriptional control of β-F1-ATPase gene expression during mitochondrial biogenesis in liver. J Biol Chem. 270:10342–50

57. Schieber GL, O'Brien TW (1985) Site of synthesis of the proteins of mammalian mitochondrial ribosomes. Evidence from cultured bovine cells. J Biol Chem 260:6367–72

58. O'Brien TW (2002) Evolution of a protein-rich mitochondrial ribosome: Implications for human genetic disease. Gene 286:73–9

59. Matthews DE, Hessler RA, Denslow ND, Edwards JS, O'Brien TW (1982) Protein composition of the bovine mitochondrial ribosome. J Biol Chem 257:8788–94

60. Goldschmidt-Reisin S, Kitakawa M, Herfurth E, Wittmann-Liebold B, Grohmann L, Graack HR (1998) Mammalian mitochondrial ribosomal proteins. N-terminal amino acid sequencing, characterization, and identification of corresponding gene sequences. J Biol Chem 273:34828–36

61. Mariottini P, Shah ZH, Toivonen JM, Bagni C, Spelbrink JN, Amaldi F, Jacobs HT (1999) Expression of the gene for mitoribosomal protein S12 is controlled in human cells at the levels of transcription, RNA splicing, and translation. J Biol Chem 274: 31853–62

62. Koc EC, Burkhart W, Blackburn K, Moseley A, Koc H, Spremulli LL (2000) A proteomics approach to the identification of mam-

malian mitochondrial small subunit ribosomal proteins. J Biol Chem 275:32585–91

63. Graack HR, Bryant ML, O'Brien TW (1999) Identification of mammalian mitochondrial ribosomal proteins (MRPs) by N-terminal sequencing of purified bovine MRPs and comparison to data bank sequences: The large subribosomal particle. Biochemistry 38: 16569–77

64. O'Brien TW, Fiesler SE, Denslow ND, Thiede B, Wittmann-Liebold B, Mougey EB, Sylvester JE, Graack HR (1999) Mammalian mitochondrial ribosomal proteins (2). Amino acid sequencing, characterization, and identification of corresponding gene sequences. J Biol Chem 274:36043–51

65. Koc EC, Burkhart W, Blackburn K, Moyer MB, Schlatzer DM, Moseley A, Spremulli LL (2001) The large subunit of the mammalian mitochondrial ribosome. Analysis of the complement of ribosomal proteins present. J Biol Chem 276:43958–69

66. Kenmochi N, Suzuki T, Uechi T, Magoori M, Kuniba M, HigaS, Watanabe K, Tanaka T (2001) The human mitochondrial ribosomal protein genes: Mapping of 54 genes to the chromosomes and implications for human disorders. Genomics 77:65–70

67. Liu M, Spremulli L (2000) Interaction of mammalian mitochondrial ribosomes with the inner membrane. J Biol Chem 2000 275:29400–6

68. Bunn CL, Wallace DC, Eisenstadt JM (1974) Cytoplasmic inheritance of chloramphenicol resistance in mouse tissue culture cells. Proc Natl Acad Sci USA 71:1681–5

69. Sylvester JE, Fischel-Ghodsian N, Mougey EB, O'Brien TW (2004) Mitochondrial ribosomal proteins: Candidate genes for mitochondrial disease. Genet Med 6:73–80

70. Spirina O, Bykhovskaya Y, Kajava AV, O'Brien TW, Nierlich DP, Mougey EB, Sylvester JE, Graack HR, Wittmann-Liebold B, Fischel-Ghodsian N (2000) Heart-specific splice-variant of a human mitochondrial ribosomal protein (mRNA processing; tissue specific splicing). Gene 261:229–34

71. Cahill A, Cunningham CC (2000) Mammalian mitochondrial ribosomal proteins: N-terminal amino acid sequencing, characterization, and identification of corresponding gene sequences. Electrophoresis 21:3420–6

72. Coleman WB, Cunningham CC (1991) Effect of chronic ethanol consumption on hepatic mitochondrial transcription and translation. Biochim Biophys Acta 1058:178–86

73. Liao HX, Spremulli LL (1989) Interaction of bovine mitochondrial ribosomes with messenger RNA. J Biol Chem. 264:7518–22

74. Ma J, Farwell MA, Burkhart WA, Spremulli LL (1995) Cloning and sequence analysis of the cDNA for bovine mitochondrial translational initiation factor 2. Biochim Biophys Acta 1261:321–4

75. Koc EC, Spremulli LL (2002) Identification of mammalian mitochondrial translational initiation factor 3 and examination of its role in initiation complex formation with natural mRNAs. J Biol Chem 277:35541–9

76. Woriax VL, Burkhart W, Spremulli LL (1995) Cloning and sequence analysis and expression of mammalian mitochondrial protein synthe-sis elongation factor Tu. Biochim Biophys Acta 1264:347–56

77. Xin H, Woriax V, Burkhart W, Spremulli LL (1995) Cloning and expression of mitochondrial translational elongation factor Ts from bovine and human liver. J Biol Chem 270:17243–9

78. Gao J, Yu L, Zhang P, Jiang J, Chen J, Peng J, Wei Y, Zhao S (2001) Cloning and characterization of human and mouse mitochondrial elongation factor G, GFM and Gfm, and mapping of GFM to human chromosome 3q25.1-q26.2. Genomics 74:109–14

79. Bogenhagen DF (1999) Repair of mtDNA in vertebrates. Am J Hum Genet 64:1276–81

80. Bohr VA, Dianov GL (1999) Oxidative DNA damage processing in nuclear and mtDNA. Biochimie 81:155–60

81. Driggers WJ, Holmquist GP, LeDoux SP, Wilson GL (1997) Mapping frequencies of endogenous oxidative damage and the kinetic response to oxidative stress in a region of rat mtDNA. Nucleic Acids Res 25:4362–9

82. Anderson CT, Friedberg EC (1980) The presence of nuclear and mitochondrial uracil-DNA glycosylase in extracts of human KB cells. Nucleic Acids Res 8:875–88

83. Slupphaug G, Markussen FH, Olsen LC, Aasland R, Aarsaether N, Bakke O, Krokan HE, Helland DE (1993) Nuclear and mitochondrial forms of human uracil-DNA glycosylase are encoded by the same gene. Nucleic Acids Res 21:2579–84

84. Caradonna S, Ladner R, Hansbury M, Kosciuk M, Lynch F, Muller S (1996) Affinity purification and comparative analysis of two distinct human uracil-DNA glycosylases. Exp Cell Res 222:345–59

85. Tomkinson AE, Bonk RT, Kim J, Bartfeld N, Linn S (1990) Mammalian mitochondrial endonuclease activities specific for ultraviolet-irradiated DNA. Nucleic Acids Res 18:929–35

86. Croteau DL, ap Rhys CM, Hudson EK, Dianov GL, Hansford RG, Bohr VA (1997) An oxidative damage-specific endonuclease from rat liver mitochondria. J Biol. Chem 272:27338–44

87. Cote J, Ruiz-Carrillo A (1993) Primers for mitochondrial DNA replication generated by endonuclease G. Science 261:765–9

88. Ikeda S, Ozaki K (1997) Action of mitochondrial endonuclease G on DNA damaged by L-ascorbic acid, peplomycin, and cis-diamminedichloroplatinum (II). Biochem Biophys Res Commun 235:291–4

89. Gerschenson M, Low RL, Loehr J (1994) Levels of the mitochondrial endonuclease during rat cardiac development implicate a role for the enzyme in repair of oxidative damage in mitochondrial DNA. J Mol Cell Cardiol 26:31–40

90. Davies AM, Hershman S, Stabley GJ, Hoek JB, Peterson J, Cahill A (2003) A Ca2+-induced mitochondrial permeability transition causes complete release of rat liver endonuclease G activity from its exclusive location within the mitochondrial intermembrane space: Identification of a novel endo-exonuclease activity residing within the mitochondrial matrix. Nucleic Acids Res 31:1364–73

91. Ohsato T, Ishihara N, Muta T, Umeda S, Ikeda S, Mihara K, Hamasaki N, Kang D (2002) Mammalian mitochondrial endonuclease G. Digestion of R-loops and localization in intermembrane space. Eur J Biochem 269:5765–70

92. Li LY, Luo X Wang X (2001) Endonuclease G is an apoptotic DNase when released from mitochondria. Nature 412: 95–9

93. Souza-Pinto NC, Croteau DL, Hudson EK, Hansford RG, Bohr VA (1999) Age-associated increase in 8-oxo-deoxyguanosine glycosylase/AP lyase activity in rat mitochondria. Nucleic Acids Res 27:1935–42

94. Druzhyna N, Smulson ME, LeDoux SP, Wilson GL (2000) Poly (ADP-ribose) polymerase facilitates the repair of N-methylpurines in mitochondrial DNA. Diabetes 49:1849–55

95. Stierum RH, Dianov GL, Bohr VA (1999) Single-nucleotide patch base excision repair of uracil in DNA by mitochondrial protein extracts. Nucleic Acids Res 27:3712–9

96. Grishko VI, Druzhyna N, LeDoux SP, Wilson GL (1999) Nitric oxide-induced damage to mtDNA and its subsequent repair. Nucleic Acids Res 15:4510–16

97. Ledoux SP, Shen CC, Grishko VI, Fields PA, Gard AL, Wilson GL (1998) Glial cell-specific differences in response to alkylation damage. Glia 24:304–12

98. Thyagarajan B, Padua RA, Campbell C (1996) Mammalian mitochondria possess homologous DNA recombination activity. J Biol Chem 271:27536–43

99. LeDoux SP, Driggers WJ, Hollensworth BS, Wilson GL (1999) Repair of alkylation and oxidative damage in mitochondrial DNA. Mutat Res 434:149–59

100. Kajander OA, Karhunen PJ, Holt IJ, Jacobs HT (2001) Prominent mitochondrial DNA recombination intermediates in human heart muscle. EMBO Rep 2:1007–12

101. Pascucci B, Versteegh A, van Hoffen A, van Zeeland AA, Mullenders LH, Dogliotti E (1997) DNA repair of UV photoproducts and mutagenesis in human mtDNA. J Mol Biol 273:417–27

102. Clayton DA, Doda JN, Friedberg EC (1974) The absence of a pyrimidine dimer repair mechanism in mammalian mitochondria. Proc Natl Acad Sci USA 71:2777–81

103. Kalinowski DP, Illenye S, Van Houten B (1992) Analysis of DNA damage and repair in murine leukemia L1210 cells using a quantitative polymerase chain reaction assay. Nucleic Acids Res 20:3485–94

104. Yasui A, Yajima H, Kobayashi T, Eker AP, Oikawa A (1992) Mitochondrial DNA repair by photolyase. Mutat Res 273:231–6

105. Chung AB, Stepien G, Haraguchi Y, Li K, Wallace DC (1992) Transcriptional control of nuclear genes for the mitochondrial muscle ADP/ATP translocator and the ATP synthase beta subunit. J Biol Chem 267:21154–61

106. Li K, Hodge JA, Wallace DC (1990) OXBOX, a positive transcriptional element of the heart-skeletal muscle ADP/ATP translocator gene. J Biol Chem 265;20585–8

107. Haragushi Y, Chung AB, Neill S, Wallace DC (1994) OXBOX and REBOX overlapping promoter elements of the mitochondrial F0F1-ATP synthase β subunit gene. J Biol Chem 269;9330–4

108. Suzuki H, Suzuki S, Kumar S, Ozawa T (1995) Human nuclear and mitochondrial Mt element-binding proteins to regulatory regions

of the nuclear respiratory genes and to the mitochondrial promoter region. Biochem Biophys Res Commun 213:204–10

109. Zhang C, Wong-Riley MT (2000) Depolarizing stimulation upregulates GA-binding protein in neurons: A transcription factor involved in the bigenomic expression of cytochrome oxidase subunits. Eur J Neurosci 12:1013–23

110. Virbasius JV, Scarpulla RC (1994) Activation of thehuman mitochondrial transcription factor A gene by nuclear respiratory factors: A potential regulatory link between nuclear and mitochondrial gene expression in organelle biogenesis. Proc Natl Acad Sci USA 91: 1309–13

111. Gugneja S, Virbasius JV, Scarpulla RC (1995) Four structurally distinct, non-DNA-binding subunits of human nuclear respiratory factor 2 share a conserved transcriptional activation domain. Mol Cell Biol 15:102–11

112. Li B, Holloszy JO, Semenkovich CF (1999) Respiratory uncoupling induces delta-aminolevulinate synthase expression through a nuclear respiratory factor-1-dependent mechanism in HeLa cells. J Biol Chem 274:17534–40

113. Wu Z, Puigserver P, Andersson U, Zhang C, Adelmant G, Mootha V, Troy A, Cinti S, Lowell B, Scarpulla RC, Spiegelman BM (1999) Mechanisms controlling mitochondrial biogenesis and respiration through the thermogenic coactivator PGC-1. Cell 98: 115–24

114. Gilde AJ, Van Der Lee KA, Willemsen PH, Chinetti G, Van Der Leij FR, Van Der Vusse GJ, Staels B, Van Bilsen M (2003) Peroxisome proliferator-activated receptor (PPAR) alpha and PPARbeta/delta, but not PPARgamma, modulate the expression of genes involved in cardiac lipid metabolism. Circ Res 92:518–24

115. Wiesner RJ, Aschenbrenner V, Ruegg JC, Zak R (1994) Coordination of nuclear and mitochondrial gene expression during the development of cardiac hypertrophy in rats. Am J Physiol 267: C229–35

116. Wiesner RJ, Kurowski TT, Zak R (1992) Regulation by thyroid hormone of nuclear and mitochondrial genes encoding subunits of cytochrome-c oxidase in rat liver and skeletal muscle. Mol Endocrinol 6:1458–67

117. Luciakova K, Li R, Nelson BD (1992) Differential regulation of the transcript levels of some nuclear-encoded and mitochondrial-

encoded respiratory-chain components in response to growth activation. Eur J Biochem 207:253–7

118. Wrutniak C, Cassar-Malek I, Marchal S, Rascle A, Heusser S, Keller JM, Rochard P, Flechon J, Dauca M, Samarut J, Ghysdael J, Cabello G (1995) A 43-kDa protein related to c-erb A a1 is located in the mitochondrial matrix of rat liver. J Biol Chem 270:16347–54

119. Casas F, Rochard P, Rodier A, Cassar-Malek I, Marchal-Victorion S, Wiesner RJ, Cabello G, Wrutniak C (1999) A variant form of the nuclear triiodothyronine receptor c-ErbAalpha1 plays a direct role in regulation of mitochondrial RNA synthesis. Mol Cell Biol 19:7913–24

120. Scheller K, Sekeris CE, Krohne G, Hock R, Hansen IA, Scheer U (2000) Localization of glucocorticoid hormone receptors in mitochondria of human cells. Eur J Cell Biol 79:299–307

121. Demonacos C, Djordjevic-Markovic R, Tsawdaroglou N, Sekeris CE (1995) The mitochondrion as a primary site of action of glucocorticoids: The interaction of the glucocorticoid receptor with mitochondrial DNA sequences showing partial similarity to the nuclear glucocorticoid responsive elements. J Steroid Biochem Mol Biol 55:43–55

122. Cassar-Malek I, Marchal S, Altabef M, Wrutniak C, Samarut J, Cabello G (1994) V-erb A stimulates quail myoblast differentiation in a T3 independent cell-specific manner. Oncogene 9:2197–6

123. Glick BS, Beasley EM, Schatz G (1992) Protein sorting in mitochondria. Trends Biochem Sci 17:453–9

124. Meisinger C, Brix J, Model K, Pfanner N, Ryan MT (1999) The preprotein translocase of the outer mitochondrial membrane: receptors and a general import pore. Cell Mol Life Sci 56:817–24

125. Hernandez JM, Giner P, Hernandez-Yago J (1999) Gene structure of the human mitochondrial outer membrane receptor Tom20 and evolutionary study of its family of processed pseudogenes. Gene 239:283–91

126. Schleiff E, Khanna R, Orlicky S, Vrielink A (1999) Expression, purification, and in vitro characterization of the human outer mitochondrial membrane receptor human translocase of the outer mitochondrial membrane 20. Arch Biochem Biophys 67:95–103

127. Craig EE, Chesley A, Hood DA (1998) Thyroid hormone modifies mitochondrial phenotype by increasing protein import without altering degradation. Am J Physiol 275:C1508–15

128. Hood DA (2001) Invited review: Contractile activity-induced mitochondrial biogenesis in skeletal muscle. J Appl Physiol 90:1137–57

129. Heddi A, Stepien G, Benke PJ, Wallace DC (1999) Coordinate induction of energy gene expression in tissue of mitochondrial disease patients. J Biol Chem 274:22968–76

# Chapter 4

# ROS Generation, Antioxidants, and Cell Death

## Overview

All cell types including cardiomyocytes are capable of generating reactive oxidative species (ROS), and the major sources of production include mitochondria, xanthine oxidases, and the NADPH oxidases. Under pathophysiological conditions, ROS levels increase and cause cellular damage and dysfunction targeting primarily the mitochondria. The cardiomyocyte and mainly its mitochondria can neutralize ROS with an array of scavenging enzymes and antioxidants. In addition to its damaging effect, ROS play a role in a number of signal transduction pathways in the cardiomyocyte. Whether the effects of this signaling role are beneficial or harmful may depend on the site, source, and amount of ROS produced, as well as the overall redox status of the cell. ROS have been implicated in the development of cardiac hypertrophy, cardiomyocyte apoptosis, and remodeling of the heart, largely by up-regulating proapoptotic proteins and the mitochondrial-dependent pathways. Cardiomyocyte apoptosis has been reported in a variety of cardiovascular diseases, including myocardial infarction, ischemia/reperfusion, end-stage heart failure, and aging.

## Introduction

Both the generation of ROS and the onset of apoptotic cell death are important and often connected events in cell homeostasis. Mitochondria are essential players in the physiology of the cardiomyocyte and play a dominant role in redox signaling pathways, stress response, myocardial ischemia, heart failure, hypertrophy, and aging. This chapter includes a discussion about ROS generation, outlining both its critical role in cell damage and signal transduction, its regulation by cellular and mitochondrial antioxidants, and its involvement in the onset of cell apoptosis and cardiac pathophysiology. Signaling pathways involved in the development and progression of apoptosis are also presented, and their significance in cardiac disease is discussed.

# The significance of ROS

## *Generation of ROS*

The major ROS are the superoxide radical $O_2^{\bullet-}$, hydrogen peroxide ($H_2O_2$), and the hydroxyl radical $OH^{\bullet}$. The superoxide anion ($O_2^{\bullet-}$) is formed when oxygen accepts an electron. Superoxide is in equilibrium with its more reactive protonated form, $\bullet HO_2$, which is favored in acidosis (such as occurs with ischemia). The rates of mitochondrial $O_2^{\bullet-}$ generation are known to be inversely correlated with the maximum life-span potential of different mammalian species [1]. The production of the hydroxyl radical (which is the most reactive form of ROS) is primarily responsible for the damage to cellular macromolecules such as proteins, DNA, and lipids. Formation of the highly reactive hydroxyl radical comes from reactions involving the other ROS species (e.g., the Fenton reaction) in which ubiquitous metal ions, such as Fe (II) or Cu (I), react with $H_2O_2$. The high reactivity of the hydroxyl radical and its extremely short physiological half-life of $10^{-9}$ sec restrict its damage to a small radius from where it is generated, since it is too short-lived to diffuse far from its origin [2]. The location of free metal ions can determine the initiation of free radical damage. In contrast, the less reactive superoxide radicals produced in mitochondria can be delivered to the cytosol through anion channels (e.g., VDAC) and thereby may impact sites far from their generation, including activation of transcription factors such as NF-κB among other effects [3]. Similarly, the freely diffusible $H_2O_2$ generated in mitochondria can be delivered to the cytosol, where it contributes to increased levels of cellular ROS. An accurate quantification of mitochondrial ROS flux inside living cells is very difficult since the turnover of several ROS species (particularly the $OH^{\bullet}$ radical) is extremely rapid. Indirect strategies, including the use of gene knockout and overexpression studies [4], have been used to demonstrate the presence and involvement of mitochondrial ROS.

Under normal physiological conditions, the primary source of ROS is the mitochondrial ETC, where oxygen can be activated to superoxide radical by a nonenzymatic process. This production of ROS is a by-product of normal metabolism and occurs from electrons produced (or leaked) from the ETC at complexes I, III, and IV. There is evidence that semiquinones generated within complexes I and III are the most likely donors of electrons to molecular oxygen, providing a constant source of superoxide [5–6]; however, a supportive role for complex II in ROS production has also been suggested [7]. Mitochondrial ROS generation can be amplified in cells with abnormal respiratory chain function as well as, under physiological and pathological conditions, where oxygen consumption is increased.

Besides mitochondria, other cellular sources for generating superoxide radicals include the reactions of oxygen with microsomal cytochrome p450 and with reduced flavins (e.g., NADPH), usually in the presence of metal ions. In addition, xanthine oxidase (XO), a primarily cytosolic enzyme involved in purine metabolism, is also a source of the superoxide radical. Notably, XO activity and its superoxide generation are markedly increased in the heart after postischemia/reperfusion damage. Its location within the human myocardium is primarily in the endothelial cells of capillaries and smaller vessels [8–9]. Multiple studies have shown that that the XO inhibitor allopurinol provides protection against the cardiac damage resulting from anoxia. Recently, Cappola and coworkers demonstrated a provocative link between XO activity and abnormal cardiac energy metabolism in patients with idiopathic DCM, since inhibition of XO with allopurinol significantly improved myocardial function [10].

In the presence of the enzyme superoxide dismutase (SOD), superoxide radicals can be converted to $H_2O_2$, which can further react via the Fenton reaction to form the hydroxyl radical. Superoxide can also react with nitric oxide (NO) to form peroxynitrite, which is also a highly reactive and deleterious free radical species (Figure 4.1).

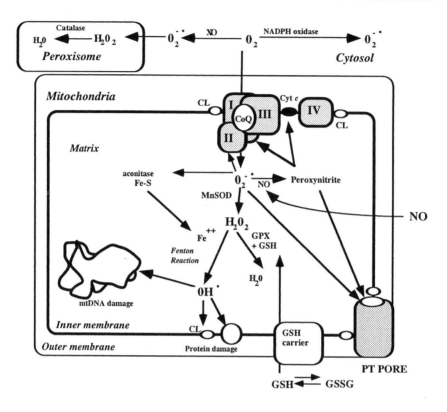

**Figure 4.1. Cellular ROS generation and metabolism.** *Sites of mitochondrial superoxide $O_2^{\cdot-}$ radical (via respiratory complexes I, II, and III) and cytosolic $O_2^{\cdot-}$. generation (by NADPH oxidase or xanthine oxidase) are depicted. Also shown are reactions of the $O_2^{\cdot-}$ radical with NO to form the highly reactive peroxynitrite, which can target PT pore opening and the inactivation of mitochondrial aconitase by $O_2^{\cdot-}$. MnSOD (in mitochondria) and CuSOD (in cytosol) to form $H_2O_2$ are also displayed. The $H_2O_2$ is then either further neutralized in the mitochondria by glutathione peroxidase (GPx) and glutathione, in the peroxisome by catalase, or in the presence of $Fe^{++}$ via the Fenton reaction,which forms the highly reactive $OH^{\cdot}$ radical, which can cause severe lipid peroxidation and extensive oxidative damage to proteins and mtDNA.*

## Negative effects of ROS

ROS cause deleterious effects on cells including extensive peroxidative damage to membrane phospholipids and proteins. Protein modifications, such as carbonylation, nitration, and the formation of lipid peroxidation adducts (e.g., 4-hydroxynonenal [HNE]), are products of oxidative damage secondary to ROS [11].

Significantly, changes in the myocardial respiratory complexes I to V by ROS-mediated nitration, carbonylation, and HNE adduct, with associated decline in their enzymatic activity, have been reported in both *in vitro* and *in vivo* studies [12]. Superoxide is also especially damaging to the Fe-S centers of enzymes (e.g., complex I, aconitase, and succinate dehydrogenase). Moreover, the inactivation of mitochondrial aconitase by superoxide, which generates Fe (II) and $H_2O_2$, also increases hydroxyl radical formation through the Fenton reaction [13]. Lipids and in particular the mitochondrial-specific cardiolipin serve as a focal target for free radical damage. A large accumulation of superoxide radicals produced *in vitro,* with sub-mitochondrial particles from heart resulted in extensive cardiolipin peroxidation with a parallel loss of cytochrome *c* oxidase activity [14–15]. Oxidative damage also affects nucleic acids and in particular mtDNA by the induction of single- and double-strand breaks, base damage, and modification (including 8-oxoguanosine formation), resulting in the generation of point mutations and deletions [16–18].

In addition, the highly reactive peroxynitrite irreversibly impairs mitochondrial respiration [19] since it inhibits complex I activity, largely by tyrosine nitration of several targeted subunits [20–21], modifies cytochrome *c* structure and function [22], affects cytochrome *c* oxidase activity, inhibits mitochondrial aconitase [23], and causes induction of the PT pore [24]. Some of the effects of peroxynitrite on its mitochondrial targets (e.g., the PT pore) are potentiated by increased calcium levels [25]. The effects of peroxynitrite on mitochondria can be clearly distinguished from the effects of NO, which often are reversible [19].

Taken together, mitochondria (which are the primary site of intracellular ROS generation) are also a primary locus of its damaging effects. In particular, damage to mtDNA induces abnormalities in the mtDNA-encoded polypeptides of the respiratory complexes located in the inner membrane, with consequent decrease of electron transfer and further production of ROS, thus establishing a vicious cycle of oxidative stress, mitochondrial function, and bioenergetic decline.

## Antioxidant defense

The powerful cell-damaging ROS oxidants can be neutralized by an array of protective antioxidant scavenger enzymes, as well as by various lipid and water-soluble compounds including ascorbic acid, glutathione, thioredoxin, and $\alpha$-tocopherol. The antioxidant enzymes are located in a variety of cellular compartments including the mitochondria (e.g., MnSOD, glutathione peroxidase, thioredoxin reductase), peroxisomes (e.g., catalase), microsomes (e.g., cytochrome P450) and in the cytosol (e.g., CuSOD and cytosolic thioredoxin reductase). In general, there are significantly lower levels of antioxidants in myocardial mitochondria than in liver mitochondria, but the consensus opinion is that the antioxidant capacity of the heart is generally sufficient to handle the normal levels of ROS production, although insufficient to meet the greater ROS accumulation that occurs during stress, myocardial disease, and ischemia [26].

A mitochondrial isoform of catalase with low specific activity has been found in rat [27–28]. This mitochondrial catalase activity was detected in the heart but not in liver or skeletal muscle and it appears to increase during caloric-restricted diets and in the diabetic heart [29–31]. The role that this enzyme plays has not been fully determined although there is evidence of its participation in the prevention of excess lipid peroxidation in myocardial ischemia [32]. On the other hand, a mitochondria-specific catalase has not been found in the heart of transgenic mice even after overexpression of the catalase gene [33].

While superoxide dismutases catalyze the removal of superoxide radicals by the formation of $H_2O_2$, glutathione peroxidase (GPx) catalyzes the breakdown of $H_2O_2$ to water and oxidized glutathione (GSSG) by using reduced glutathione (GSH) as shown in Figure 4.1. Since GPx is located in both the mitochondria and cytosol, $H_2O_2$ can be removed from either compartment depending on the availability of glutathione. A small fraction of the total cellular pool of GSH is sequestered in mitochondria by the action of a carrier that transports GSH from cytosol to the mitochondrial matrix [34]. On exposure to increased exogenous ROS, isolated, perfused rat hearts are rapidly depleted of their antioxidant reserves, including those of SOD and GSH, rendering them more vulnerable to the action of oxidative injury [35].

Another important mechanism in the antioxidant reactions is the sequestering of iron and copper ions to keep them from reacting with superoxide or $H_2O_2$. The antioxidant dexrazoxane prevents site-specific iron-based oxygen radical damage by chelating free and loosely bound iron. It has been used as a cardioprotective drug against doxorubicin-induced oxidative damage to myocardial mitochondria in both humans and animals [36–37]. The antioxidant metal-binding protein metallothionein (MT) also provides cardioprotection by directly reacting with ROS produced by ischemia/reperfusion and doxorubicin treatment, as demonstrated by studies with a cardiac-specific, MT-overexpressing transgenic mouse model [38]. MT expression is also inducible within the heart (and other tissues) by TNF-α, IL-6, doxorubicin, and metals such as cadmium and Zn [38–40], although its cardioprotective role in those studies was not determined

The uncoupling of mitochondrial respiration from OXPHOS ATP production—by either artificial uncouplers such as 2,4-dinitrophenol (e.g., DNP) or natural uncouplers (e.g., laurate), fatty acids, and mitochondrial uncoupling (UCP) proteins—strongly inhibits $O_2^{\bullet-}$ and $H_2O_2$ formation in mitochondria [41–43]. ROS production is favored when the mitochondrial membrane potential is above a specific threshold. Under conditions where the mitochondrial membrane potential is at its peak (e.g., state 4 respiration), ROS production is augmented. Significantly, increased mitochondrial membrane potential slows electron transport through the respiratory chain, resulting in increased half-life of the ubiquinone free radical and increasing the likelihood that electrons will interact with oxygen to form ROS [44]. Uncouplers prevent the transmembrane electrochemical $H^+$ potential difference ($\Delta \mu_H$) from being above a threshold critical for ROS formation by respiratory complexes I and III. This has been corroborated in transgenic mice in which UCP3 protein is lacking, resulting in enhanced ROS production and increased oxidative stress in the heart and skeletal muscle [45]; in transgenic mice with UCP1 overexpresssion [46]; and in cardiomyocytes with UCP2 overexpression in which ROS is markedly attenuated [47].

## Role of ROS in cell signaling

In addition to the cell-damaging effects of ROS, mitochondrial ROS generation and the oxidative stress they engender play a major role in cell regulation and signaling. Oxidative species such as $H_2O_2$ and the superoxide anion can be used as potent signals sent from mitochondria to other cellular sites rapidly and reversibly, triggering an array of intracellular cascades leading to diverse physiological end-points for the cardiomyocyte, some negative (e.g., apoptosis and necrosis) and others positive (e.g., cardioprotection and cell proliferation). $H_2O_2$ produced by mitochondria and sent to the cytosol is involved in several signal transduction pathways, including the activation of c-Jun N-terminal kinase (JNK1) and mitogen-activated protein kinases (MAPK) activities [48–50], and can impact the regulation of redox-sensitive $K^+$ channels affecting arteriole constriction [51]. The release of $H_2O_2$ from mitochondria and its subsequent cellular effects are increased in cardiomyocytes treated with antimycin and high $Ca^{++}$ and further enhanced by treatment with CoQ. CoQ plays a dual role in the mitochondrial generation of intracellular redox signaling, by acting both as a prooxidant involved in ROS generation and as an antioxidant by inhibiting the PT pore and cytochrome c release and also by increasing ATP synthesis [52]. Increased mitochondrial $H_2O_2$ generation and signaling occur with NO modulation of the respiratory chain [49, 53], as well as with the induction of myocardial mitochondrial NO production, resulting from treatment with enalapril [54]. ROS play a fundamental role in the cardioprotective signaling pathways of ischemic preconditioning, in critical oxygen sensing, and in the induction of stress responses that promote cell survival. These phenomena are further examined in Chapters 5 and 10.

## ROS and cardiac pathology

ROS generation increases in the aging heart, myocardial ischemia and reperfusion, inflammation, and in general, the presence of impaired antioxidant defenses. It is known that a burst of ROS occurs during the first moments of reperfusion and is associated with changes in mitochondria (e.g., PT pore opening) and myocardial injury [55]. The source of ROS generation during early reperfusion has not been determined and may be of either mitochondrial or cytoplasmic origin. In contrast, the source of ROS generated during ischemia (and likely in the early/acute pathway of ischemic preconditioning) more clearly involves the mitochondrial ETC and may be different than the source of ROS generated in early reperfusion [56–57].

In the canine model of pacing-induced DCM and heart failure, there is a marked increase in left ventricular tissue aldehyde levels, suggesting elevated free radical-induced damage [58–59]. The increased levels of oxidative stress correlated with the onset of reduced cardiac complex III and V activities. This has been corroborated by measurements of ROS levels in paced compared to unpaced dogs, revealing that both $O_2^{\bullet-}$ and $OH^{\bullet}$ radicals generated from mitochondrial-produced $H_2O_2$ are increased in the failing myocardium and correlated with the severity of left ventricular dysfunction [60–61].

Oxidative stress also appears to be involved in the generation of large-scale myocardial mtDNA deletions demonstrated in pacing-induced cardiac failure [58] as well as in studies of ameroid constriction-mediated myocardial ischemia in the dog [62]. In addition, neonatal cardiac myocytes treated with TNF-$\alpha$ displayed a significant increase in ROS levels, accompanied by an overall decline in mtDNA copy number and decreased complex III activity [63]. The TNF-$\alpha$ mediated decline in mtDNA copy number might result from an increase in mtDNA deletions.

ROS-induced mtDNA damage, resulting in respiratory complex enzyme dysfunction, contributes to the progression of left ventricular (LV) remodeling and failure after myocardial infarction (MI). In a murine model of MI and remodeling created by ligation of the left anterior descending coronary artery, increased ROS production (e.g., $OH^{\bullet}$ level) was found in association with decreased levels of mtDNA and ETC activities, suggesting impairment of mitochondrial function [64].

Recently, the chronic release of ROS has been linked to the development of left ventricular hypertrophy and progressive heart failure. Chronic ROS generation can derive both from mitochondria and from nonmitochondrial NADPH oxidase, which in endothelial cells is activated by cytokines, neurohormones, and growth factors (e.g., angiotensin II, norepinephrine, and TNF-$\alpha$) [65–66].

Long-term abnormalities in cardiac phenotype can be driven by redox-sensitive gene expression, and in this way ROS may act as potent intracellular second messengers. In cardiac myocytes, NADPH oxidase plays a prominent role in the hypertrophic pathway [67–69]. In addition, NADPH oxidase activity is significantly increased in the failing versus nonfailing myocardium [70]. Recently, it has been reported that statins (i.e., 3-hydroxyl-3-methylglutaryl coenzyme A [HMG-CoA] reductase inhibitors), by modulating the ROS-generating activity of NADPH oxidase, can inhibit cardiac hypertrophy by cholesterol-independent mechanisms [71–72]. Statins block the isoprenylation and activation of members of the Rho guanosine triphosphatase (GTPase) family such as Rac1, an essential component of NADPH oxidase. Thus, it appears that blocking ROS production with statins may be beneficial to patients with myocardial hypertrophy and chronic heart failure.

## *ROS and apoptosis*

Increased oxidative stress and ROS accumulation can lead to apoptosis. Apoptosis can be blocked or delayed by treatment with antioxidants and thiol reductants [73]. Moreover, overexpression of antioxidant proteins (e.g., MnSOD, glutathione peroxidase, and metallothionein) can block apoptotic progression [74–76]. Attenuation of apoptosis by overexpression of the antiapoptotic protein Bcl-2 was associated with protection against ROS and oxidative stress [77]. Cells from transgenic mice containing ablated genes encoding antioxidant proteins (e.g., glutathione peroxidase) have both increased oxidative stress levels and increased apoptosis [78–79].

Agents that induce apoptosis (e.g., TNF-$\alpha$) also promote high levels of mitochondrial-generated ROS [80]. In addition, ROS production can target an array of signal transducers (e.g. JNK, TNF-$\alpha$, and MAPK), which interface with the apoptotic machinery described in detail below. This includes both activation of the proapoptotic Bcl-2 family and mediators (e.g., TNF-$\alpha$), as well as the modulation of their gene expression by activation of specific transcription factors (e.g., NF-$\kappa$B).

Recently, an important model system has emerged to study the induction of oxidative stress and apoptosis by employing the treatment of cultured cardiomyocytes with $H_2O_2$ [81]. This approach has permitted a molecular and biochemical appraisal of the cellular and mitochondrial events presaging, accompanying and following the induction of cardiomyocyte apoptosis. In addition, it has allowed the study of short-lived signaling intermediates, as well as various treatments (e.g., antioxidants) to stem the development of cardiomyocyte oxidative stress and apoptotic progression [82–83].

It is also important to point out that not all cardiomyocyte apoptosis is triggered by oxidative stress and ROS generation. Recent reports have shown no evidence of ROS (or NO) involvement in the palmitate-mediated induction of apoptosis in neonatal rat cardiomyocytes [84], illustrating the complex, multiforked, and parallel nature of signals in the apoptotic pathway.

## Apoptosis and cell death

It is well established that mitochondria play a pivotal role in the early events of apoptosis. An early event in the mitochondrial apoptotic pathway (as shown in Figure 4.2) is the release from the intermembrane space into the cytosol of a group of proteins (e.g., cytochrome *c*, Smac/diablo, AIF, and endonuclease G) [85]. These mitochondrial proteins are involved in triggering the subsequent activation of downstream cysteine-aspartate proteases (caspases), initiating cell self-digestion (e.g., cytochrome *c* and Smac/diablo), and nuclear DNA fragmentation by endonucleases (e.g., endonuclease G and AIF) leading to apoptotic cell death [86]. Caspases, which are normally inactive enzymes, require specific proteolytic cleavage for their activation. This is achieved by the formation in the cytosol of large protein complexes termed *apoptosomes,* which incorporate released cytochrome *c*, Apaf-1, and recruited caspases (e.g., caspase-9). The assembly and function of the apoptosome are regulated by Smac/diablo, intracellular $K^+$ levels, and a class of proteins termed *IAPs* [87]. The release of the mitochondrial intermembrane peptides to the cytosol occurs primarily as a result of the disruption of the mitochondrial outer membrane [88].

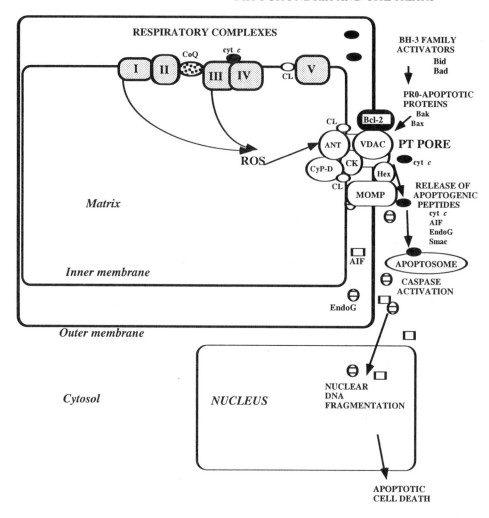

**Figure 4.2. The mitochondrial pathway of apoptosis.** *An array of cellular signals, including ROS and UV-induced DNA damage, trigger the apoptotic pathway regulated by proapoptotic proteins (e.g., Bax, Bid and Bad) binding to outer mitochondrial membrane leading to mitochondrial outer-membrane permeabilization (MOMP) and PT pore opening. Elevated levels of mitochondrial Ca^{++} as well as ETC-generated ROS also promote PT pore opening. This is followed by the release of cytochrome c (Cyt c), Smac, endonuclease G (Endo G), and apoptosis-inducing factor (AIF) from the mitochondrial intermembrane space to the cytosol, and apoptosome formation leading to caspase and endonuclease activation, DNA fragmentation, and cell death. Association of Bax with mitochondria is prevented by antiapoptogenic proteins (e.g., Bcl-2). Also shown are major proteins comprising the PT pore including hexokinase (Hex), adenine nucleotide translocator (ANT), creatine kinase (CK), cyclophilin D (CyP-D), and porin (VDAC) as well as the inner membrane phospholipid cardiolipin (CL).*

This change in mitochondrial membrane integrity is regulated by the complex and dynamic interactions of different members of the Bcl-2 family, including Bax, Bid, Bcl-2, and Bcl-X$_L$. Proteins of the Bcl-2 family share one or several Bcl-2 homology (BH) regions and behave as either pro- or antiapoptotic proteins. The highly conserved BH domains (BH1-4) are essential for homo- and heterocomplex formation, as well as to induce cell death. Proapoptotic homologues can be subdivided into 2 major subtypes, the multidomain Bax subfamily (e.g., Bax and Bak) which possesses BH1-3 domains, and the BH3-only subfamily (e.g., Bad and Bid). Both proapoptotic subtypes promote cell-death signaling by targeting mitochondrial membranes, albeit by different mechanisms [89]. Proapoptotic membrane-binding proteins (e.g., Bax) on translocation from the cytosol to mitochondria, potentiate cytochrome *c* release, presumably by forming channels in the outer membrane. This is supported by data showing that Bax can form channels and release cytochrome *c* from artificial membranes or liposomes [90]. The BH3-only proteins (e.g., Bid) act by activating the multidomain proapoptotic proteins or by binding and antagonizing the antiapoptotic proteins. Activation of proapoptotic proteins such as Bax to oligomerize, translocate, and bind to the mitochondria represents a critical control point for apoptosis. It requires extensive conformational changes, in response to a multitude of death signals involving the binding of several factors (e.g., BH3-only proteins) and phosphorylation by several kinases including P38 MAP kinase. Cytoplasmic p53 can directly activate Bax and trigger apoptosis by functioning similarly to the BH3-only proteins [91]. The antiapoptotic proteins Bcl-2 and Bcl-X$_L$ display conservation in all four BH1-4 domains and act to preserve mitochondrial outer membrane integrity by binding and sequestering proapoptotic activating factors (e.g., Bad or Bid), antagonizing the events of channel formation and cytochrome *c* release. Bcl-2 prevents the functional association of Bax with the mitochondria and interferes with the release of apoptogenic peptides (e.g., cytochrome *c* and AIF) from the mitochondria.

Protein release from the cristae, where the majority of cytochrome *c* is located, may be associated with the opening of the membrane mitochondrial megachannel, the PT pore located at contact sites between the inner and outer membranes [92]. However, the role of the transient opening of the PT pore in the release of cytochrome *c* is not yet fully understood, since cytochrome *c* release occurs prior to any discernable mitochondrial swelling. Nevertheless, PT pore opening is an early requisite feature of apoptosis preceding the activation of caspases and is promoted by elevated $Ca^{++}$ influx into mitochondria, excessive mitochondrial ROS production (primarily from respiratory complex I and III), prooxidants, fatty acids, and nitric oxide [86].

Opening of the PT pore causes a number of important changes in mitochondrial structure and metabolism, including increased mito-chondrial matrix volume, leading to mitochondrial swelling, release of matrix calcium, altered cristae, and cessation of ATP production, due to uncoupling of ETC and dissipation of the mitochondrial membrane potential. Both Bax and Bcl-2 directly interact with the voltage-dependent anion channel protein VDAC/porin, both a component of the PT pore as well as a major contributor to the mitochondrial outer membrane permeability [93]. The efflux of cytochrome *c* is therefore coordinated with the activation of a mitochondrial remodeling pathway characterized by changes in inner membrane morphology and organization, ensuring the complete release of cytochrome *c* and the onset of mitochondrial dysfunction [94].

## *Myocardial apoptosis*

In the last decade, there was increasing support from both animal models and clinical studies that myocardial apoptosis progressively increases and is a significant feature of cardiac failure. Apoptotic processes are pivotally involved in the remodeling of the heart, which accompanies or precedes the development of heart failure. The loss of cardiac cells (by inappropriate cell death) might take on particular significance during conditions of increased hemodynamic cardiac loading and in myocardial infarct. In addition, inappropriate loss of atrial cells has been suggested as a mechanism for cardiac arrhythmias [95]. Myocardial apoptosis has been documented in patients with end-stage DCM [96–97]. Cytochrome *c* release from mitochondria was found to also occur in the failing human heart and in cardiomyopathy [98]. Critical issues that remain to be elucidated include identification of the molecular triggers for cardiac apoptosis, the precise quantification of apoptotic cells, and the time of apoptosis onset and completion. The overall role of apoptosis in cardiac failure (while highly attractive as a theoretical construct) is not yet known. Findings from *in vitro* systems and animal models suggest that myocardial apoptosis occurs in response to a variety of insults, including ischemia-reperfusion, myocardial infarction, atrial pacing, and mechanical stretch, and following aortic constriction-pressure overload. Apoptotic induction has also been described in pacing-induced cardiac failure in dogs [99–100].

A large number of factors present in the failing myocardium have been shown to caused or be involved with apoptosis, including catecholamines, angiotensin, inflammatory cytokines, ROS, NO, hypoxia, peptide growth factors (e.g., TGF and cardiotrophin), and mechanical stress. A subset of these factors are involved in the mediation of hypertrophic growth of cardiac myocytes [67, 101–102]; some factors (e.g., ROS) contribute to both pathways (apoptosis and cell growth) [67], while others clearly favor 1 pathway and antagonize the other. For instance, the activation of phosphoinositide-3 kinase (PI3K) and its downstream serine-threonine effector Akt is a pivotal transducing event in cell proliferation, cardiomyocyte survival, and myocardial hypertrophy [103] and a potent antagonist to the apoptotic pathway (and vice versa).

In the adult heart, several of the signaling cascades mediating myocyte growth and hypertrophy also function to enhance cardiomyocyte survival, in response to pleiotropic death stimuli [104]. The modulation of myocardial growth by blocking intracellular apoptotic signaling pathways may have potential value in the prevention and treatment of heart failure.

# References

1. Sohal RS, Svensson l, Sohal BH, Brunk UT (1989) Superoxide anion radical production in different animal species. Mech Ageing Dev 49:129–35

2. Pryor WA (1986) Oxy-radicals and related species: Their formation, lifetimes, and reactions. Annu Rev Physiol 48:657–67

3. Han D, Antunes F, Canali R, Rettori D, Cadenas E (2003) Voltage-dependent anion channels control the release of the superoxide anion from mitochondria to cytosol. J Biol Chem 278:5557–63

4. Wallace DC (2002) Animal models for mitochondrial disease. Methods Mol Biol 197:3–54

5.  Chen Q, Vazquez EJ, Moghaddas S, Hoppel CL, Lesnefsky EJ (2003) Production of reactive oxygen species by mitochondria: Central role of complex III. J Biol Chem 278:36027–31

6.  Herrero A, Barja G (2000) Localization of the site of oxygen radical generation inside the complex I of heart and nonsynaptic brain mammalian mitochondria. J Bioenerg Biomembr 32:609–15

7.  McLennan HR, Degli Esposti M (2000) The contribution of mitochondrial respiratory complexes to the production of reactive oxygen species. J Bioenerg Biomembr 32:153–62

8.  Hellsten-Westing Y (1993) Immunohistochemical localization of xanthine oxidase in human cardiac and skeletal muscle. Histochemistry 100:215–22

9.  Moriwaki Y, Yamamoto T, Suda M, Nasako Y, Takahashi S, Agbedana OE, Hada T, Higashino K (1993) Purification and immunohistochemical tissue localization of human xanthine oxidase. Biochim Biophys Acta 1164:327–30

10. Cappola TP, Kass DA, Nelson GS, Berger RD, Rosas GO, Kobeissi ZA, Marban E, Hare JM (2001) Allopurinol improves myocardial efficiency in patients with idiopathic dilated cardiomyopathy. Circulation 104:2407–11

11. Stadtman ER, Berlett BS (1998) Reactive oxygen-mediated protein oxidation in aging and disease. Drug Metab Rev 30:225–43

12. Choksi KB, Boylston WH, Rabek JP, Widger WR, Papaconstantinou J (2004) Oxidatively damaged proteins of heart mitochondrial electron transport complexes. Biochim Biophys Acta 1688:95–101

13. Vasquez-Vivar J, Kalyanaraman B, Kennedy MC (2000) Mitochondrial aconitase is a source of hydroxyl radical. An electron spin resonance investigation. J Biol Chem 275:14064–9

14. Petrosillo G, Ruggiero FM, Pistolese M, Paradies G (2001) Reactive oxygen species generated from the mitochondrial electron transport chain induce cytochrome c dissociation from beef-heart submitochondrial particles via cardiolipin peroxidation: Possible role in the apoptosis. FEBS Lett 509:435–8

15. Paradies G, Petrosillo G, Pistolese M, Ruggiero FM (2002) Reactive oxygen species affect mitochondrial electron transport complex I activity through oxidative cardiolipin damage. Gene 286:135–41

16. Shen Z, Wu W, Hazen SL (2000) Activated leukocytes oxidatively damage DNA, RNA, and the nucleotide pool through halide-dependent formation of hydroxyl radical. Biochemistry 39:5474–82

17. LeDoux SP, Wilson GL (2001) Base excision repair of mito-chondrial DNA damage in mammalian cells. Prog Nucleic Acid Res Mol Biol 68:273–84

18. Yakes FM, Van Houten B (1997) Mitochondrial DNA damage is more extensive and persists longer than nuclear DNA damage in human cells following oxidative stress. Proc Natl Acad Sci USA 94: 514–9

19. Brown GC (1999) Nitric oxide and mitochondrial respiration. Biochim Biophys Acta 1411:351–69

20. Riobo NA, Clementi E, Melani M, Boveris A, Cadenas E, Moncada S, Poderoso JJ (2001) Nitric oxide inhibits mitochondrial NADH:ubiquinone reductase activity through peroxynitrite formation. Biochem J 359:139–45

21. Murray J, Taylor SW, Zhang B, Ghosh SS, Capaldi RA (2003) Oxidative damage to mitochondrial complex I due to peroxynitrite: Identification of reactive tyrosines by mass spectrometry. J Biol Chem 278:37223–30

22. Cassina AM, Hodara R, Souza JM, Thomson L, Castro L, Ischiropoulos H, Freeman BA, Radi R (2000) Cytochrome c nitration by peroxynitrite. J Biol Chem 275:21409–15

23. Castro L, Rodriguez M, Radi R (1994) Aconitase is readily inactivated by peroxynitrite, but not by its precursor, nitric oxide. J Biol Chem 269:29409–15

24. Packer MA, Scarlett JL, Martin SW, Murphy MP (1997) Induction of the mitochondrial permeability transition by peroxy-nitrite. Biochem Soc Trans 25:909–14

25. Brookes PS, Darley-Usmar VM (2004) Role of calcium and superoxide dismutase in sensitizing mitochondria to peroxynitrite-induced permeability transition. Am J Physiol Heart Circ Physiol 286:H39–46

26. Chen Y, Saari JT, Kang YJ (1994) Weak antioxidant defenses make the heart a target for damage in copper-deficient rats. Free Radic Biol Med 17:529–36

27. Radi R, Turrens JF, Chang LY, Bush KM, Crapo JD, Freeman BA (1991) Detection of catalase in rat heart mitochondria. J Biol Chem 266:22028–34

28. Antunes F, Han D, Cadenas E (2002) Relative contributions of heart mitochondria glutathione peroxidase and catalase to $H_2O_2$ detoxification in in vivo conditions. Free Radic Biol Med 33:1260–7

29. Phung CD, Ezieme JA, Turrens JF (1994) Hydrogen peroxide metabolism in skeletal muscle mitochondria. Arch Biochem Biophys 315:479–82

30. Judge S, Judge A, Grune T, Leeuwenburgh C (2004) Short-term CR decreases cardiac mitochondrial oxidant production but increases carbonyl content. Am J Physiol Regul Integr Comp Physiol 286:R254–9

31. Turko IV, Murad F (2003) Quantitative protein profiling in heart mitochondria from diabetic rats. J Biol Chem 278:35844–9

32. Radi R, Bush KM, Freeman BA (1993) The role of cytochrome c and mitochondrial catalase in hydroperoxide-induced heart mitochondrial lipid peroxidation. Arch Biochem Biophys 300:409–15

33. Zhou Z, Kang YJ (2000) Cellular and subcellular localization of catalase in the heart of transgenic mice. J Histochem Cytochem 48:585–94

34. Fernandez-Checa JC, Garcia-Ruiz C, Colell A, Morales A, Mari M, Miranda M, Ardite E (1998) Oxidative stress: Role of mitochondria and protection by glutathione. Biofactors 8:7–11

35. Vaage J, Antonelli M, Bufi M, Irtun O, DeBlasi RA, Corbucci GG, Gasparetto A, Semb AG (1997) Exogenous reactive oxygen species deplete the isolated rat heart of antioxidants. Free Radic Biol Med 22:85–92

36. Hasinoff BB, Schnabl KL, Marusak RA, Patel D, Huebner E (2003) Dexrazoxane protects cardiac myocytes against doxorubicin by preventing damage to mitochondria. Cardiovasc Toxicol 3:89–99

37. Lipshultz SE, Rifai N, Dalton VM, Levy DE, Silverman LB, Lipsitz SR, Colan SD, Asselin B, Barr RD, Clavell LA, Hurwitz CA, Moghrabi A, Samson Y, Schorin MA, Gelber RD, Sallan SE (2004) The effect of dexrazoxane on myocardial injury in doxorubicin-treated children with acute lymphoblastic leukemia. N Engl J Med 351:145–53

38. Kang YJ (1999) The antioxidant function of metallothionein in the heart. Proc Soc Exp Biol Med 222:263–73

39. Nath R, Kumar D, Li T, Singal PK (2000) Metallothioneins, oxidative stress and the cardiovascular system. Toxicology 2000 155:17–26

40. Ali MM, Frei E, Straub J, Breuer A, Wiessler M (2002) Induction of metallothionein by zinc protects from daunorubicin toxicity in rats. Toxicology 179:85–93

41. Okuda M, Lee HC, Kumar C, Chance B (1992) Comparison of the effect of a mitochondrial uncoupler, 2,4-dinitrophenol and adrenaline on oxygen radical production in the isolated perfused rat liver. Acta Physiol Scand 145:159–68

42. Korshunov SS, Korkina OV, Ruuge EK, Skulachev VP, Starkov AA (1998) Fatty acids as natural uncouplers preventing generation of $O_2^-$ and $H_2O_2$ by mitochondria in the resting state. FEBS Lett 435:215–8

43. Casteilla L, Rigoulet M, Penicaud L (2001) Mitochondrial ROS metabolism: modulation by uncoupling proteins. IUBMB Life 52:181–8

44. Papa S, Skulachev VP (1997) Reactive oxygen species, mitochondria, apoptosis and aging. Mol Cell Biochem 174:305–19

45. Vidal-Puig AJ, Grujic D, Zhang CY, Hagen T, Boss O, Ido Y, Szczepanik A, Wade J, Mootha V, Cortright R, Muoio DM, Lowell BB (2000) Energy metabolism in uncoupling protein 3 gene knockout mice. J Biol Chem 275:16258–66

46. Hoerter J, Gonzalez-Barroso MD, Couplan E, Mateo P, Gelly C, Cassard-Doulcier AM, Diolez P, Bouillaud F (2004) Mitochondrial uncoupling protein 1 expressed in the heart of transgenic mice protects against ischemic-reperfusion damage. Circulation 110:528–33

47. Teshima Y, Akao M, Jones SP, Marban E (2003) Uncoupling protein-2 overexpression inhibits mitochondrial death pathway in cardiomyocytes. Circ Res 93:192–200

48. Nemoto S, Takeda K, Yu ZX, Ferrans VJ, Finkel T (2000) Role for mitochondrial oxidants as regulators of cellular metabolism. Mol Cell Biol 20:7311–8

49. Cadenas E (2004) Mitochondrial free radical production and cell signaling. Mol Aspects Med 25:17–26

50. Bogoyevitch MA, Ng DC, Court NW, Draper KA, Dhillon A, Abas L (2000) Intact mitochondrial electron transport function is essential for signalling by hydrogen peroxide in cardiac myocytes. J Mol Cell Cardiol 32:1469–80

51. Archer SL, Wu XC, Thebaud B, Moudgil R, Hashimoto K, Michelakis ED (2004) O2 sensing in the human ductus arteriosus: redox-sensitive K+ channels are regulated by mitochondria-derived hydrogen peroxide. Biol Chem 385:205–16

52. Yamamura T, Otani H, Nakao Y, Hattori R, Osako M, Imamura H, Das DK (2001) Dual involvement of coenzyme Q10 in redox

signaling and inhibition of death signaling in the rat heart mitochondria. Antioxid Redox Signal 3:103–12

53. Brookes PS, Levonen AL, Shiva S, Sarti P, Darley-Usmar VM (2002) Mitochondria: Regulators of signal transduction by reactive oxygen and nitrogen species. Free Radic Biol Med 33:755–64

54. Boveris A, D'Amico G, Lores-Arnaiz S, Costa LE (2003) Enalapril increases mitochondrial nitric oxide synthase activity in heart and liver. Antioxid Redox Signal 5:691–7

55. Hess ML, Manson NH (1984) Molecular oxygen: Friend and foe. The role of the oxygen free radical system in the calcium paradox, the oxygen paradox and ischemia/reperfusion injury. J Mol Cell Cardiol 16:969–85

56. Becker LB (2004) New concepts in reactive oxygen species and cardiovascular reperfusion physiology. Cardiovasc Res 61:461–70

57. Becker LB, vanden Hoek TL, Shao ZH, Li CQ, Schumacker PT (1999) Generation of superoxide in cardiomyocytes during ischemia before reperfusion. Am J Physiol 277:H2240–6

58. Marin-Garcia J, Goldenthal MJ, Moe GW (2001) Anormal cardiac and skeletal muscle mitochondrial function in pacing-induced cardiac failure. Cardiovasc Res 52:103–10

59. Moe GW, Marin-Garcia J, Konig A, Goldenthal M, Lu X, Feng Q (2004) In vivo tumor necrosis factor alpha inhibition ameliorates cardiac mitochondrial dysfunction, oxidative stress and apoptosis in experimental heart failure. Am J Physiol Heart Circ Physiol 287:H1813–20

60. Ide T, Tsutsui H, Kinugawa S, Suematsu N, Hayashidani S, Ichikawa K, Utsumi H, Machida Y, Egashira K, Takeshita A (2000) direct evidence for increased hydroxyl radicals originating from superoxide in the failing myocardium. Circ Res 86:152–7

61. Ide T, Tsutsui H, Kinugawa S, Utsumi H, Kang D, Hattori N, Uchida K, Arimura K, Egashira K, Takeshita A (1999) Mitochondrial electron transport complex I is a potential source of oxygen free radicals in the failing myocardium. Circ Res 85:357–63

62. Marin-Garcia J, Goldenthal MJ, Ananthakrishnan R, Mirvis D (1996) Specific mitochondrial DNA deletions in canine myocardial ischemia. Biochem Mol Biol Int 40:1057–65

63. Suematsu N, Tsutsui H, Wen J, Kang D, Ikeuchi M, Ide T, Hayashidani S, Shiomi T, Kubota T, Hamasaki N, Takeshita A (2003) Oxidative stress mediates tumor necrosis factor-alpha-induced

mitochondrial DNA damage and dysfunction in cardiac myocytes. Circulation 107:1418–23

64. Ide T, Tsutsui H, Hayashidani S, Kang D, Suematsu N, Nakamura K, Utsumi H, Hamasaki N, Takeshita A (2001) Mitochondrial DNA damage and dysfunction associated with oxidative stress in failing hearts after myocardial infarction. Circ Res 88:529–35

65. Sorescu D, Griendling K (2002) Reactive oxygen species, mitochondria, and NAD(P)H oxidases in the development and progression of heart failure. Congest Heart Fail 8:132–40

66. Griendling KK, Sorescu D, Ushio-Fukai M (2000) NAD(P)H oxidase: Role in cardiovascular biology and disease. Circ Res 86:494–501

67. Sabri A, Hughie HH, Lucchesi PA (2003) Regulation of hypertrophic and apoptotic signaling pathways by reactive oxygen species in cardiac myocytes. Antioxid Redox Signal 5:731–40

68. Li JM, Gall NP, Grieve DJ, Chen M, Shah AM (2002) Activation of NADPH oxidase during progression of cardiac hypertrophy to failure. Hypertension 40:477–84

69. Xiao L, Pimentel DR, Wang J, Singh K, Colucci WS, Sawyer DB (2002) Role of reactive oxygen species and NAD(P)H oxidase in alpha(1)-adrenoceptor signaling in adult rat cardiac myocytes. Am J Physiol Cell Physiol 282:C926–34

70. Heymes C, Bendall JK, Ratajczak P, Cave AC, Samuel JL, Hasenfuss G, Shah AM (2003) Increased myocardial NADPH oxidase activity in human heart failure. J Am Coll Cardiol 41:2164–71

71. Nakagami H, Liao JK (2004) Statins and myocardial hypertrophy. Coron Artery Dis 15:247–50

72. Maack C, Kartes T, Kilter H, Schafers HJ, Nickenig G, Bohm M, Laufs U (2003) Oxygen free radical release in human failing myocardium is associated with increased activity of rac1-GTPase and represents a target for statin treatment. Circulation 108:1567–74

73. Kannan K, Jain SK (2000) Oxidative stress and apoptosis. Pathophysiology 7:153–63

74. Keller JN, Kindy MS, Holtsberg FW, St Clair DK, Yen HC, Germeyer A, Steiner SM, Bruce-Keller AJ, Hutchins JB, Mattson MP (1998) Mitochondrial manganese superoxide dismutase prevents neural apoptosis and reduces ischemic brain injury: Suppression of peroxynitrite production, lipid peroxidation, and mitochondrial dysfunction. J Neurosci 18:687–97

75. Shiomi T, Tsutsui H, Matsusaka H, Murakami K, Hayashidani S, Ikeuchi M, Wen J, Kubota T, Utsumi H, Takeshita A (2004) Overexpression of glutathione peroxidase prevents left ventricular remodeling and failure after myocardial infarction in mice. Circulation 109:544–9

76. Kang YJ, Zhou ZX, Wu H, Wang GW, Saari JT, Klein JB (2000) Metallothionein inhibits myocardial apoptosis in copper-deficient mice: Role of atrial natriuretic peptide. Lab Invest 80:745–57

77. Lud Cadet J, Harrington B, Ordonez S (2000) Bcl-2 overexpression attenuates dopamine-induced apoptosis in an immortalized neural cell line by suppressing the production of reactive oxygen species. Synapse 35:228–33

78. Kokoszka JE, Coskun P, Esposito LA, Wallace DC (2001) Increased mitochondrial oxidative stress in the Sod2 (+/-) mouse results in the age-related decline of mitochondrial function culminating in increased apoptosis. Proc Natl Acad Sci USA 98:2278–83

79. Fu Y, Porres JM, Lei XG (2001) Comparative impacts of glutathione peroxidase-1 gene knockout on oxidative stress induced by reactive oxygen and nitrogen species in mouse hepatocytes. Biochem J 359:687–95

80. Goossens V, Stange G, Moens K, Pipeleers D, Grooten J (1999) Regulation of tumor necrosis factor-induced, mitochondria- and reactive oxygen species-dependent cell death by electron flux through electron transport chain complex I. Antioxid Redox Signal 1:285–95

81. von Harsdorf R, Li PF, Dietz R (1999) Signaling pathways in reactive oxygen species-induced cardiomyocyte apoptosis. Circulation 99:2934–41

82. Akao M, O'Rourke B, Teshima Y, Seharaseyon J, Marban E (2003) Mechanistically distinct steps in the mitochondrial death pathway triggered by oxidative stress in cardiac myocytes. Circ Res 92:186–94

83. Long X, Goldenthal MJ, Wu GM, Marin-Garcia J (2004) Mitochondrial Ca2+ flux and respiratory enzyme activity decline are early events in cardiomyocyte response to H(2)O(2). J Mol Cell Cardiol 37:63–70

84. Hickson-Bick DL, Sparagna GC, Buja LM, McMillin JB (2002) Palmitate-induced apoptosis in neonatal cardiomyocytes is not dependent on the generation of ROS. Am J Physiol Heart Circ Physiol 282:H656–64

85. Regula KM, Ens K, Kirshenbaum LA (2003) Mitochondria-assisted cell suicide: A license to kill. J Mol Cell Cardiol 35:559–67
86. Kroemer G (2003) Mitochondrial control of apoptosis: An introduction. Biochem Biophys Res Commun 304:433–5
87. Acehan D, Jiang X, Morgan DG, Heuser JE, Wang X, Akey CW (2002) Three-dimensional structure of apoptosome: Implications for assembly, procaspase-9 binding, and activation. Mol Cell 9:423–32
88. Green DR, Reed JC (1998) Mitochondria and apoptosis. Science 281:1309–12
89. Danial NN, Korsmeyer SJ (2004) Cell death: Critical control points. Cell 116:205–19
90. Epand RF, Martinou JC, Montessuit S, Epand RM, Yip CM (2002) Direct evidence for membrane pore formation by the apoptotic protein Bax. Biochem Biophys Res Commun 298:744–9
91. Chipuk JE, Kuwana T, Bouchier-Hayes L, Droin NM, Newmeyer DD, Schuler M, Green DR (2004) Direct activation of Bax by p53 mediates mitochondrial membrane permeabilization and apoptosis. Science 303:1010–4
92. Scorrano L, Ashiya M, Buttle K, Weiler S, Oakes S, Mannella CA, Korsmeyer SJ (2002) A distinct pathway remodels mitochondrial cristae and mobilizes cytochrome c during apoptosis. Dev Cell 2:55–67
93. Belzacq AS, Vieira HL, Verrier F, Vandecasteele G, Cohen I, Prevost MC, Larquet E, Pariselli F, Petit PX, Kahn A, Rizzuto R, Brenner C, Kroemer G (2003) Bcl-2 and Bax modulate adenine nucleotide translocase activity. Cancer Res 63:541–6
94. Scorrano L, Korsmeyer SJ (2003) Mechanisms of cytochrome c release by proapoptotic BCL-2 family members. Biochem Biophys Res Commun 304:437–44
95. James TN (1998) Normal and abnormal consequences of apoptosis in the human heart. Annu Rev Physiol 60:309–25
96. Olivetti G, Abbi R, Quaini F, Kajstura J, Cheng W, Nitahara JA, Quaini E, Di Loreto C, Beltrami CA, Krajewski S, Reed JC, Anversa P (1997) Apoptosis in the failing human heart. N Engl J Med 336:1131–41
97. Anversa P, Kajstura J, Olivetti G (1996) Myocyte death in heart failure. Curr Opin Cardiol 11:245–51
98. Narula J, Pandey P, Arbustini E, Haider N, Narula N, Kolodgie FD, Dal Bello B, Semigran MJ, Bielsa-Masdeu A, Dec GW, Israels S, Ballester M, Virmani R, Saxena S, Kharbanda S (1999) Apoptosis in

heart failure: Release of cytochrome c from mitochondria and activation of caspase-3 in human cardiomyopathy. Proc Natl Acad Sci USA 96:8144–9

99. Liu Y, Cigola E, Cheng W, Kajstura J, Olivetti G, Hintze TH, Anversa P (1995) Myocyte nuclear mitotic division and programmed myocyte cell death characterize the cardiac myopathy induced by rapid ventricular pacing in dogs. Lab Invest 73:771–87

100. Cesselli D, Jakoniuk I, Barlucchi L, Beltrami AP, Hintze TH, Nadal-Ginard B, Kajstura J, Leri A, Anversa P (2001) Oxidative stress-mediated cardiac cell death is a major determinant of ventricular dysfunction and failure in dog dilated cardiomyopathy. Circ Res 89:279–86

101. Hunter JJ, Chien KR (1999) Signaling pathways for cardiac hypertrophy and failure. N Engl J Med 341:1276–83

102. Colucci WS (1997) Molecular and cellular mechanisms of myocardial failure. Am J Cardiol 80:15L–25L

103. Oudit GY, Sun H, Kerfant BG, Crackower MA, Penninger JM, Backx PH (2004) The role of phosphoinositide-3 kinase and PTEN in cardiovascular physiology and disease. J Mol Cell Cardiol 7:449–71

104. Van Empel VP, De Windt LJ (2004) Myocyte hypertrophy and apoptosis: a balancing act. Cardiovasc Res 63:487–99

# Chapter 5

# Myocardial Ischemia and Cardioprotection

## Overview

Acute ischemia and myocardial infarct as a consequence of coronary artery disease remain major public health problems. The incidence of heart failure secondary to myocardial ischemia/myocardial infarct is increasing, and in the United States alone, more than a half million new cases are diagnosed each year in adults and aging individuals. Moreover, after myocardial infarction, patients are at high risk for recurrent cardiovascular events, new onset heart failure, and increased mortality. Data so far accumulated using ischemic preconditioning (IPC) and cardioprotection (CP) in animal models suggest that these interventions may be a desirable alternative to the currently available drug armamentarium and surgical interventions for coronary artery disease.

## Introduction

When exposed to an insult, cardiomyocytes are able to mount a cardioprotective response. Until recently, reperfusion of the ischemic myocardium was the only intervention available to restore the various cellular functions affected by myocardial ischemia, including preventing cell death by necrosis or apoptosis. Unfortunately, reperfusion may result in extensive myocardial damage, including myocardial stunning, and the functional recovery of the heart may appear only after a period of cardiac contractile dysfunction that may last for several hours or days. Understanding the damage that ischemia produce in mitochondrial structure and function as well as the cellular and molecular mechanisms of IPC-CP is essential in developing new therapies to improve the welfare of so many patients with myocardial diseases. Unequivocal data and more refined techniques to evaluate the molecular events occurring in ischemia and CP are required prior to clinical trials with drugs and regimens whose specificity of action, including their overall metabolic and physiological role, and potential benefits are not absolutely clear.

## Mitochondrial dysfunction in myocardial ischemia

### Oxidation-phosphorylation decline in ischemia

When the supply of oxygen becomes limited as occurs with myocardial ischemia, OXPHOS and mitochondrial ETC flux decline. Data collected from the porcine model of myocardial ischemia demonstrated significant reduction in mitochondrial respiratory complex I activity (35%) and in state 3 mitochondrial respiration supported by NAD-linked substrates, glutamate and malate [1–2]. These studies also found that in addition to complex I, complex V (oligomycin-sensitive $F_0$-$F_1$ATPase) was a critical target of early myocardial ischemia, exhibiting severe activity reduction (>45%). These findings have since been confirmed in rat and human myocardium [3]. As ischemia progresses, rat hearts also display a moderate decrease (25%) in complex IV activity level, in parallel with significantly depleted levels of the mitochondrial inner membrane phospholipid, cardiolipin, which as previously noted plays an integral role in promoting the stability and activity of complexes I and IV [4–6]. Additional evidence supports the notion that a functionally distinct subpopulation of myocardial mitochondria (i.e., subsarcolemmal mitochondria) are preferentially affected during ischemia displaying discernible damage in complex IV [7–8]. Also, complex III deficiency occurs during the progression of myocardial ischemia [9].

Despite evidence that specific mitochondrial OXPHOS and ETC functions are affected following myocardial ischemia, the molecular and biochemical basis of that dysfunction has not yet been fully established. Considerable experimental data support the hypothesis that there is not a common mechanism for ischemia-mediated decline in enzymatic activity for the different respiratory complexes [10]. Ischemia-related damage to complex III results in highly targeted injury to the Fe-S cluster of the Rieske protein subunit of complex III [9]. Evolutionarily conserved cysteine and histidine residues in the Rieske subunit responsible for $Fe^{++}$ binding and for the integrity of the cluster are the proposed targets for ischemic impairment of the complex III activity; the level of the Rieske subunit itself is not affected in myocardial ischemia. In contrast, neither qualitative nor quantitative defects in complex IV protein subunits have been detected in myocardial ischemia. The loss of the inner membrane lipid cardiolipin, which has been demonstrated in both *in vivo* and *in vitro* models of myocardial ischemia, has been proposed as the probable explanation for the specific dysfunction of complex IV activity. Cardiolipin depletion with its attendent decrease in membrane fluidity might also impact other inner-membrane transporters and ETC complexes.

The loss of complex I activity has been attributed to depletion of both flavin mononucleotide [2] and, more recently, cardiolipin [5], although the precise mechanism has not yet been determined. Supplementation of ischemic cells with exogenous cardiolipin has been shown to largely restore both complex I and IV activities after ischemic insult [4–5]. If this is true, the mechanism of how cardiolipin is disturbed in ischemia needs to be determined. This mechanism must also take into account both the rapidity of the ischemic insult and its differential effect on respiratory enzymes. Essentially 30 minutes of ischemic insult is required for the decline in complex III and IV activity and discernible cardiolipin depletion, while complex I activity decline is detectable within 10 minutes.

Other potential explanations for the impact of myocardial ischemia on mitochondrial respiratory enzymes have been considered. These include altered mitochondrial protein import during ischemia, mitochondrial transcription, and protein synthesis [10]. Evidence for altered protein import to mitochondria is presently scant and does not provide an explanation of why many cytoplasmically synthesized mitochondrial proteins are not affected in ischemia. The notion that mitochondrial transcription and protein synthesis are affected is consistent with the loss of specific respiratory complex activities whose subunits are encoded by mtDNA (i.e., I, III, IV, and V). However, data on ischemia-mediated decreases in mitochondrial-specific transcript and peptide levels (e.g., COXI and ATPase6) are not available.

On the other hand, mtDNA damage has been reported in association with ischemia. Data from clinical studies of patients with ischemic heart disease have shown that large-scale mtDNA deletions are prevalent in myocardium [11]. Studies from dogs undergoing ameroid constriction also found a significant elevation in the level of myocardial mtDNA deletions (with a concomitant decline in respiratory enzyme activities) in ischemia-affected myocardium compared to controls [12]. These findings support a loss of mtDNA integrity with chronic ischemic insult and are unlikely to explain the rapid and differential loss of specific respiratory enzymatic activities found in acute myocardial ischemia. Parenthetically, similar findings were not demonstrated using the rat model of myocardial ischemia described above.

In addition to mitochondrial OXPHOS and ETC, other mitochondrial bioenergetic pathways are significantly affected in ischemic myocardium. Levels of creatine phosphate are rapidly depleted along with progressive decline in mitochondrial creatine kinase activity, reducing the export of high-energy phosphates from mitochondria [13]. During the development of myocardial ischemia in rats, in addition to a progressive decline in respiratory enzyme activities there is an increase in proton leak across the mitochondrial inner membrane [14–15].

Ischemia promotes a cellular bioenergetic substrate selection shift in the myocyte, with a switch to glycolytic/glucose pathway from FAO/ aerobic metabolic pathways, underlying the mitochondrial plasticity concept [16]. Impaired oxidation of fatty acids results in the accumulation of long-chain fatty acids that inhibit PDH and that can result in cardiac arrhythmias. The hydrolysis of glycolytically derived ATP, accumulation of lactate, and a marked decline in pyruvate oxidation lead to a decrease in intracellular pH and intracellular acidosis, which has a direct inhibitory effect on contractile function. AMP and other intermediates accumulate, and subsequent mitochondrial swelling and progressive degeneration occur.

## Myocardial ischemia and oxidative stress

Ischemia results in oxidative damage to proteins, including the oxidation of carbonyl and sulfhydryl groups; the latter occurs concomitantly with a severe depletion in glutathione levels [17]. Mitochondrial proteins are readily targeted as they are close to the site of free radical generation. Ischemia triggers protease activity and also mediates the peroxidation of lipids; in addition to a marked loss in cardiolipin, there is loss of membrane fluidity and movement within the mitochondrial membranes [18]. Also, the mitochondrial antioxidant response appears to be hampered by the ischemic insult [17-19]. Besides a marked reduction in the levels of reduced compared to oxidized glutathione, the ischemic myocardium also exhibits a decrease in mitochondrial-localized MnSOD and GPx activities. In contrast, the levels of cytoplasmic antioxidants (e.g., CuSOD and catalase) are unchanged.

Sustained myocardial ischemia can lead to pronounced ATP depletion and either apoptotic or necrotic cell death. The selection of apoptosis as compared to necrosis centers on the availability of ATP; higher levels of ATP furnish energy needed for the apoptotic events to occur, whereas low levels of ATP promote necrosis. The release of cytochrome $c$ is also predisposed by the events of ischemia [20]. The relationship of cytochrome $c$ loss, oxidative stress, and myocardial apoptosis have been previously discussed.

## *Myocardial ischemia and mitochondrial calcium flux*

Mitochondrial $Ca^{++}$ flux represents an early pivotal event in ischemia/anoxia-induced cardiomyocyte damage, preceding and presumably leading to reduced mitochondrial respiratory activity levels followed by an accumulation of intracellular oxidation, mitochondrial membrane depolarization, and cell death. What remains unclear at this time is the critical sequence of early mitochondrial-related events, including mitochondrial membrane depolarization and its functional consequences, particularly with respect to mitochondrial bioenergetic function, cytochrome $c$ release, and the role of the opening of the mitochondrial PT pore. In addition, calcium flux into mitochondria has a potentially important regulatory role in this response, since it is well established that calcium overload promotes mitochondrial PT pore opening and agents that block PT pore opening inhibit apoptosis [21].

As a surrogate of ischemia/reperfusion cardiac damage, the model of $H_2O_2$-treated cardiomyocytes has been recently used in the assessment of mitochondrial oxidative damage and cardioprotective mechanisms, with potential clinical application [22]. By using a variety of cardioprotective agents the modulation of various stages in the cardiomyocyte $H_2O_2$ response was tested [23]. These studies demonstrated that the activation of mitoK$_{ATP}$ channels (proposed as a central event in cardioprotective IPC) targeted and suppressed the mitochondrial morphological changes that require matrix $Ca^{++}$ overload, preceding changes in the mitochondrial membrane potential. A representative illustration depicting mitochondrial $Ca^{++}$ flux in neonatal rat cardiomyocytes in response to $H_2O_2$ treatment is shown in Figure 5.1.

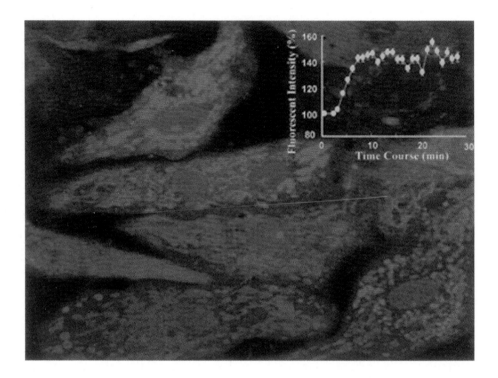

**Figure 5.1. Fluorescent imaging of mitochondrial calcium in cultured neonatal rat cardiomyocytes.** *Cells were loaded with rhod-2, a fluorescent indicator of mitochondrial calcium level at 4°C for 60 min followed by incubation at 37°C for 30 min. The graph inside shows the time-lapse increases in mitochondrial-localized rhod-2 fluorescence in cardiomyocytes subjected to $H_2O_2$ treatment.*

## Gene expression

Myocardial ischemia can also elicit a marked and rapid activation of myocardial gene expression affecting mitochondrial function [24–25]. The current availability of microarray technology may allow the identification of changes in the overall myocardial transcriptional programming at the onset and progression of ischemia. This technology may also allow assessment of the role that ischemia plays in modulating transcriptional expression of genes involved in a plurality of mitochondrial functions including OXPHOS/ETC, the TCA cycle, FAO, mitochondrial PT pore and antioxidant responses, mtDNA transcription and maintenance, as well as nuclear transcription factors known to be involved in mitochondrial biogenesis.

## *Reperfusion*

Paradoxically, functional mitochondria can exacerbate ischemic damage, especially at the onset of reperfusion. A pronounced increase in fatty acid influx and unbalanced FAO predominates during reperfusion, producing an excess of acetyl CoA saturating the TCA cycle at the expense of glucose and pyruvate oxidation, which is eventually inhibited. Increased OXPHOS causes elevated ROS accumulation with increased lipid peroxidation; this results in lower cardiolipin levels in the inner membrane with consequent effect on complex IV activity. Normal respiratory activity can be restored by adding exogenous cardiolipin [4–5]. At present, there is evidence that reperfusion injury involves apoptotic cell death in contrast to ischemic injury, which primarily involves necrotic cell death [26].

## Cardioprotection

Hyperthermic stress can protect against myocardial dysfunction after ischemia/reperfusion injury [27]. Improved levels of complex I to V activities, heat-shock protein expression (i.e., HSP32, HSP60, and HSP72), and ventricular function were attained in heat-stressed hearts. In comparison to untreated reperfused myocardium, in which mitochondria were severely disrupted, the reperfused heat-stressed myocardium exhibited higher respiratory enzyme activities and displayed mitochondria with intact membranes, packed with parallel lamellar cristae. These findings provided evidence that heat-stress-mediated enhancement of the mitochondrial energetic capacity is associated with increased tolerance to ischemia-reperfusion injury.

## *Ischemic cardioprotection*

IPC is a phenomenon in which single or multiple brief periods of ischemia have been shown to protect the heart against a more prolonged ischemic insult (index ischemia), resulting in the reduction in myocaridial infarct size, severity of stunning, and incidence of cardiac arrhythmias. IPC was first demonstrated by Murry [28] in a canine model, showing that brief periods of ischemia and reperfusion provided cardioprotection to a prolonged ischemic insult. Subsequent studies have demonstrated CP in all animals studied and have also shown that IPC-like effects occur in cultured cells exposed to hypoxia and metabolic inhibition, impacting both the structure and function of mitochondria. A key rationale for IPC is to prevent ischemia-driven myocardial necrosis [29].

Information about IPC has also been derived from the use of potassium channel openers (KCOs) such as nicorandil, diazoxide, pinacidil, and cromakalin and also by the use of $K_{ATP}$ channel blockers (e.g., glibenclamide and 5-hydroxydecanoic acid (5-HD), which diminish the beneficial effects of short ischemic events on cardiac tissue [29]. Initially, sarcolemmal $K_{ATP}$ (sarc$K_{ATP}$) channels were thought to be implicated in IPC but more recently the focus has shifted to the mito$K_{ATP}$ channels. Garlid and associates have shown that the KCO diazoxide was 1,000 to 2,000 times more potent in opening the mito$K_{ATP}$ channel than the sarc$K_{ATP}$ channel [30]. The negative effect of 5-HD (abolishing diazoxide's protective effect entirely) further suggested that mito$K_{ATP}$ mediated IPC, since 5-HD is highly selective in interacting with the mito$K_{ATP}$, as compared to the sarcolemmal channel. However, 5-HD treatment has been recently shown to also modulate mitochondrial respiration and fatty acid $\beta$-oxidation independently of its interaction with the mito$K_{ATP}$ channel [31]. Nevertheless, recent data support the view that both the mito$K_{ATP}$ and sarc$K_{ATP}$ channels have contributory roles in cardioprotection [32–33]. Under specific conditions, diazoxide and 5-HD can modulate sarc$K_{ATP}$ channel opening [32], whereas mito$K_{ATP}$ can bind molecules previously thought to interact solely with sarc$K_{ATP}$ channels and in some species (e.g., dogs) both the mitochondrial and sarc$K_{ATP}$ channels must be blocked to entirely abolish IPC cardioprotection [33]. Another ion channel previously thought to be exclusive to the myocardial sarcolemmal membrane (i.e., the calcium-activated $K^+$ channel) has recently been located on the mitochondrial inner membrane and demonstrated to be functionally cardioprotective against myocardial infarct [34].

Biochemical structural analysis of the proteins comprising the $K_{ATP}$ channels has been performed with functional channels isolated from both myocardial sarcolemmal and mitochondrial membranes [35–36]. The channel activities of these preparations have been reconstituted in liposomes and shown to be regulated by the same ligands as *in vivo*, in both heart and brain. While the sarc$K_{ATP}$ channels are heteromultimeric complexes of sulfonylurea receptors (SUR) and potassium inward rectifier (Kir) gene products [37], the precise molecular composition of the mitoK$_{ATP}$ channel has yet to be identified [38]. Using immunoblot analysis, no evidence for the presence of either known sulfonylurea receptors (SUR1 or SUR2) in mitochondria has been found [39]. While there is evidence for the presence of Kir6.1 and 6.2 in cardiac mitochondria [40], gene knockout studies demonstrated no discernible functional role for these proteins in the mitoK$_{ATP}$ channel [38]. A recent study has indicated that a multiprotein complex can be purified from the mitochondrial inner membrane, which functions as a mitoK$_{ATP}$ channel, fully sensitive to channel activators and blockers on reconstitution into proteoliposomes and lipid bilayers [41]. This complex contains 5 mitochondrial proteins, including ANT, the mitochondrial ATP-binding cassette protein 1 (mABC1), the phosphate carrier (PIC), ATP synthase, and SDH. However, at this time, the pore-forming component of the mitoK$_{ATP}$ channel remains undetermined as do the potential identity of other proteins within this complex. The identity of major bioenergetic proteins (ATP synthase and SDH) within the mitoK$_{ATP}$ channel and their overlap with structural components of the PT pore (e.g., ANT) have important ramifications for the mechanism of cardioprotection and its relatedness to both bioenergetic function and apoptosis regulation.

## Cascade of mitochondrial events in IPC

Treatment with KCOs causes a reduction in mitochondrial Ca$^{++}$ influx [42–43]. Korge et al. [42] performed experiments with isolated mitochondria that are anoxic and "deenergized", simulating the ischemic state. Under these conditions, a mild depolarization of the mitochondrial membrane potential occurs, which prevents the uptake into the matrix of extramitochondrial Ca$^{++}$ (preventing mitochondrial Ca$^{++}$ overload, which could ensue during ischemia or reperfusion) and also results in inhibition in the opening of the PT pore. If isolated mitochondria are previously loaded with Ca$^{++}$ and subsequently depolarized (with diazoxide), the PT pore is opened [44–45]. Other studies have found that the PT pore opens in the first minutes of reperfusion following ischemia [46], in association with elevated levels of mitochondrial Ca$^{++}$, increased oxidative stress, and increased matrix pH [47]. Opening the PT pore allows H$_2$O and solutes to enter the mitochondria, increasing matrix volume and rupturing the outer membrane and can result in cell death by either apoptosis or necrosis.

Inhibiting PT pore opening at reperfusion using cyclosporin A has been reported to be cardioprotective [48].

IPC not only protects against necrotic cell death but blunts the progression of myocyte apoptosis. Apoptosis occurs as a consequence of ischemia/reperfusion, and the predominant view is that myocyte apoptosis, occurring as a result of ischemia/reperfusion (I/R), is in fact reperfusion-triggered [49]. This may be because reperfusion rapidly restores intracellular ATP levels that are required to allow the progression of the apoptotic pathway. Reduction of apoptosis by IPC is elicited by the inhibition of inflammatory cell activation and by altering the expression of apoptogenic proteins (e.g., Bax) and protein kinase C activity. Early hallmark events of apoptosis occur at the mitochondrial inner membrane and include opening of the PT pore and release of cytochrome $c$ from mitochondria. With CP, cytochrome $c$ release is inhibited along with PT pore opening, and the $Ca^{++}$ flux into mitochondria is stemmed. The IPC-modulation of myocardial apoptotic events has been documented in early but not delayed IPC [50].

The connection of mitochondrial respiratory activity and ATP levels to IPC and to the opening of mito$K_{ATP}$ channels has been proposed to be critical in the overall regulation of myocardial bioenergetics, as well as in the survival of the ischemic cell. A modest but significant level of uncoupling of respiration and OXPHOS occurs with IPC [16]. The uncoupling of OXPHOS, under certain circumstances, can allow the fine-tuning of cellular bioenergetic efficiency in accord with cell needs, proposed as a primary reason for mitochondrial uncoupling proteins. The importance of uncoupling has been further supported by studies in which treatment with uncouplers (e.g., DNP) mimics IPC [48]. Moreover, it has been demonstrated in myocytes that a crucial determinant in opening of both sarc$K_{ATP}$ and mito$K_{ATP}$ channels is the cytoplasmic ATP pool, mainly produced by mitochondrial OXPHOS. Either uncoupling of mitochondrial OXPHOS or inhibition of COX results in the opening of cardiac $K_{ATP}$ channels, even in the presence of glucose [51]. Modulation of COX activity by NO should be expected to impact directly on the opening of $K_{ATP}$ channels and may be contributory to the known effect of NO on IPC [52]. In addition, increased myocardial ATP levels have been reported in rat hearts treated with IPC and with diazoxide (in comparison to levels in untreated animals) [53–54]. There is evidence that IPC and KCO treatment causes the inhibition of cardiac mitochondrial ATPase and reduction of ATP depletion during the early stages of sustained ischemia, and this effect persists during the critical early phase of reperfusion [55]. The inhibition of ATP hydrolysis will allow the conservation of high-energy phosphates, improve the energy state of the heart during ischemia, and may contribute to postischemic recovery. Similarly, in isolated mitochondria subjected to anoxia, diazoxide (if present during the anoxic insult) preserved ADP-stimulated respiration and ATP levels, relative to untreated anoxic-stressed mitochondria [56]. On the other hand, it is important to note that mitochondrial ATP depletion and decreased mitochondrial ATPase activity are unlikely to be responsible for the cardioprotective effects of IPC. These conclusions are supported by findings that ATP depletion can remain unchanged and even be enhanced during IPC cardioprotection [57–58].

Differential compartmentation of ATP within the cardiomyocyte may also contribute to CP since ATP located near the sarcolemmal membrane would be more readily available for the membrane trans-porters and ion pumps needed for cardiomyocyte function [16].

It is generally accepted that the mitoK$_{ATP}$ channels close when the mitochondrial ATP level is high and open under conditions of low ATP levels (responding to ATP/ADP ratio, as well as to localized changes in adenosine content derived from adenine nucleotide metabolism). Contributory roles have been proposed for ANT, VDAC, and creatine kinase, important factors both in the control and cellular distribution of mitochondria ATP and as components of the PT pore [59]. The opening of mitoK$_{ATP}$ channels either by KCOs or by ischemic preconditioning modulates the PT pore opening, although it has not yet been determined whether the PT pore is a upstream target of the cardioprotective stimuli or a downstream end-effector [60]. In addition, the role of K$_{ATP}$ channel opening in mediating VDAC activity and outer mitochondrial membrane permeability to regulate both the efflux and influx of mitochondrial adenine nucleotide levels may be critical in cardioprotection and remains to be fully elucidated. In this regard, it is noteworthy to mention that VDAC is a pivotal control site in the triggering of myocardial apoptosis with high affinity for both the proapoptotic and antiapoptotic proteins of the Bcl-2 family and for kinases such as PKCε [61]. Another important aspect of respiratory and OXPHOS regulation is the pivotal role played by ROS generation (a by-product of OXPHOS), which as discussed below represents a critical downstream mediator of preconditioning. Recently, it has been reported that ROS induces a significant decrease in mitochondrial NADH-supported respiration, which can be reproduced by pharmacologically inhibiting the activity of complex I, a primary site of mitochondrial ROS generation [62].

IPC and treatment with KCOs significantly increase cardiomyocyte mitochondrial volume, presumably due to the influx of $K^+$ [63]. Induced mitochondrial matrix swelling may result in improved mitochondrial energy production by the activation of FAO, mitochondrial respiration, and ATP production [64]. In experiments with isolated mitochondria, $K^+$-induced mitochondrial swelling was not necessary for the increased ROS production mediated by diazoxide, suggesting that diazoxide may modulate ROS by a mechanism independent of the $K^+$ channel opening [56]. However, controversy exists concerning both the extent, cause, and significance of matrix changes during IPC [65]. Other effects of mito$K_{ATP}$ channel opening include the maintenance of the tight structure of the intermembrane space required to preserve the normal low outer-membrane permeability to adenine nucleotides and cytochrome *c*, beneficial effects elicited by diaxoxide treatment which are abrogated by the mito$K_{ATP}$ channel inhibitor 5-HD [66]. Consequently, the mito$K_{ATP}$ channel opening is considered both a signaling trigger and a mediator/effector of the CP pathway [67].

## Signaling pathways

### *Adenosine and other ligands*

Adenosine and its G-protein coupled receptors represent an important positive stimulus, as well as a locus for feedback control of IPC [68]. Adenosine is generated at high levels during myocardial ischemia from ATP metabolism, which is produced primarily in mitochondria. IPC-induced cardioprotection is abrogated by treatment with adenosine receptor antagonists, suggesting that adenosine, produced during

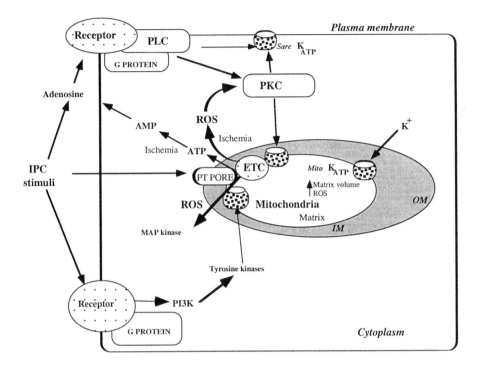

**Figure 5.2. Schematic representation depicting cellular events occurring in early ischemic preconditioning.** *Adenosine, produced by the breakdown of adenine nucleotides during ischemia, leads to the activation of phospholipase C (PLC), which in turn activates and translocates protein kinase C (PKC) to target mitochondrial membranes modulating the opening of mitoK$_{ATP}$ and to a lesser extent sarcK$_{ATP}$ channels. Other agonists of G-protein coupled receptors also stimulate parallel signaling pathways with either PKC-dependent or tyrosine kinase-dependent and phosphoinositide-3 kinase (PI3K) cascades. Multiple mitochondrial events are integral to cardioprotection including increased mitochondrial ROS generation, modulation of permeability transition (PT) pore opening, and mitochondrial ETC activity, albeit the temporal sequence of these events is presently undetermined. MitoK$_{ATP}$ channel opening also provides positive feedback by altering components such as ROS, mitogen-activated protein kinase (MAPK) or PKC activation.*

IPC, acts on cell-surface receptors, the most important being the A1 adenosine receptor [69]. Other ligands (including bradykinin, acetylcholine, and endothelin) have been identified that bind specific G-protein coupled receptors, mediate mitoK$_{ATP}$ channel opening, and elicit IPC cardioprotection. These receptors represent parallel and likely redundant pathways [70]. At least 3 surface receptors, acting in parallel, can trigger preconditioning (PC). This redundancy also appears to extend to the signal transduction pathways, involved with at least two independent parallel pathways, with consequent kinase activation [71–73]. Whether these multiple receptor pathways act in concert or synergistically holds great significance for developing more effective therapeutic approaches, including reduced drug dosages that may avoid side-effect reactions. The binding of specific ligands to their membrane-bound receptors leads to subsequent activation of phospholipase C and production of diacylglycerol, which in turn stimulates the pivotal signal transducer protein kinase C (PKC) as depicted in Figure 5.2. Alternatively, the activation of phosphoinositide-3-kinase (PI3K) and several tyrosine kinases have been implicated as signaling cardioprotective responses, in conjunction with different stimuli [70–73]. Recently, it has been proposed that the sphingolipid signaling pathway can also have a contributory role in IPC-mediated CP [74]. Activation of these kinases can be cardioprotective by altering energy metabolic pathways as well as by directly modulating cell-death mechanisms as discussed in the previous chapter.

## *Activation and translocation of PKC as a pivotal signaling event in IPC and CP*

With IPC, two isoforms of PKC, PKCε, and PKCδ can translocate and become active in mitochondria. Several studies support the view that PKC activation likely precedes mitoK$_{ATP}$ channel opening in the CP pathway [75–76]. Moreover, in ischemia-induced damaged cardiomyocytes and in transgenic mice, PKCε and PKCδ have been shown to have strikingly opposing effects on CP. Specifically, activation of PKCε caused increased CP, whereas activation of PKCδ increased the damage induced by ischemia *in vitro* and *in vivo* [77]. PKCε activation has been implicated in mitoK$_{ATP}$ channel activation [78], and PKCε can also directly form complexes with components of the PT pore [79], although the role of this interaction in either modulating PT pore opening or in conferring CP has not been established.

Activation of ERK and JNK subfamilies of the mitogen-activated protein kinase (MAPK) can play a contributory role in the signal transduction cascade(s) involved in IPC-mediated cardioprotection, with much attention directed to the role of p38 MAPK. While the opening of mitoK$_{ATP}$ channels was shown to activate p38 MAPK [80–81], currently there is controversy concerning its role in IPC, although a downstream role seems plausible [82–83]. Further support for P38 MAPK providing a downstream function in the CP signaling process comes from studies of hypoxic cardiomyocytes demonstrating that mitochondrial ROS generation (at complex I and III) is a necessary prerequisite leading to the downstream activation of P38 MAPK [84–85].

## Reactive oxygen species

That ROS is involved in CP appears unquestionable. Diazoxide-mediated CP results in ROS production and blocking of ROS production with antioxidants blunts CP [86]. Moreover, it has been established that mitochondrial ROS production occurs downstream and as a consequence of mitoK$_{ATP}$ channel opening [87]. A further link between the signaling pathways, ROS generation and mito-chondrial bioenergetic function has been confirmed by the recent discovery that the second messenger, ceramide directly targets complex III activity, which is a pivotal site of mitochondrial ROS generation [88].

ROS generation functions in the CP pathway(s) as a downstream intracellular signal or second messenger which can lead to further protein kinase and G-protein activation, activation of the nuclear poly (ADP-ribose) polymerase (PARP) or direct modulation of the mitoK$_{ATP}$ channel [89–91]. However, the large ROS accumulation that occurs in ischemic cardiomyocytes in response to reperfusion is reduced either by diazoxide or by hypoxic PC [92–93]. Moreover, ROS levels are reduced in preconditioned tissues following index ischemia, at the time of reperfusion, which is considered to be a consequence of PC preventing PT pore opening [94]. These findings have prompted the characterization of ROS as dual-sided with respect to CP, both involved in signaling or triggering of preconditioning and, as a consequence of ischemia/reperfusion damage, mediating ischemic cell death (which cardioprotection can stem). While it is accepted that the initial signaling mechanism of ROS generation lies downstream of mitoK$_{ATP}$ channel opening, further research is necessary to precisely delineate its temporal place within the order of events comprising the cardioprotective pathway, as well as to explain how ROS generation occurs as a consequence of $K_{ATP}$ channel opening [95].


# Cardioprotection: An emerging field

In the relatively new field of CP, a number of conflicting findings have been noted. Data frequently don't translate among different models (or species) used in the experimental studies, which may limit their utility. Also, some of the difficulties encountered are related to the common definition of cellular events using a variety of pharmaceutical reagents (e.g., inhibitors of specific protein kinases, ROS scavengers and mimetics, channel openers and inhibitors, metabolic uncouplers, etc.). Moreover, the signaling protein kinases have multiple isoforms, some with demonstrably opposing effects on CP, as well as markedly different affinities for the inhibitors used [96]. A subset of the pharmacological treatments used (particularly at high dosage) may have compromised "specificity" impacting on more than a single cellular event, thereby complicating the interpretation. Recent findings that both diazoxide and 5-HD have distinctive effects on mitochondria, independent of the mitoK$_{ATP}$ channel targets [97–100], have made the evaluation of upstream and downstream events rather difficult. For example, respiratory complex II (SDH) activity appears to be directly inhibited by some KCOs (e.g., diazoxide) [101], which may complicate the interpretation of experiments utilizing diazoxide to elicit mitoK$_{ATP}$ channel opening (a standard procedure in this field). This finding, however, takes on added significance with the recent discovery that SDH is likely a primary component of the mitoK$_{ATP}$ channel [41]. This is also consistent with the finding that specific SDH inhibitors such as 3-nitropropionic acid (3-NPA) can result in increased $K^+$ transport by the mitoK$_{ATP}$ channel and can mimic the CP provided by ischemic preconditioning [41, 102]. Moreover, $K_{ATP}$ channel blockers, which entirely abolish the cardioprotective effect of diazoxide, also reverse the effect of complex II inhibitors [41].

Another question raised with CP experiments has been the use of anesthesia in some animal models. A number of anesthetics have marked influence on CP, presumably through targeting mitoK$_{ATP}$ channels [103] as well as several mitochondrial metabolic processes, including reduction of mitochondrial complex I activity [104] and mitochondrial membrane potential [105]. Contradictory results have also emerged when comparing studies and findings from isolated mitochondria from cultured cells, organs, or whole animal.

Another confounding variable that may impact CP studies is gender, as suggested by a recent report showing that testosterone can induce cytoprotection by specifically activating the mitoK$_{ATP}$ channel in rat cardiomyocytes [106]. Further studies will be needed to confirm these findings in the *in vivo* heart and to assess their clinical implications.

## *Early and late IPC pathways*

Two distinct pathways of IPC cardioprotection have been demonstrated. Acute protection occurs as a result of a brief period of ischemia applied 1 to 2 hr before a longer ischemic insult. The resulting early CP occurs within a few minutes after the initial stimulus and lasts for 2 to 3 hr and is considered the model of classic preconditioning. A later pathway of delayed preconditioning, often referred to as a second window of protection, appears about 12 to 24 hr after the preconditioning event and lasts several days [107]. The events of delayed preconditioning have generally been recognized as having greater clinical relevance, since the protective phase is longer and appears to be effective against both myocardial infarction and stunning.

While the delayed preconditioning process involves a similar spectrum of stimuli (e.g., adenosine and bradykinin), the involvement of their receptors and transducers (e.g., the mitoK$_{ATP}$ channels and protein kinases), and pathophysiological mediators (e.g., ROS) utilized by the acute IPC pathway, there appears to be a greater complexity in its regulation since a number of effectors of delayed CP need to be synthesized entirely *de novo*, a response involving the coordinated regulation of expression of multiple genes. Previously, it was thought that the acute preconditioning pathway did not involve protein synthesis since blockades at either the transcription or translational levels had no effect on IPC. However, new studies show that actinomycin D-transcriptional inhibition abolished IPC-induced CP with dramatic reductions in the activation of several MAP kinases and subsequent transcription and phosphorylation of specific transcription factors [108]. Unlike the acute protection pathway, the delayed IPC pathway appears to be more dependent on the involvement of NO and its synthase (NOS), heat-shock proteins (e.g.,

HSP27 and HSP72), MnSOD and cytokine induction [109–113] (as shown in Figure 5.3) than the acute protection pathway, although the involvement of NO in concert with the acute protection pathway has been recently reported [87]. The ability of NO to act in concert with ROS signaling (generated in the CP after cell exposure to KCOs and other preconditioning stimuli) may be a critical factor in targeting the mitochondrial respiratory chain and modulating mitoK$_{ATP}$ channels to provide protection against ischemia [114]. This is supported by data showing that (1) inhibitors of NOS abrogate delayed IPC-mediated protection [112]; (2) NO donors can mimic IPC in conferring CP [114] and (3) free radical scavengers can reduce NOS activation, NO generation, and the induction of cardioprotective signaling [107].

As noted with early preconditioning, delayed preconditioning also promotes CP by augmenting cardiomyocyte bioenergetic capacity in response to ischemic and anoxic insult. The modulation of mito-chondrial respiration in response to delayed preconditioning has recently been shown to occur primarily as a consequence of the induction of ETC and ANT transcription, promoted by the ROS-dependent up-regulation of nuclear transcription factors NRF-1 and PGC-1α [115].

The role of mitochondria in both types of IPC and CP therefore appears to be critical. In addition to the contributory roles that the mitoK$_{ATP}$ channels, mitochondrial-generated ROS, and ETC induction play in the events of both types of PC, a mitochondrial-specific antioxidant response has been demonstrated, primarily with respect to the events of delayed preconditioning [110]. The time course of MnSOD induction, a mitochondrial-specific protective response to ROS mediated damage, correlates well with the appearance of ischemic tolerance. The activities of other cellular antioxidants (i.e., catalase and CuSOD) were not similarly affected. That MnSOD induction plays a role in delayed IPC is further supported by findings that treatment with antisense oligonucleotides to MnSOD, immediately after IPC, completely abolished both the IPC cardioprotective effects as well as MnSOD induction [110]. MnSOD induction is likely downstream of both ROS generation and ROS-mediated activation of specific transcription factors (e.g., NF-KB), and the subsequent induction of cytokines (e.g., TNF–α and IL-1β) [74, 116]. It is noteworthy that the myocyte intracellular pathways af-

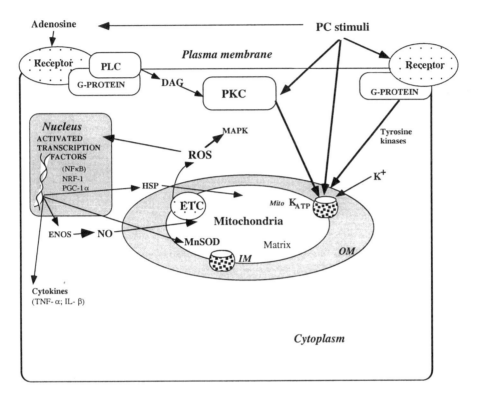

**Figure 5.3. Schematic representation depicting cellular events occurring in delayed ischemic preconditioning.** *The contributions of mitoK$_{ATP}$ channels and the parallel signal transduction pathways utilizing a variety of agonists, G-coupled proteins, and protein kinases are depicted as found with the early preconditioning model. Also, a protein kinase-mediated activation (with ROS involvement) of specific nuclear transcription factors (e.g,. NF-kB, NRF-1, and PGC-1α) is involved, leading to increased gene expression and synthesis of protective proteins, enabling sustained CP. These include mitochondrial MnSOD, ETC and ANT proteins, eNOS, and several stress-activated heat-shock proteins (HSPs) as well as activation of cytokines (including TNF-α and IL-1β). These proteins provide several levels of CP by acting at a variety of cellular sites, including mitochondria.*

fected by TNF-α include the rapid activation of the sphingolipid-ceramide signaling pathway generating endogenous second-messengers ceramide and sphingosine [74].

Thus, in the delayed IPC pathway, the mitochondrial response to relatively short-term metabolic stresses contributes to a dynamic intracellular cross-talk and signaling between multiple cellular compartments, enabling the cardiomyocyte to adopt a stress-tolerant state. Moreover, in addition to IPC, several physical stresses can serve to promote MnSOD-associated delayed cardioprotective induction including, whole body hyperthermia and exercise [110, 116].

## Potential applications to clinical medicine

Understanding the molecular and biochemical mechanism of CP offers great potential in the clinical treatment of myocardial diseases. Given the increasing number of individuals affected with myocardial ischemia, novel therapeutic interventions would appear of interest, even if effective only in a limited number of cases. Nevertheless, in this chapter, we have noted a number of methodological limitations presently associated with a number of the IPC studies. Most researchers are aware of these limitations and are vigorously attempting to circumvent them. Unequivocal data and more refined techniques for the precise evaluation of the molecular events of CP are required prior to treatment with drugs and regimens whose specificity of action and overall metabolic and physiological role (as well as potential benefit) are not absolutely clear. These new data will be instrumental in further understanding the temporal pathway of mitochondrial-mediated CP and will allow the development of new, more effective drugs with increased specificity of action, as well as the acquisition of the critical information needed to know when to apply CP. For instance, the addition of specific cardioprotective agents at the immediate onset of reperfusion has been found to significantly reduce infarct size [117–119]. Exploration of alternative methods to improve mitochondrial cardioprotective responses seems warranted. For example, the finding that PT pore opening during reperfusion can be modulated by either mitochondrial $Ca^{++}$ levels or oxidative stress suggests that regulation of mitochondrial $Ca^{++}$ and/or ROS levels prior to reperfusion might be effective in exerting CP. Moreover, the use of gene therapy in animal models of myocardial ischemia [120–121] has shown promising results with the upregulation of cardioprotective genes (e.g., iNOS and heme oxygenase); human studies are underway. Notwithstanding, further research is needed to understand the role that mitochondria play in the protection against the cell damage that may occur with transient ischemia and reperfusion, such as hypercontracture and swelling finally leading to sarcoplasmic rupture and cell death.

As a corollary, it is important to understand that the IPC events examined so far took place primarily in the healthy heart of experimental animals [122–123]. We need to consider that PC may behave differently and may be less effective in humans with compromised cardiac function secondary to cardiac failure/ cardiomyopathies. While the application of PC in human cardiovascular diseases has been generally limited thus far, there is evidence that CP may be a useful adjunct in the management of cardiovascular diseases. Several clinical studies have shown that the IPC-mediated cardioprotection [124] or the careful use of stress or pharmacological stimuli (e.g., exercise, nitroglycerin and adenosine) can be of benefit in patients who have angina or who are undergoing coronary angioplasty or open heart surgery [124–127]. Moreover, recent clinical trials suggest that chronic administration of the KCO nicorandil improves the cardiovascular prognosis in patients with coronary artery disease [128].

Also, screening of potential PC-mimetic candidates in patients undergoing angioplasty appears feasible, as is the evaluation of PC-based strategies in clinical trials of heart transplant and bypass surgery. However, definitive evidence of their beneficial effects must be established prior to be used in the aged and diseased heart [129].


# References

1. Rouslin W, Millard RW (1981) Mitochondrial inner membrane enzyme defects in porcine myocardial ischemia. Am J Physiol 240:H308–13

2. Rouslin W (1983) Mitochondrial complexes I, II, III, IV and V in myocardial ischemia and autolysis. Am J Physiol 244:H743–8

3. Ylitalo K, Ala-Rami A, Vuorinen K, Peuhkurinen K, Lepojarvi M, Kaukoranta P, Kiviluoma K, Hassinen I (2001) Reversible ischemic inhibition of F(1)F(0)-ATPase in rat and human myocardium. Biochim Biophys Acta 1504:329–39

4. Paradies G, Petrosillo G, Pistolese M, Di Venosa N, Serena D, Ruggiero FM (1999) Lipid peroxidation and alterations to oxidative metabolism in mitochondria isolated from rat heart subjected to ischemia and reperfusion. Free Radic Biol Med 27:42–50

5. Paradies G, Petrosillo G, Pistolese M, Di Venosa N, Federici A, Ruggiero FM (2004) Decrease in mitochondrial complex I activity in ischemic/reperfused rat heart: Involvement of reactive oxygen species and cardiolipin. Circ Res 94:53–9

6. Lesnefsky EJ, Slabe TJ, Stoll MS, Minkler PE, Hoppel CL (2001) Myocardial ischemia selectively depletes cardiolipin in rabbit heart sub-sarcolemmal mitochondria. Am J Physiol Heart Circ Physiol 280:H2770–8

7. Lesnefsky EJ, Tandler B, Ye J, Slabe TJ, Turkaly J, Hoppel CL (1997) Myocardial ischemia decreases oxidative phosphorylation through cytochrome oxidase in subsarcolemmal mitochondria. Am J Physiol 273:H1544–54

8. Lesnefsky EJ, Chen Q, Slabe TJ, Stoll MS, Minkler PE, Hassan MO, Tandler B, Hoppel CL (2004) Ischemia, rather than reperfusion, inhibits respiration through cytochrome oxidase in the isolated, perfused rabbit heart: role of cardiolipin. Am J Physiol Heart Circ Physiol 287:H258–67

9. Lesnefsky EJ, Gudz TI, Migita CT, Ikeda-Saito M, Hassan MO, Turkaly PJ, Hoppel CL (2001) Ischemic injury to mitochondrial electron transport in the aging heart: Damage to the iron-sulfur protein subunit of electron transport complex III. Arch Biochem Biophys 385:117–28

10. Lesnefsky EJ, Moghaddas S, Tandler B, Kerner J, Hoppel CL (2001) Mitochondrial dysfunction in cardiac disease: Ischemia-reperfusion, aging, and heart failure. J Mol Cell Cardiol 33:1065–89

11. Corral-Debrinski M, Stepien G, Shoffner JM, Lott MT, Kanter K, Wallace DC (1991) Hypoxemia is associated with mitochondrial DNA damage and gene induction. Implications for cardiac disease. JAMA 266:1812–6

12. Marin-Garcia J, Goldenthal MJ, Ananthakrishnan R, Mirvis D (1996) Specific mitochondrial DNA deletions in canine myocardial ischemia. Biochem Mol Biol Int 40:1057–65

13. Ventura-Clapier R, Veksler V (1994) Myocardial ischemic contracture: Metabolites affect rigor tension development and stiffness. Circ Res 74:920–9

14. Borutaite V, Mildaziene V, Brown GC, Brand MD (1995) Control and kinetic analysis of ischemia-damaged heart mitochondria: Which parts of the oxidative phosphorylation system are affected by ischemia? Biochim Biophys Acta 1272:154–8

15. Pepe S (2000) Mitochondrial function in ischaemia and reperfu-

sion of ageing heart. Clin Exp Pharmacol Physiol 27:745–50

16. Opie LH, Sack MN (2002) Metabolic plasticity and the promotion of cardiac protection in ischemia and ischemic preconditioning. J Mol Cell Cardiol 34:1077–89

17. Ferrari R, Guardigli G, Mele D, Percoco GF, Ceconi C, Curello S (2004) Oxidative stress during myocardial ischaemia and heart failure. Curr Pharm Des 10:1699–711

18. Rouslin W, MacGee J, Gupte S, Wesselman A, Epps DE (1982) Mitochondrial cholesterol content and membrane properties in porcine myocardial ischemia. Am J Physiol 242:H254–9

19. Venditti P, Masullo P, Di Meo S (2001)Effects of myocardial ischemia and reperfusion on mitochondrial function and susceptibility to oxidative stress. Cell Mol Life Sci 58:1528–37

20. Czerski LW, Szweda PA, Szweda LI (2003) Dissociation of cytochrome c from the inner mitochondrial membrane during cardiac ischemia. J Biol Chem 278:34499–504

21. Crompton M, Costi A, Hayat L (1987) Evidence for the presence of a reversible Ca2+-dependent pore activated by oxidative stress in heart mitochondria. Biochem J 245:915–18

22. Long X, Goldenthal MJ, Wu GM, Marin-Garcia J (2004) Mitochondrial Ca(2+) flux and respiratory enzyme activity decline are early events in cardiomyocyte response to H(2)O(2). J Mol Cell Cardiol 37:63–70

23. Akao M, O'Rourke B, Kusuoka H, Teshima Y, Jones SP, Marban E (2003) Differential actions of cardioprotective agents on the mitochondrial death pathway. Circ Res 92:195–202

24. Szendrei L, Turoczi T, Kovacs P, Vecsernyes M, Das DK, Tosaki A (2002) Mitochondrial gene expression and ventricular fibrillation in ischemic/reperfused nondiabetic and diabetic myocardium. Biochem Pharmacol 63:543–52

25. Ferrari R (1995) The role of mitochondria in ischemic heart disease. J Cardiovasc Pharmacol 1272:154–8

26. Gottlieb RA, Burleson KO, Kloner RA, Babior BM, Engler RL (1994) Reperfusion injury induces apoptosis in rabbit cardiomyocytes. J Clin Invest 94:1621–8

27. Sammut IA, Jayakumar J, Latif N, Rothery S, Severs NJ, Smolenski RT, Bates TE, Yacoub MH (2001) Heat stress contributes to the enhancement of cardiac mitochondrial complex activity. Am J Pathol 158:1821–31

28.  Murry CE, Jennings RB, Reimer KA (1986) Preconditioning with ischemia: A delay of lethal cell injury in ischemic myocardium. Circulation 74:1124–36

29.  O'Rourke B (2000) Myocardial KATP channels in preconditioning. Circ Res 87:845–55

30.  Garlid KD, Paucek P, Yarov-Yarovoy V, Murray HN, Darbenzio R, D'Alonzo AJ, Lodge NJ, Smith MA, Grover GJ (1997) Cardioprotective effect of diazoxide and its interaction with mitochondrial ATP-sensitive K+ channels. Circ Res 81:1072-82

31.  Hanley PJ, Mickel M, Loffler M, Brandt U, Daut J (2002) K(ATP) channel-independent targets of diazoxide and 5-hydroxy-decanoate in the heart. J Physiol 542:735–41

32.  D'hahan N, Moreau C, Prost AL, Jacquet H, Alekseev AE, Terzic A, Vivaudou M (1999) Pharmacological plasticity of cardiac ATP-sensitive potassium channels toward diazoxide revealed by ADP. Proc Natl Acad Sci USA 96:12162–7

33.  Sanada S, Kitakaze M, Asanuma H, Harada K, Ogita H, Node K, Takashima S, Sakata Y, Asakura M, Shinozaki Y, Mori H, Kuzuya T, Hori M (2001) Role of mitochondrial and sarcolemmal K(ATP) channels in ischemic preconditioning of the canine heart. Am J Physiol Heart Circ Physiol 280:H256–63

34.  Xu W, Liu Y, Wang S, McDonald T, Van Eyk JE, Sidor A, O'Rourke B (2002) Cytoprotective role of Ca2+- activated K+ channels in the cardiac inner mitochondrial membrane. Science 298:1029–33

35.  Paucek P, Mironova G, Mahdi F, Beavis AD, Woldegiorgis G, Garlid KD (1992) Reconstitution and partial purification of the glibenclamide-sensitive, ATP-dependent K+ channel from rat liver and beef heart mitochondria. J Biol Chem 267:26062–9

36.  Bajgar R, Seetharaman S, Kowaltowski AJ, Garlid KD, Paucek P (2001) Identification and properties of a novel intracellular (mitochondrial) ATP-sensitive potassium channel in brain. J Biol Chem 276:33369–74

37.  Babenko AP, Gonzalez G, Aguilar-Bryan L, Bryan J (1998) Reconstituted human cardiac KATP channels: Functional identity with the native channels from the sarcolemma of human ventricular cells. Circ Res 83:1132–43

38.  Seharaseyon J, Ohler A, Sasaki N, Fraser H, Sato T, Johns DC, O'Rourke B, Marban E (2000) Molecular composition of mitochon-

drial ATP-sensitive potassium channels probed by viral Kir gene transfer. J Mol Cell Cardiol 32:1923–30

39. Lacza Z, Snipes JA, Kis B, Szabo C, Grover G, Busija DW (2003) Investigation of the subunit composition and the pharmacology of the mitochondrial ATP-dependent K+ channel in the brain. Brain Res 994:27–36

40. Lacza Z, Snipes JA, Miller AW, Szabo C, Grover G, Busija DW (2003) Heart mitochondria contain functional ATP-dependent K+ channels. J Mol Cell Cardiol 35:1339–47

41. Ardehali H, Chen Z, Ko Y, Mejia-Alvarez R, Marban E (2004) Multiprotein complex containing succinate dehydrogenase confers mitochondrial ATP-sensitive K+ channel activity. Proc Natl Acad Sci USA 101:11880–5

42. Korge P, Honda HM, Weiss JN (2002) Protection of cardiac mitochondria by diazoxide and protein kinase C: Implications for ischemic preconditioning. Proc Natl Acad Sci USA 99:3312–7

43. Murata M, Akao M, O'Rourke B, Marban E (2001) Mitochondrial ATP-sensitive potassium channels attenuate matrix Ca (2+) overload during simulated ischemia and reperfusion: Possible mechanism of cardioprotection. Circ Res 89:891–8

44. Katoh H, Nishigaki N, Hayashi H (2002) Diazoxide opens the mitochondrial permeability transition pore and alters Ca2+ transients in rat ventricular myocytes. Circulation 105:2666–71

45. Xu M, Wang Y, Ayub A, Ashraf M (2001) Mitochondrial K (ATP) channel activation reduces anoxic injury by restoring mito-chondrial membrane potential. Am J Physiol Heart Circ Physiol 281:H1295–303

46. Griffiths EJ, Halestrap AP (1995) Mitochondrial non-specific pores remain closed during cardiac ischaemia, but open upon reperfu-sion. Biochem J 307:93–8

47. Crompton M, Costi A (1988) Kinetic evidence for a heart mito-chondrial pore activated by $Ca^{2+}$, inorganic phosphate and oxidative stress. Potential mechanism for mitochondrial dysfunction during cellular $Ca^{2+}$ overload. Eur J Biochem 178:489–501

48. Minners J, van den Bos EJ, Yellon DM, Schwalb H, Opie LH, Sack MN (2000) Dinitrophenol, cyclosporin A, and trimetazidine modulate preconditioning in the isolated rat heart: Support for a mitochondrial role in cardioprotection. Cardiovasc Res 47:68–73

49. Zhao ZQ, Nakamura M, Wang NP, Wilcox JN, Shearer S,Ronson RS, Guyton RA, Vinten-Johansen J (2000) Reperfusion induces myocardial apoptotic cell death. Cardiovasc Res 45:651–60
50. Zhao ZQ, Vinten-Johansen J (2002) Myocardial apoptosis and ischemic preconditioning. Cardiovasc Res 55:438–55
51. Knopp A, Thierfelder S, Doepner B, Benndorf K (2001) Mitochondria are the main ATP source for a cytosolic pool controlling the activity of ATP-sensitive K(+) channels in mouse cardiac myocytes. Cardiovasc Res 52:236–45
52. Trochu JN, Bouhour JB, Kaley G, Hintze TH (2000) Role of endothelium-derived nitric oxide in the regulation of cardiac oxygen metabolism: Implications in health and disease. Circ Res 87:1108–17
53. Miura T, Liu Y, Kita H, Ogawa T, Shimamoto K (2000) Roles of mitochondrial ATP-sensitive K channels and PKC in anti-infarct tolerance afforded by adenosine A1 receptor activation. J Am Coll Cardiol 35:238–45
54. Kobara M, Tasumi T, Matoba S, Yamahara Y, Nakagawa C, Ohta B, Matsumoto T, Inoue D, Asayama J, Nakagawa M (1997) Effect of ischemic preconditioning on mitochondrial oxidative phosphorylation and high energy phosphates in rat hearts. J Mol Cell Cardiol 28:417–28
55. Bosetti F, Yu G, Zucchi R, Ronca-Testoni S, Solaini G (2000) Myocardial ischemic preconditioning and mitochondrial F1F0-ATPase activity. Mol Cell Biochem 215:31–7
56. Ozcan C, Holmuhamedov EL, Jahangir A, Terzic A (2001) Diazoxide protects mitochondria from anoxic injury: implications for myopreservation. J Thorac Cardiovasc Surg 121:298–306
57. Green DW, Murray HN, Sleph PG, Wang FL, Baird AJ, Rogers WL, Grover GJ (1998) Preconditioning in rat hearts is independent of mitochondrial F1F0 ATPase inhibition. Am J Physiol 274:H90–7
58. Asimakis GK, Inners-McBride K, Medellin G, Conti VR (1992) Ischemic preconditioning attenuates acidosis and postischemic dysfunction in isolated rat heart. Am J Physiol 263:H887–94
59. Laclau MN, Boudina S, Thambo JB, Tariosse L, Gouverneur G, Bonoron-Adele S, Saks VA, Garlid KD, Dos Santos P (2001) Cardioprotection by ischemic preconditioning preserves mitochondrial function and functional coupling between adenine nucleotide translocase and creatine kinase. J Mol Cell Cardiol 33:947–56

60. Weiss JN, Korge P, Honda HM, Ping P (2003) Role of the mitochondrial permeability transition in myocardial disease. Circ Res 93: 292–301

61. Baines CP, Zhang J, Wang GW, Zheng YT, Xiu JX, Cardwell EM, Bolli R, Ping P (2002) Mitochondrial PKCepsilon and MAPK form signaling modules in the murine heart: Enhanced mitochondrial PKCepsilon-MAPK interactions and differential MAPK activation in PKCepsilon-induced cardioprotection. Circ Res 90:390–7

62. Da Silva MM, Sartori A, Belisle E, Kowaltowski AJ (2003) Ischemic preconditioning inhibits mitochondrial respiration, increases $H_2O_2$ release and enhances K+ transport. Am J Physiol Heart Circ Physiol 285:H154–62

63. Garlid KD (2000) Opening mitochondrial K(ATP) in the heart: What happens, and what does not happen. Basic Res Cardiol 95:275–9

64. Halestrap AP (1989) The regulation of the matrix volume of mammalian mitochondria *in vivo* and *in vitro* and its role in the control of mitochondrial metabolism. Biochim Biophys Acta 973: 355–82

65. Halestrap AP, Clarke SJ, Javadov SA (2004) Mitochondrial permeability transition pore opening during myocardial reperfusion: A target for cardioprotection. Cardiovasc Res 61:372–85

66. Dos Santos P, Kowaltowski AJ, Laclau MN, Seetharaman S, Paucek P, Boudina S, Thambo JB, Tariosse L, Garlid KD (2002) Mechanisms by which opening the mitochondrial ATP- sensitive K(+) channel protects the ischemic heart. Am J Physiol Heart Circ Physiol 283:H284–95

67. Oldenburg O, Cohen M, Yellon D, Downey J (2002) Mitochondrial K(ATP) channels: Role in cardioprotection. Cardiovasc Res 55:429–37

68. Mubagwa K, Flameng W (2001) Adenosine, adenosine receptors and myocardial protection: An updated overview. Cardiovasc Res 52:25–39

69. Liu GS, Thornton J, Van Winkle DM, Stanley AW, Olsson RA, Downey JM (1991) Protection against infarction afforded by preconditioning is mediated by A1 adenosine receptors in rabbit heart. Circulation 84:350–6

70. Cohen MV, Baines CP, Downey JM (2000) Ischemic preconditioning: From adenosine receptor of KATP channel. Annu Rev Physiol 62:79–109

71.  Murphy E (2004) Primary and secondary signaling pathways in early preconditioning that converge on the mitochondria to produce cardioprotection. Circ Res 94:7–16

72.  Qin Q, Downey JM, Cohen MV (2003) Acetylcholine but not adenosine triggers preconditioning through PI3-kinase and a tyrosine kinase. Am J Physiol Heart Circ Physiol 284:H727–34

73.  Krieg T, Qin Q, McIntosh EC, Cohen MV, Downey JM (2002) ACh and adenosine activate PI3-kinase in rabbit hearts through transactivation of receptor tyrosine kinases. Am J Physiol Heart Circ Physiol 283:H2322–30

74.  Lecour S, Smith RM, Woodward B, Opie LH, Rochette L, Sack MN (2002) Identification of a novel role for sphingolipid signaling in TNF alpha and ischemic preconditioning mediated cardioprotection. J Mol Cell Cardiol 34:509–18

75.  Wang Y, Hirai K, Ashraf M (1999) Activation of mitochondrial ATP-sensitive K(+) channel for cardiac protection against ischemic injury is dependent on protein kinase C activity. Circ Res 85:731–41

76.  Ping P, Song C, Zhang J, Guo Y, Cao X, Li RC, Wu W, Vondriska TM, Pass JM, Tang XL, Pierce WM, Bolli R (2002) Formation of protein kinase C(epsilon)-Lck signaling modules confers cardioprotection. J Clin Invest 109:499–507

77.  Chen L, Hahn H, Wu G, Chen CH, Liron T, Schechtman D, Cavallaro G, Banci L, Guo Y, Bolli R, Dorn GW, Mochly-Rosen D (2001) Opposing cardioprotective actions and parallel hypertrophic effects of delta PKC and epsilon PKC. Proc Natl Acad Sci USA 98:11114–19

78.  Sato T, O'Rourke B, Marban E. (1998) Modulation of mitochondrial ATP-dependent K+ channels by protein kinase C. Circ Res 83:110–4

79.  Baines CP, Song CX, Zheng YT, Wang GW, Zhang J, Wang OL, Guo Y, Bolli R, Cardwell EM, Ping P (2003) Protein kinase Cepsilon interacts with and inhibits the permeability transition pore in cardiac mitochondria. Circ Res 92:873–80

80.  Zhao TC, Hines DS, Kukreja RC (2001) Adenosine-induced late preconditioning in mouse hearts: Role of p38 MAP kinase and mitochondrial K(ATP) channels. Am J Physiol Heart Circ Physiol 280:H1278–85

81.  Fryer RM, Schultz JE, Hsu AK, Gross GJ (1999) Importance of PKC and tyrosine kinase in single or multiple cycles of preconditioning in rat hearts. Am J Physiol Heart Circ Physiol 276:

H1229–35

82. Schulz R, Cohen MV, Behrends M, Downey JM, Heusch G (2001) Signal transduction of ischemic preconditioning. Cardiovasc Res 52:181–98

83. Steenbergen C (2002) The role of p38 mitogen-activated protein kinase in myocardial ischemia/reperfusion injury: Relationship to ischemic preconditioning. Basic Res Cardiol 97:276–85

84. Kulisz A, Chen N, Chandel NS, Shao Z, Schumacker PT (2002) Mitochondrial ROS initiate phosphorylation of p38 MAP kinase during hypoxia in cardiomyocytes. Am J Physiol Lung Cell Mol Physiol 282:L1324–9

85. Das DK, Maulik N, Sato M, Ray PS (1999) Reactive oxygen species function as second messenger during ischemic preconditioning of heart. Mol Cell Biochem 196:59–67

86. Pain T, Yang XM, Critz SD, Yue Y, Nakano A, Liu GS, Heusch G, Cohen MV, Downey JM (2000) Opening of mitochondrial K(ATP) channels triggers the preconditioned state by generating free radicals. Circ Res 87:460–6

87. Lebuffe G, Schumacker PT, Shao ZH, Anderson T, Iwase H, Vanden Hoek TL (2003) ROS and NO trigger early preconditioning: relationship to mitochondrial KATP channel. Am J Physiol Heart Circ Physiol 284:H299–308

88. Gudz T, Tserng K, Hoppel CL (1997) Direct inhibition of mitochondrial respiratory chain complex III by cell-permeable ceramide. J Biol Chem 272:24154–8

89. Krenz M, Oldenburg O, Wimpee H, Cohen MV, Garlid KD, Critz SD, Downey JM, Benoit JN (2002) Opening of ATP-sensitive potassium channels causes generation of free radicals in vascular smooth muscle cells. Basic Res Cardiol 97:365–73

90. Cohen MV, Yang XM, Liu GS, Heusch G, Downey JM (2001) Acetylcholine, bradykinin, opioids, and phenylephrine, but not adenosine, trigger preconditioning by generating free radicals and opening mitochondrial K(ATP) channels. Circ Res 89:273–8

91. Halmosi R, Berente Z, Osz E, Toth K, Literati-Nagy P, Sumegi (2001) Effect of poly(ADP-ribose) polymerase inhibitors on the ischemia-reperfusion-induced oxidative cell damage and mitochondrial metabolism in Langendorff heart perfusion system. Mol Pharmacol 59:1497–505

92. Van den Hoek TL, Becker LB, Shao Z, Li C, Schumacker PT (1998) Reactive oxygen species released from mitochondria during

brief hypoxia induce preconditioning in cardiomyocytes. J Biol Chem 273:18092–8

93. Ozcan C, Bienengraeber M, Dzeja PP, Terzic A (2002) Potassium channel openers protect cardiac mitochondria by attenuating oxidant stress at reoxygenation. Am J Physiol Heart Circ Physiol 282:H531–9

94. Hausenloy DJ, Maddock HL, Baxter GF, Yellon DM (2002) Inhibiting mitochondrial permeability transition pore opening: A new paradigm for myocardial preconditioning? Cardiovasc Res 55:534–43

95. Yue Y, Qin Q, Cohen MV, Downey JM, Critz SD (2002) The relative order of mitoK(ATP) channels, free radicals and p38 MAPK in preconditioning's protective pathway in rat heart. Cardiovasc Res 55:681–9

96. Ping P, Murphy E (2000) Role of p38 mitogen-activated protein kinases in preconditioning: A detrimental factor or a protective kinase? Circ Res 86:921–2

97. Hanley PJ, Gopalan KV, Lareau RA, Srivastava DK, von Meltzer M, Daut J (2003) Beta-oxidation of 5-hydroxydecanoate, a putative blocker of mitochondrial ATP-sensitive potassium channels. J Physiol 547:387–93

98. Lim KH, Javadov SA, Das M, Clarke SJ, Suleiman MS, Halestrap AP (2002) The effects of ischaemic preconditioning, diazoxide and 5-hydroxydecanoate on rat heart mitochondrial volume and respiration. J Physiol 545:961–74

99. Das M, Parker JE, Halestrap AP (2003) Matrix volume measurements challenge the existence of diazoxide/glibencamide-sensitive KATP channels in rat mitochondria. J Physiol 547:893–902

100. Javadov SA, Clarke S, Das M, Griffiths EJ, Lim KH, Halestrap AP (2003) Ischaemic preconditioning inhibits opening of mitochondrial permeability transition pores in the reperfused rat heart. J Physiol 549:513–24.

101. Grimmsmann T, Rustenbeck I (1998) Direct effects of diazoxide on mitochondria in pancreatic B-cells and isolated liver mitochondria. Br J Pharmacol 123:781–8

102. Akao M, O'Rourke B, Kusuoka H, Teshima Y, Jones SP, Marban E (2003) Differential actions of cardioprotective agents on the mitochondrial death pathway. Circ Res 92:195–202

103. Zaugg M, Lucchinetti E, Spahn DR, Pasch T, Garcia C, Schaub MC (2002) Differential effects of anesthetics on mitochondrial K(ATP) channel activity and cardiomyocyte protection. Anesthesiology 97:15–23

104. Hanley PJ, Ray J, Brandt U, Daut J (2002) Halothane, isoflurane and sevoflurane inhibit NADH:ubiquinone oxidoreductase (complex I) of cardiac mitochondria. J Physiol 544:687–93

105. Szewczyk A, Wojtczak (2002) Mitochondria as a pharmacological target. Pharmacol Rev 54:101–27

106. Er F, Michels G, Gassanov N, Rivero F, Hoppe UC (2004) Testosterone induces cytoprotection by activating ATP-sensitive K+ channels in the cardiac mitochondrial inner membrane. Circulation 110:3100–7

107. Bolli R (2000) The late phase of preconditioning. Circ Res 87: 972–83

108. Strohm C, Barancik M, von Bruehl M, Strniskova M, Ullmann C, Zimmermann R, Schaper W (2002) Transcription inhibitor actinomycin-D abolishes the cardioprotective effect of ischemic re-conditioning. Cardiovasc Res 55:602–18

109. Zhao TC, Kukreja RC (2002) Late preconditioning elicited by activation of adenosine A (3) receptor in heart: Role of NF- kB, iNOS and mitochondrial K(ATP) channel. Mol Cell Cardiol 34:263–77

110. Hoshida S, Yamashita N, Otsu K, Hori M (2002) The importance of manganese superoxide dismutase in delayed preconditioning. Involvement of reactive oxygen species and cytokines. Cardiovasc Res 55:495–505

111. Wang Y, Kudo M, Xu M, Ayub A, Ashraf M (2001) Mitochondrial K(ATP) channel as an end effector of cardioprotection during late preconditioning: Triggering role of nitric oxide. Mol Cell Cardiol 33:2037–46

112. Ockaili R, Emani VR, Okubo S, Brown M, Krottapalli K, Kukreja RC (1999) Opening of mitochondrial KATP channel induces early and delayed cardioprotective effect: Role of nitric oxide. Am J Physiol 277:H2425–34

113. Latchman DS (2001) Heat shock proteins and cardiac protection. Cardiovasc Res 51:637–46

114. Rakhit RD, Mojet MH, Marber MS, Duchen MR (2001) Mitochondria as targets for nitric oxide-induced protection during simulated ischemia and reoxygenation in isolated neonatal cardiomyocytes. Circulation 103:2617–23

115. McLeod CJ, Jeyabalan AP, Minners JO, Clevenger R, Hoyt RF Jr, Sack MN (2004) Delayed ischemic preconditioning activates nuclear-encoded electron-transfer-chain gene expression in parallel with enhanced postanoxic mitochondrial respiratory recovery.

Circulation 110:534–9

116. Yamashita N, Hoshida S, Otsu K, Taniguchi N, Kuzuya T, Hori M (2000) The involvement of cytokines in the second window of ischaemic preconditioning. Br J Pharmacol 131:415–22

117. Inagaki K, Chen L, Ikeno F, Lee F, Imahashi K, Bouley D, Rezaee M, Yock P, Murphy E, Mochly-Rosen D (2003) Inhibition of protein kinase C protects against reperfusion injury of the ischemic heart. Circulation 108:2304–7

118. Zhao ZQ, Corvera JS, Halkos ME, Kerendi F, Wang NP, Guyton RA, Vinten-Johansen J (2003) Inhibition of myocardial injury by ischemic postconditioning during reperfusion: comparison with ischemic preconditioning. Am J Physiol 285:H579–88

119. Xu Z, Jiao Z, Cohen MV, Downey JM (2002) Protection from AMP 579 can be added to that from either cariporide or ischemic preconditioning in ischemic rabbit heart. J Cardiovasc Pharmacol 40: 510–8

120. Li Q, Guo Y, Xuan Y-T, Lownestein CJ, Stevenson SC, Prabhu SD, Wu W-J, Zhu Y, Bolli R (2003) Gene therapy with inducible nitric oxide synthase protects against myocardial infarction via a cyclooxygenase-2–dependent mechanism. Circ Res 92:741–8

121. Melo LG, Agrawal R, Zhang L, Rezvani M, Mangi AA, Ehsan A, Griese DP, Dell'Acqua G, Mann MJ, Oyama J, Yet SF, Layne MD, Perrella MA, Dzau VJ (2002) Gene therapy strategy for long-term myocardial protection using adeno-associated virus-mediated delivery of heme oxygenase gene. Circulation 105: 602–7

122. Ferdinandy P, Szilvassy Z, Baxter GF (1998) Adaptation to myocardial stress in disease states: Is preconditioning a healthy heart phenomenon? Trends Pharmacol Sci 19:223–9

123. Ghosh S, Standen NB, Galinianes M (2001) Failure to precondition pathological human myocardium. J Am Coll Cardiol 37:711–8

124. Leesar MA, Stoddard MF, Xuan YT, Tang XL, Bolli R (2003) Nonelectrocardiographic evidence that both ischemic preconditioning and adenosine preconditioning exist in humans. J Am Coll Cardiol 42:437–45

125. Leesar MA, Stoddard MF, Dawn B, Jasti VG, Masden R, Bolli R (2001) Delayed preconditioning-mimetic action of nitroglycerin in patients undergoing coronary angioplasty. Circulation 103:2935–41

126. Crisafulli A, Melis F, Tocco F, Santoboni UM, Lai C, Angioy G, Lorrai L, Pittau G, Concu A, Pagliaro P (2004) Exercise-induced and nitroglycerin-induced myocardial preconditioning improves

hemodynamics in patients with angina. Am J Physiol Heart Circ Physiol 287:H235–42

127. Mikhail P, Verma S, Fedak PW, Weisel RD, Li RK (2003) Does ischemic preconditioning afford clinically relevant cardioprotection? Am J Cardiovasc Drugs 3:1–11

128. Argaud L, Ovize M (2004) How to use the paradigm of ischemic preconditioning to protect the heart? Med Sci (Paris) 20:521-5

129. Kloner R, Speakman M, Przyklenk K (2002) Ischemic preconditioning: a plea for rationally targeted clinical trials. Cardiovasc Res 55:526–33

# Chapter 6

# Mitochondria Dysfunction in Cardiomyopathy and Heart Failure

## Overview

Cardiac failure is an endemic health problem of great magnitude in the Western world. In spite of considerable clinical and research efforts during the last decade and the development of new drugs and surgical modalities of therapy, mortality and morbidity remain high. Clinical cardiologists and basic researchers have shown great interest in mitochondria research, not only in their structure and function but also in the multiple roles that the organelle plays in cell homeostasis and in particular in programmed cell death and necrosis during cardiac failure, myocardial ischemia, and aging. The focus of an increasing number of publications, mitochondria are being intensively examined in the search for answers to outstanding questions in the pathogenesis and pathophysiology of a myriad of cardiovascular diseases and in particular in cardiac failure. This chapter focuses on the progress made in our understanding of the biochemistry and molecular analysis of mitochondria in cardiomyopathy and cardiac failure and on future directions in mitochondrial-directed therapies.

## Introduction

Broadly used, the term *heart failure* (HF) refers to a pathophysiologic state where the heart is unable to meet the metabolic requirements of the body. A chronic disorder, HF is the principal cause of hospitalization in patients over 65 years of age. It has a progressive clinical course resulting in high morbidity and mortality and poses a tremendous burden for the health-care delivery system.

Taking advantage of the remarkable fusion recently achieved by genetics and biochemistry in molecular biology, mitochondrial research is accelerating its application to cardiovascular pathologies. In this chapter, a discussion of how mitochondrial dysfunction may be related to other critical cellular and molecular changes found in cardiac hypertrophy and failure—including dysfunctional structural and cytoskeletal proteins, apoptosis, calcium flux and handling, and signaling pathways—is presented. Moreover, the biochemical and molecular changes occurring in severe HF secondary to primary cardiomyopathy (dilated/hypertrophic) in humans and in animal models of HF secondary to volume or pressure overload are examined. Finally, the available evidence that mitochondrial dysfunction plays a pivotal role in cardiac failure is presented.

## Mitochondria are the major source of bioenergy in the cardiac cell

The heart is highly dependent for its function on oxidative energy generated in mitochondria, primarily by fatty acid β-oxidation, ETC, and OXPHOS (Figure 6.1). Mitochondria are abundant in energy-demanding cardiac tissue constituting over one-third of the cardiomyocyte cellular volume (i.e., a greater proportion than found in skeletal muscle). Energy production in mitochondria depends on genetic factors that modulate normal mitochondrial function, including enzyme activity and cofactor availability and on environmental factors such as the availability of fuels (e.g., sugars, fats, and proteins) and oxygen. In the postnatal and adult heart, fatty acids are the primary energy substrate for heart muscle ATP generation by OXPHOS and the mitochondrial respiratory chain, the most important supply of cardiac energy, whereas the fetal heart derives energy primarily from the oxidation of glucose and lactate supplied by the glycolytic pathway. The phosphotransferase enzymes, creatine kinase, and to a lesser extent adenylate kinase play a pivotal role in the distribution of ATP from its site of synthesis in the mitochondria to spatially distinct sites of ATP utilization within the cytosol [1].

During contraction and relaxation, over 75% of the cardiomyocyte ATP is utilized by actomyosin ATPase and various ion pumps. More-

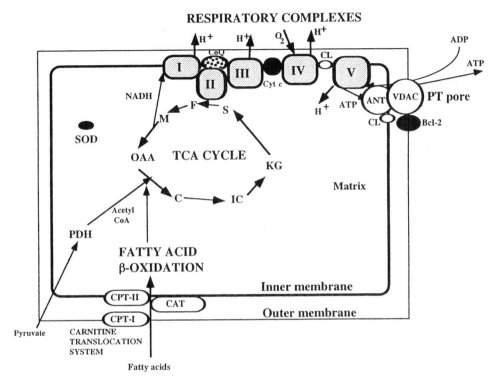

**Figure 6.1. Mitochondrial bioenergetic pathways in heart failure.** *Mitochondri-al inner-membrane localized respiratory complexes I to V with asso-ciated electron-transfer components, CoQ and Cyt c, are depicted as are the matrix-localized NADH and acetyl-CoA-generating fatty acid β-oxidation and TCA cycle pathways. Several inner-membrane transporters (CAT, CPT-I, and CPT-II) for carnitine/fatty acids and the adenine nucleotide transporter (ANT) are shown. Key markers of apoptotic processes are shown, including cyt c, the PT pore with its constituent proteins ANT, VDAC and associated phospholipid cardiolipin (CL), Bcl-2 in the outer membrane, and matrix-localized mitochondrial superoxide dismutase (SOD).*

over, decreased cellular ATP levels (due to mitochondrial dysfunc-tion) can markedly lower the threshold of plasma membrane depolarization [2] and therefore potentially   influence impulse generation and conduction in the myocardium. As the amount of ATP in the heart is relatively small compared to the demand, the cardiomyocyte must continually and rapidly resynthesize ATP to maintain normal contractility, pump function, and cell viability. Cardiac mitochondrial dysfunction leads to reduced ATP generation and causes diminished myocardial contractile function, which can lead to cardiac failure and death.

## What is the evidence for myocardial dependency on mitochondrial function?

### Mitochondrial dysfunction and cardiomyopathy: Support from human studies

Both DCM and HCM are frequently accompanied by changes in one or more of the OXPHOS/ respiratory enzyme activities [3–8]. Disorders of mitochondrial OXPHOS are typically biochemically and clinically heterogenous, often displaying a wide spectrum of clinical presentations, including myopathy and cardiomyopathy.

Significantly reduced activity levels of myocardial respiratory complexes I, III, IV, and V have been reported in patients in which HCM or DCM is the only clinical manifestation, as well as in patients with cardiac involvement in addition to a wide and variable spectrum of primarily neurological presentations associated with mitochondrial disorders (such as MELAS, MERRF, and PEO). While no relationship has been established with either patient age or cardiac phenotype (e.g., HCM or DCM) to the type or extent of respiratory enzyme affected, older patients tend to have an increase in the number of respiratory enzymes involved [9]. Specific gene defects (usually in mtDNA) have been identified in a relatively small number of patients with significant enzyme deficiencies, and these are described below. Recently, a study of terminally failing myocardium from a series of 43 explanted failing hearts demonstrated significantly decreased levels of complex I activity with no detectable mtDNA abnormalities in either structure or level [10].

Specific pathogenic point mutations in mtDNA have been demonstrated in a number of patients with cardiomyopathy, mainly in HCM [11–27]. Most of the pathogenic mtDNA mutations were found in highly conserved nucleotides, frequently present in a heteroplasmic fashion (a mixed population of both mutant and wildtype mtDNA genomes) and accompanied by decreased levels of respiratory enzyme activity(s). Some of the pathogenic mtDNA mutations, identified in association with cardiomyopathy, are in mitochondrial tRNA genes (Table 6.1) with particularly high incidence in tRNAs for Leu, Lys, and Ile. The location of the mutation within the generic tRNA clover-

**Table 6.1. Specific mitochondrial tRNA and rRNA point mutations in cardiomyopathy**

| Gene | Site | Cardiac Phenotype | References |
|------|------|-------------------|------------|
| Leu | 3243 (A→G) | DCM | [19] |
| Leu | 3260 (A→G) | Tachycardia | [17] |
| Leu | 3303 (C→T ) | Fatal infantile CM | [13] |
| Ile | 4300 (A→G) | HCM- adult onset | [18] |
| Ile | 4317 (A→G) | Fatal infantile CM | [11] |
| Ile | 4320 (C→T) | Fatal infantile CM | [14] |
| Ile | 4269 (A→G) | HF at 18 years | [12] |
| Ile | 4295 (A→G) | HCM | [27] |
| Ile | 4284 (G→A) | Fatal CM | [22] |
| Lys | 8334 (A→G) | HCM | [19] |
| Lys | 8363 (G→A) | HCM | [15] |
| Lys | 8348 (A→G) | HCM/DCM | [20] |
| Lys | 8296 (A→G) | Fatal HCM | [21] |
| Gly | 9997 (T→C) | Arrhythmia/HCM | [16] |
| Ala | 5587 (T→C) | DCM | [33] |
| Arg | 10415 (T→C) | DCM | [33] |
| Arg | 10424 (T→C) | Fatal DCM | [34] |
| 16S rRNA | 3093 (C→G | MELAS/CM | [30] |
| 12S rRNA | 1555 (A→G) | CM | [31] |
| Cys | 5814 (A→G) | HCM | [23] |
| Val | 1644 (G→A) | HCM/MELAS | [24] |
| Val | 1624 (C→T) | HCM | [25] |
| Leu | 12297 (T→C) | DCM | [26] |

leaf may relate to the severity of the phenotypic effect and possibly to its tissue specificity [28]. For example, severe cardiomyopathies have been diagnosed in patients harboring mutations in nucleotides at similar positions in their respective tRNAs (e.g., 4269/9997 and 3303/8363).

Mitochondrial protein synthesis and specific respiratory enzyme activities are negatively affected by pathogenic mutations in tRNA genes. Cardiomyopathy-associated mtDNA mutations have also been found in mitochondrial rRNAs [29–30]. Additional mtDNA point mutations have been reported in patients with cardiomyopathy and HF and were not detected in normal individuals. Some reside in other

**Table 6.2. Mitochondrial structural gene mutations in cardiomyopathy**

| Gene | Site | AA change | Cardiac Phenotype | References |
|------|------|-----------|-------------------|------------|
| Cytb | 14927 (A→G) | Thr→Ala | DCM, HCM | [32, 45] |
| Cytb | 15236 (A→G) | Ile→Val | DCM | [45] |
| Cytb | 15508 (C→G) | Asp→Glu | DCM | [34] |
| Cytb | 15509 (A→C) | Asn→His | FPCM | [46] |
| Cytb | 15498 (G→A) | Gly→Asp | HiCM | [47] |
| Cytb | 15243 (G→A) | Gly→Glu | HCM | [48] |
| COII | 7923 (A→G) | Tyr→Cys | DCM | [34] |
| COIII | 9216 (A→G) | Gln→Glu | DCM | [34] |
| COI | 6860 (A→C) | Lys→Asn | DCM | [31] |
| ND1 | 3310 (C→T) | Pro→Ser | HCM | [49] |
| ND5 | 14609 (C→T) | Ser→Leu | DCM | [34] |
| ATPase6 | 8993 (T→G) | Leu→Arg | LS /HCM | [41] |

*Note:* LS = Leigh syndrome; HiCM = Histiocytoid cardiomyopathy; FPCM = Fatal postpartum cardiomyopathy.

tRNA genes, while other mutations occur in mtDNA protein-encoding or structural genetic loci as shown in Table 6.2. These mtDNA mutations are primarily heteroplasmic and reside in highly conserved sequences [31–34]. Recent studies have also implicated specific homoplasmic mutations in mtDNA as a possible if not frequent cause of cardiomyopathy [35–36]. Whether heteroplasmic or homoplasmic, the rigorous assignment of many of these mutations as truly the primary cause of cardiomyopathy remains to be established.

Evidence of the relationship of cardiac cellular damage and mtDNA mutations has been further confirmed from cybrid experiments. Experiments with mutant alleles at nt 3243, 3260, and 9997 show that cells harboring these point mutations have diminished mitochondrial protein synthesis and respiratory enzyme activities [37–39]. Similarly, large-scale deletions in mtDNA have also been shown to adversely effect mitochondrial protein synthesis and respiratory function(s) in cells in which they have been introduced [40]. A limitation of these type of studies (which involve single cells in culture) is that they confirm that there is a relationship between a defect in mtDNA and mitochondrial dysfunction but not necessarily one with the cardiac dysfunction/phenotype.

In addition to mitochondrial cardiomyopathy, many cases of systemic mitochondrial diseases with cardiac involvement have been reported. These disorders tend to have a variable spectrum of neurological manifestations. Some are maternally inherited (due to mtDNA mutation) and may present a variable cardiac phenotype including ventricular hypertrophy, cardiomegaly, and dysrhythmias) [19, 28, 41–42]. Examples include Leigh, MELAS, and MERRF syndromes.

One of the more puzzling aspects in the area of mtDNA pathogenesis relates to the frequent finding that specific mtDNA mutations found in association with primary cardiomyopathy can also be found in patients with different arrays of neurological disorders. For instance, the 8363 mutation has been found in several cases of HCM; however, the same mutation has also been detected in patients and relatives with severe encephalomyopathies, including Leigh syndrome [43], ataxia, or sensorineural deafness with or without the cardiomyopathy [15]. Similarly, a mutation at nt 3423 in tRNA$^{Leu}$ (probably the best characterized and more often mtDNA mutation reported in mitochondrial disorders), which in the past has been associated only with the MELAS phenotype, was recently detected in patients with isolated cardiomyopathy without neuromuscular involvement [44]. A potential explanation for this challenging situation correlating genotypic mutation to phenotypic manifestation, is the involvement of other genetic or environmental cofactors, which may modulate the effect of mtDNA mutations.

In addition to maternally inherited disorders, a number of the mitochondrial abnormalities with associated cardiac manifestations are sporadic (in general, due to somatic large-scale mtDNA deletions), including KSS in which patients may display cardiomyopathy, mitral valve prolapse, and/or cardiac conduction abnormalities. The majority of KSS mtDNA deletions are of a single type, are not inherited, and have been found primarily in skeletal muscle [50]. In contrast, defects in autosomal nuclear loci are thought to be the cause of multiple mtDNA deletion phenotypes. However, the precise genetic defect has not yet been identified [51] and can be either dominantly or recessively inherited [52–53]. The mtDNA deletion events detected in KSS and in autosomal disorders tend to be highly abundant (ranging up to 95% of the total mtDNA) either as discrete single-sized deletions or in the aggregate [32]. Due to their abundance, these deletions are often detected by southern blot analysis. A second type of large-scale mtDNA deletion has been found in cardiac tissue of many primary cardiomyopathies. These mtDNA deletions tend to be less abundant (<0.1%) and are often detectable only by PCR analysis. Their significance in cardiac pathogenesis is not yet clear; they may be evidence of specific mtDNA damage and tend to occur in an age-dependent manner [54–56]. Whether mtDNA deletions are primary to cardiomyopathic disease or whether they represent secondary somatic mutations arising from cardiac dysfunction and resulting metabolic changes (e.g., increased ROS-mediated damage to mtDNA) remains unresolved [32, 54]. Evidence that increased levels of oxidative stress can result in increased levels of myocardial mtDNA deletions, in association with elevated ROS production, has been provided by studies in transgenic mice containing defective ANT1 alleles [57] and in patients with specific ANT1 mutations [58].

As discussed in Chapter 4, increased ROS can promote extensive mtDNA damage, which can lead to defects in mitochondrial encoded gene expression and respiratory chain enzymes and contribute to the progression of HF. In a murine model of myocardial infarct and HF, mtDNA copy number significantly decreased by 44% compared to sham animals [59]. In addition, this study found a parallel decrease in steady-state levels of several mtDNA-encoded transcripts, including subunits of complexes I, III, and IV as well as 12S and 16S rRNAs. Moreover, the enzymatic activity of respiratory complexes I, III, and IV (each containing subunits encoded by mtDNA) were decreased, while the complexes encoded only by nuclear DNA (e.g., citrate synthase and complex II) showed normal activity. These findings suggest that ROS, mtDNA damage, and defective ETC might play an important role in the development and progression of cardiac failure [59]. Transgenic mice with TNF-$\alpha$ overexpression also develop early HF and display markedly reduced cardiac mtDNA repair activity, resulting in extensive mtDNA mutations associated with mitochondrial structural and functional defects [60], suggesting that defects in mitochondrial structure and function contribute to the pathophysiological effects of TNF-$\alpha$ on the heart.

Cardiac mtDNA depletion has also been described in cardiomyopathy. Depletion of cardiac mtDNA levels with concomitant reduction in mitochondrial respiratory activities accompanies DCM in both animal models and patients treated with AZT (or zidovudine), which inhibits the activities of both the HIV-virus reverse transcriptase and mitochondrial DNA polymerase γ [61–62]. Reduced cardiac mtDNA levels have also been reported in patients with severe cardiomyopathy and reduced cardiac respiratory enzyme activities [8, 45, 63]. Moreover, reduced mtDNA levels have been found in the skeletal muscle of patients with cardiomyopathy as well as in patients with myopathy [64]. In one study of neuropathies associated with skeletal muscle mtDNA depletion, a direct relationship of mtTFA levels to mtDNA levels was suggested [65]. However, no evidence of reduced levels in cardiac mtTFA levels was found in cardiomyopathic patients with cardiac mtDNA depletion [63].

## Clinical evidence of nuclear mutations in mitochondrial components

Mutations in a wide spectrum of nuclear genes encoding mitochondrial proteins also can cause cardiomyopathy. For example, mutations in mitochondrial transport proteins (e.g., carnitine-acylcarnitine translocase), which facilitate the passage of critical metabolites across the inner mitochondrial membrane, have been shown to be involved in cardiomyopathy [66]. Friedreich ataxia (FRDA), which often presents with HCM, is caused by mutations in a nuclear-encoded mitochondrial transport protein, frataxin, implicated in mitochondrial iron accumulation and compromised respiratory enzyme activities [67–69]. Mutations in several of the 36 nuclear-encoded subunits of respiratory complex I have been identified as contributory to the onset of Leigh disease with associated cardiomyopathy and to HCM (e.g., NDUFS2) [70–71]. In addition, mutations in nuclear genes encoding factors required for the assembly and functioning of the multiple-subunit respiratory complexes have been implicated in mitochondrial-based diseases such as Leigh syndrome. These include mutations in the $SCO_2$ gene encoding a copper chaperone involved in COX assembly, which can result in fatal infantile HCM with complex IV deficiency [72]. It is noteworthy that the clinical phenotype in patients with SCO2 mutations is distinct from that found with mutations in other COX assembly factors (e.g., SURF1), which typically present without cardiac involvement. Recently, deleterious mutations in COX15, a heme A farnesyltransferase involved in the synthesis of the prosthetic heme A group in COX, were identified in HCM [73].

As is discussed in greater depth in Chapter 7, a number of nuclear gene defects in the mitochondrial fatty acid β-oxidation pathway can lead to cardiomyopathy [74]. Cardiomyopathy results from specific defects in the genes encoding very long-chain acyl-CoA dehydrogenase (VLCAD) [75] and long-chain 3-hydroxylacyl-CoA dehydrogenase (LCAD) [76] and from mutations affecting carnitine metabolism [77]. Potential causes of many of the inherited disorders of FAO and carnitine metabolism include inadequate supply of NADH and energy to the heart, as well as the accumulation and pathophysiological effects of toxic levels of free fatty acids on cardiac function. Moreover, there is evidence that mutations in the tafazzin gene results in reduced mitochondrial phospholipid levels, including cardiolipin leading to Barth syndrome, an X-linked disorder characterized by DCM and frequent presentation of cardiac arrhythmias and heart failure [78–80].

## Contribution of transgenic models to the study of mitochondria in heart dysfunction

There is increasing evidence from mouse transgenic models that disruption of mitochondrial bioenergy at specific loci or pathways can cause cardiomyopathy and HF. Gene ablation in mice (i.e., the generation of null mutations or gene knockouts) targeting a relatively wide spectrum of genes encoding specific mitochondrial proteins results in severe cardiomyopathy. Targeted genes include ANT [81], MnSOD [82], GPx [83], factors involved in fatty acid metabolism (e.g., MTP subunits) [84], mtTFA [85], and frataxin (e.g., the protein responsible for FRDA) [86]. ANT-deficient mice develop progressive HCM while MnSOD deficient mice develop DCM, yet both types of null mutation cause severe cardiac ATP deficiency, which is thought to underlie the resulting cardiac phenotype(s). Another major contribution of the transgenic mouse model has been to further our understanding of the family of transcriptional coactivators and factors (including PPAR-α, PGC-1α, NRF-1, and MEF-2), which coordinately regulate myocardial energy metabolism and of their essential role in the developing embryonic heart, and to delineate the order of biochemical and molecular events in the metabolic and transcriptional cascade governing energy regulation in both the normal and diseased heart [87].

In addition to examining the specific effects on cardiac phenotype by eliminating specific nuclear genes regulating mitochondrial function, tissue-specific knockout mice with mitochondrial cardiomyopathy have been used to identify modifying genes of potential therapeutic value [88]. At present, there is limited information about the impact on myocardium of knocking out nuclear genes involved directly in mitochondrial OXPHOS. A recent report described cardiac dysfunction in mice lacking cytochrome *c* oxidase subunit VIa-H, the heart isoform [89]. In addition, the knockout approach has not yet been accomplished with mtDNA genes due to the formidable technical difficulty involved in direct gene replacement or ablation of a multicopy gene, in the setting of a non-nuclear multicopy organelle (i.e., the mitochondrion), although several promising approaches are discussed in a later chapter.

The use of cardiac-specific overexpression of specific genes has also proved highly informative in furthering our understanding of the role of mitochondria in cardiac dysfunction. This technique involves fusing a regulatory region from a cardiac-specific gene with a candidate gene of interest and introduction into the transgenic mice, which will express the candidate gene specifically in cardiac muscle cells. Overexpression of genes that mediate the expression and control of cardiac energy metabolism (e.g., PGC-1α and PPAR-α) has been shown to lead to severe cardiac dysfunction and marked changes in mitochondrial structure and function [90–92]. Similarly, transgenic mice containing cardiac-specific overexpression of calcineurin exhibited severe cardiac hypertrophy (that progresses to heart failure), marked mitochondrial respiratory dysfunction, and superoxide generation [93].

The development of animal models of mitochondrial-based cardiac dysfunction offers the possibility of direct testing for potential treatments. For example, the demonstration that MnSOD-deficient animals developed ROS toxicity and DCM prompted speculation that effective treatment with antioxidants could ameliorate the cardiac phenotype. Indeed, peritoneal injection of MnSOD-deficient mice with the antioxidant Manganese (III) tetrakis (4-benzoic acid) porphyrin eliminated the cardiac dysfunction and reversed the ROS accumulation [94].

## Evidence from animal models that mitochondrial bioenergetic enzymes play a critical role in HF

Canine pacing-induced cardiomyopathy is a model of HF in which rapid ventricular pacing leads to an increase in chamber dimension, wall thinning, elevation in ventricular wall stress, and congestive HF, mimicking DCM in humans [95–96]. Myocardial tissues from paced dogs had markedly reduced activities of myofibrillar $Ca^{++}$ ATPase, sarcoplasmic reticulum $Ca^{++}$ ATPase, and respiratory complexes III and V [97–98]. On the other hand, paced dogs had significantly higher activities of the fatty acid oxidation enzyme hydroxylacyl-CoA dehydrogenase and the TCA cycle enzyme oxoglutarate dehydrogenase. These data suggest that in pacing-induced HF, there is an impairment of key ATP generating enzymes and down-regulation of ATP-utilizing enzymes with an increase (possibly compensatory) in FAO and TCA cycle activities [98]. The reduction in the levels of myocardial mitochondrial complex V activity was further identified as both an early and a persistent event in the development of HF [97–99]. Similar findings of reduced levels of complex V activity were also reported in a naturally occurring canine model of idiopathic DCM [100].

Several models of mechanically overloaded heart have presented further evidence of defective mitochondrial bioenergetics in HF. In both volume- and pressure-overloaded rat hearts [101], depletion of phosphocreatine occurs with left ventricular hypertrophy. Patients in HF have shown marked reductions in levels of phosphocreatine (similarly decreased in HCM and DCM) [102], and reduced mitochondrial creatine kinase activity and content were also demonstrated in a pressure-overload rat model [103]. In volume-overloaded hearts, alterations in myocardial high-energy phosphates (i.e., significantly lower myocardial creatine phosphate/ATP ratios) have been postulated to contribute to contractile/pump dysfunction occurring during exercise [104]. These mitochondrial abnormalities in function persisted despite adequate tissue oxygenation [105] and suggest that altered regulation of mitochondrial OXPHOS results in reduced phosphocreatine levels present in HF [106]. Modulation of OXPHOS activities could be achieved by differential substrate utilization, changes in ADP, inorganic phosphate, intramitochondrial NADH, and oxygen levels [107]. In recent studies using a porcine model of left ventricular infarction and remodeling (induced by ligation of the left circumflex artery), reduced systolic performance accompanied by reduced levels of high-energy phosphates, myocardial OXPHOS, ANT protein and in the β subunit of complex V were noted [108–109]. These findings suggest that specific mitochondrial inner-membrane proteins may play a critical role during the remodeling that occurs in HF. Nevertheless, the order of the myocardial molecular and biochemical events leading to abnormal regulation of OXPHOS needs to be established.

## Mitochondria dysfunction and other cellular pathways in cardiomyopathy

Numerous molecular and cellular changes leading to HF have been identified [110]. Traditionally, research has centered on abnormalities in the cardiac pump function by examining disturbances in calcium flux/homeostasis and levels of major contractile proteins (e.g., myosin, actin, ATPase, and troponin) [111]. Currently, the research focus has shifted toward hypertrophic growth and myocardium-remodeling stimuli, the elucidation of signal transduction pathways leading to cardiac hypertrophy and failure, the role of apoptosis in heart remodeling, and the extracellular matrix/cytoskeletal changes occurring in HF [112].

A number of the aforementioned cellular/molecular changes observed during HF involve mitochondria and bioenergetic production. However, this complex relationship has not been fully investigated and requires further research. It could be argued that mitochondrial dysfunction plays an integral part in the mechanism(s) of cardiac dysfunction, even when other factors are more evident, or it may represent a common downstream event in the pathways leading to HF. Nevertheless, in most cases of HF, it remains to be established whether the mitochondrial abnormalities associated with other myocardial changes (discussed below) are truly primary or secondary to other abnormalities in myocardium (e.g., hypertrophy and remodeling). In addition, further work is critically needed to measure the extent that mitochondrial abnormalities (either primary or secondary to other myocardial changes) contribute to HF pathophysiology .

## Mutations in contractile/sarcomere proteins and mitochondrial function

Genes encoding important structural and cytoskeletal myocardial proteins (located outside the mitochondria) have frequently been implicated in the pathogenesis of cardiomyopathy. Familial hypertrophic cardiomyopathy (FHCM) often is due to mutations in myofibrillar proteins, which are involved in the generation of force, including β-myosin heavy chain (β-MHC), cardiac troponin T, α-tropomyosin, and myosin-binding protein C [113–116]. The best-characterized mutations reside in β-MHC [113], and a number of these mutations are associated with poor prognosis (including sudden death). Other β-MHC mutations are associated with more moderate cardiac phenotype(s) and only mild hypertrophy.

Genes encoding important structural and cytoskeletal proteins have also recently been implicated in the pathogenesis of other types of cardiomyopathy such as DCM. These proteins (e.g., actin) organize the contractile apparatus of cardiac myocytes and in some cases (e.g., dystrophin and sarcoglycan) anchor the myocytes in their extracellular milieu, allowing the generation of force [112]. Mutations in the cardiac actin gene have been found in patients with familial DCM [117]. Moreover, mutations in the δ-sarcoglycan gene have been identified as the molecular defect responsible for the autosomal recessive cardiomyopathy found in the Syrian hamster [118]. Defects in the gene encoding dystrophin have been identified as causal in the X-linked DCM and HF associated with Duchenne syndrome [119]. Recent studies have also reported that specific point mutations as well as a null allele in the gene for desmin, a major myofibrillar structural protein involved in linking Z bands to the plasma membrane, resulted in both DCM and skeletal myopathy [120]. In mice null for desmin, the muscle-specific member of the intermediate filament gene family, a severe cardiomyopathy develops characterized by extensive cardiomyocyte death, myocardial fibrosis, calcification, and eventual HF with the earliest ultrastructural defects observed in mitochondria [121]. Overexpression of the antiapoptotic protein Bcl-2 in the desmin null heart resulted in the amelioration of the mitochondrial defects, reduced fibrotic myocardial lesions and cardiac hypertrophy, restored cardiomyocyte ultrastructure, and significantly improved cardiac function [122].

The relationship of mitochondrial bioenergetic defects with mutations in nuclear-encoded structural proteins is worthy of note. Patients with specific β-MHC mutations may develop abnormal mitochondrial number and a marked reduction in mitochondrial respiratory function [123–124]. A potential interaction of these nuclear pathogenic mutations with specific mtDNA mutations is also suggested by studies showing coexistence in some patients with HCM of mutations in both β-MHC and mtDNA [125]. In addition, the intracellular distribution of mitochondria can be profoundly altered in patients with defective structural proteins, since both the intracellular position and movement of mitochondria are mediated by cytoskeletal proteins. Defective cellular location of mitochondria, with potential downstream effects on cardiac bioenergetic function, may play a critical role in cardiac pathophysiology.

While structural gene mutations in sarcomeric contractile proteins such as myosin, myosin binding protein, cardiac troponin T and I, and tropomyosin are well recognized in FHCM, their role in cardiac pathogenesis has remained obscure despite intense investigation over the last decade. It has been proposed that cardiac energy depletion or a mismatch between ATP utilization and supply, rather than depressed sarcomeric contraction, may in fact be the underlying cause [126]. This hypothesis stems from the observation that mutations in different sarcomeric proteins leads to inefficient ATP utilization and by the demonstration of mitochondrial respiratory enzymatic dysfunction in patients containing mutations in myosin structural genes known to cause HCM, as well as in transgenic mice with missense cardiac troponin T alleles, and recently, in a transgenic mouse model of HCM with mutant myosin heavy chain alleles [123, 127–128]. In addition, several mutations in the regulatory subunit of AMP-activated protein kinase (AMPK), a key sensor and mediator in cellular energy metabolism, have been found in patients with HCM and ventricular preexcitation (Wolff-Parkinson-White syndrome) [129]. In response to activation following an increase in the AMP/ATP ratio, AMPK phosphorylates a number of downstream targets culminating in the switching off of energy (ATP)-utilizing pathways and the switching on of energy-generating pathways including mitochondrial FAO, essentially functioning as a low-fuel gauge. Although the precise mechanism by which the AMPK mutations promote cardiac disease is still undetermined, a plausible hypothesis is that they aberrantly signal cardiac energy depletion and that normal levels of AMPK serve to protect against cardiac hypertrophy [130]. The realization that mitochondrial energy deficiency may act as an initiating signal for myocardial hypertrophy can prove useful as a unifying framework and may provide further insights into a number of clinical features of HCM, such as its heterogeneity and variable onset.

The wide variability in the clinical phenotype of HCM remains unexplained, and it is likely that there are multiple contributing factors, including mitochondrial dysfunction. In two transgenic models of HCM, mitochondrial function was evaluated in mice with either a mutant myosin heavy chain gene (MyHC) or a mutant cardiac troponin T (R92Q) gene [128]. Despite mitochondrial ultrastructural abnormalities in both models, the rate of state 3 respiration was significantly decreased only in the mutant MyHC mice, and this decrease preceded the cardiac dysfunction. Also, the maximum activity of α-ketoglutarate dehydrogenase as assayed in isolated disrupted mitochondria was decreased compared with isolated control mitochondria. Moreover, respiratory activities of complexes I and IV were decreased in the mutant MyHC transgenic mice. Inhibition of β-adrenergic receptor kinase, which is elevated in mutant MyHC mouse hearts, prevented mitochondrial respiratory impairment. Therefore, mitochondria may contribute to the hemodynamic dysfunction seen in some forms of HCM and may be responsible for some of the heterogeneity of the disease phenotypes.

An informative experimental model used to study the genesis of cardiomyopathy utilizes the Syrian hamster, in which inbred sublines (derived from a common ancestor) feature either HCM or DCM, inherited as an autosomal-recessive trait [118]. As noted above, a common defect in a gene for δ-sarcoglycan (δ-SG) causes cardiomyopathy and has been identified in both HCM and DCM hamsters [131]. The δ-SG mutation results in altered sarcolemmal membrane permeability and integrity with impact on contractility (in both cardiac and skeletal muscle) and disturbed ion homeostasis (including $Ca^{++}$ levels). Mitochondria from cardiomyopathic (CM) hamsters have been shown to have altered levels of TCA cycle enymes and PDH activities (possibly as a function of different $Ca^{++}$ levels), FAO enzymes and creatine kinase. Analysis of mitochondrial respiration found a significant difference between control and CM hamsters in specific subpopulations of myocardial mitochondria. Hoppel and associates [132] reported that sarcolemmal mitochondrial respiration was largely unchanged in CM hamsters compared to controls, while interfibrillar mitochondrial state 3 respiration levels were significantly depressed in the CM hamster myocardium. Moreover, the finding that the same mutation results in HCM (in BIO 14 strains) while resulting in DCM in a second strain (TO strains) has led researchers to propose that other genetic or environmental factors might contribute to the pathogenesis and phenotype of cardiomyopathy. Indeed, a recent study found a heteroplasmic mtDNA mutation in COXIII in BIO 14 hamster strains associated with HCM but not in DCM development [133].

## Mitochondrial function and cardiac hypertrophy

Cardiac hypertrophy has been associated with increased mitochondrial number and size as well as increased mtDNA synthesis [134–136]. Studies of rat cardiac hypertrophy documented a coordination between complex IV activity, nuclear-encoded mRNA, and mitochondrial rRNA synthesis. Within 24 hr after growth stimulus, a specific decrease was found only in mitochondrial mRNA synthesis [136].

A number of studies have reported that thyroid hormone (TH) can affect mitochondrial structure and function since treatment with TH causes myocardial hypertrophy. Models of cardiac hypertrophy show TH-induced increases in total tissue RNA and ventricular weight, as well as in the levels of both cytosolic and mitochondrial ribosomes. TH can also modulate increases in mitochondrial enzyme activities. One way that TH regulates mitochondria is by modulating the transcriptional activation of nuclear genes encoding mitochondrial proteins including components of the respiratory pathway [137]. This regulatory effect occurs as a result of many of the nuclear-encoded mitochondrial genes having TH-sensitive promoter elements [138]. Recent study has also demonstrated that TH treatment *in vivo* caused elevated levels of markers of mitochondrial biogenesis including myocardial mtDNA, specific mtDNA-encoded proteins and transcripts as well as nuclear-encoded regulators including mtTFA and PPAR-α [139]. The majority of the observed TH-induced changes in myocardial mitochondria followed the onset of cardiac hypertrophy by TH.

## Calcium signaling and mitochondrial function in HF

Changes in $Ca^{++}$ transport and metabolism are known to occur in HF. At the molecular level, marked reductions in the levels of phospholamban mRNA and both sarcoplasmic reticulum $Ca^{++}$-ATPase (SERCA) mRNA and enzyme activity, as well as increased levels of sarcolemmal $Na^+$-$Ca^{++}$ exchanger have been reported [140–143]. At the physiological level, there is prolonged action potential and $Ca^{++}$ transient, decreased $Ca^{++}$ uptake and reduced $Ca^{++}$ release by the sarcoplasmic reticulum, and increased diastolic $Ca^{++}$ concentration [143]. However, it is not clear whether these are primary or secondary changes to other events happening in HF.

Mitochondria also exert a significant regulatory role as a sensor of intracellular free $Ca^{++}$. Several mechanisms of enhanced function of OXPHOS by $Ca^{++}$ have been reported, including stimulation of several dehydrogenases in the TCA cycle due to increases in mitochondrial matrix $Ca^{++}$ [144–145], and activation by $Ca^{++}$ of mitochondrial ATP synthase activity [146–147]. Acute HF generated by manipulating calcium concentrations in perfused canine hearts was accompanied by a striking decrease in mitochondrial respiratory function [148]. Of significance, the methodologies for investigating mitochondrial pool sizes and fluxes of $Ca^{++}$ using fluorescent dyes have been markedly improved and should be evaluated relative to mitochondrial respiratory activities.

## Mitochondrial function and apoptosis in HF

Apoptotic processes have been shown to be crucial in the cardiac remodeling, which accompanies or precedes HF. Myocardial apoptosis has been documented in patients with end-stage DCM [149–150], as is discussed in Chapter 4, but there are several critical issues that remain to be elucidated, including identification of the molecular triggers for cardiac apoptosis, the precise quantification of apoptotic cells, and the timing of apoptosis onset and completion. The overall role of apoptosis in HF (while highly attractive as a theoretical construct) is not yet known.

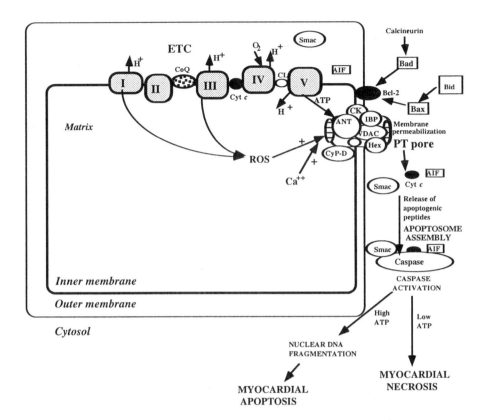

**Figure 6.2. Pathway of apoptosis.** *Cellular signals, including ROS, trigger the apoptotic pathway regulated by binding of proapoptogenic proteins to mitochondrial membranes (e.g., Bax, Bid, and Bad), leading to mitochondrial membrane permeabilization and PT pore opening. Elevated levels of mitochondrial calcium as well as ETC-generated ROS as shown also promote PT pore opening. This is followed by the release of cytochrome c (Cyt c), Smac, and apoptosis-inducing factor (AIF) from the mitochondrial intermembrane space to the cytosol, apoptosome formation leading to caspase and endonuclease activation and apoptotic cell death. Association of Bax with mitochondria is prevented by antiapoptogenic proteins (e.g., Bcl-2). The major proteins comprising the PT pore— including hexokinase (Hex), adenine nucleotide translocator (ANT), creatine kinase (CK), cyclophilin D (CyP-D), porin (VDAC), the benzodiazepine receptor (IBP), and the inner-membrane phospholipid cardiolipin (CL)—are also shown.*

Data from *in vitro* systems and animal models experiments suggest that myocardial apoptosis occurs in response to a variety of insults including ischemia-reperfusion, myocardial infarction, pacing, mechanical stretch and pressure overload (Figure 6.2). Factors present in the failing myocardium that may cause or be involved with apoptosis, include catecholamines, angiotensin, inflammatory cytokines, ROS,

NO, hypoxia, mechanical stress, and peptide growth factors (e.g., TGF and cardiotrophin). A subset of these factors also mediates hypertrophy of cardiac myocytes *in vitro*. As previously discussed, many of the major apoptotic proteins are located in mitochondria and may impact on mitochondrial function and signaling (which is discussed in depth in Chapter 10). The contribution of mitochondria to caspase activation in myocardial apoptosis, including the recent identification of several procaspases within the mitochondrial inter-membrane space, is under investigation [151]. There is also some evidence that myocardial apoptosis in response to specific stimuli may depend on the energy content of the myocyte [152].

Recent studies have examined the release of cytochrome *c* from mitochondria to the cytosol as a key hallmark and critical signaling event of apoptosis. Cytochrome *c* release from mitochondria has been reported in the failing human heart and cardiomyopathy [153]. However, to the best of our knowledge, the investigation of OXPHOS activities during HF-associated apoptosis has been inexplicably limited. Moreover, the role of the oncogenic protein Bcl-2 in human/rat cardiac apoptosis studies has been arguably equivocal, although it is a well-established and well-characterized marker of apoptosis in cell culture models. Recently, in mice that express a proofreading-deficient mitochondrial DNA polymerase in the heart, it was demonstrated that increased levels of mtDNA mutations activate the mitochondrial apoptotic pathway and cause severe DCM [154].

ROS has been implicated in apoptosis induction, as is discussed at length in Chapter 4, and evidence has been presented that the generation of free $O_2^{\bullet-}$ radicals comes largely from hypoxic mitochondria and from respiratory dysfunction. The mitochondrial apoptotic pathway is activated in cardiac myocytes in response to a variety of physiological stimuli, including oxidative stress and hypoxia as well as serum and glucose deprivation [155–157]. In addition, the mitochondrial-located MnSOD, which has a pivotal role in regulating the accumulation of mitochondrial generated ROS, can be recruited during CP to limit myocardial apoptosis [158].

## What events occurring in HF are truly tissue-specific?

Patients suffering from HF often exhibit early muscular fatigue and exercise intolerance. The finding of shared events in skeletal muscle and heart during HF has considerable prognostic implication for the clinician. Yet to date, despite considerable research efforts in this area, the relationship between cardiac and skeletal muscle events in HF at the cellular and molecular levels remains unclear. In this section, a brief overview of molecular and cellular changes occurring in cardiac and skeletal muscle is presented, focusing on the mitochondrial bioenergetic events in both tissues.

A number of changes occur in skeletal muscle during HF, including histological and electromyographic evidence of generalized myopathy and exercise intolerance. Evaluation of skeletal muscle metabolism by the noninvasive methodology of phosphorus nuclear magnetic resonance spectroscopy has demonstrated abnormal levels of phosphocreatine and inorganic phosphate in patients with HF following moderate exercise [159–160]. Also, patients with desmin and β-MHC mutations known to cause HCM and HF have defined changes in skeletal muscle fibers. Patients with specific β-MHC mutations may develop abnormal mitochondrial number and function in skeletal muscle as well as type I fiber abnormalities and atrophy [161]. Congestive HF is often accompanied by skeletal myopathy with a shift from slow aerobic fatigue-resistant fibers to fast anaerobic ones. Is the fiber atrophy mediated by apoptosis?. Evidence of apoptosis as gauged by TUNEL and by significantly reduced expression of Bcl-2 has been demonstrated in both skeletal muscle of both patients with chronic HF [162] and in rats with experimentally induced HF [163]. Evidence of increased iNOS was also noted in the patients with HF.

Structural and functional changes in skeletal muscle mitochondria have also been found in cardiomyopathy/HF [164–165]. Specific pathogenic mtDNA mutations (e.g., 3243, 3260, 4269, 8344, 8363, and 9997) and accompanying respiratory enzyme defects present in cardiomyopathy with a broad spectrum of myopathies are present at relatively high levels in skeletal muscle mtDNA. Moreover, the use of skeletal muscle biopsies (instead of endomyocardial biopsy) for the analysis of respiratory enzyme dysfunction has been recommended in the diagnostic evaluation of mitochondrial-mediated cardiac abnormalities [166]. Reductions in specific enzyme activities were found in both skeletal and cardiac muscle in a group of children with cardiomyopathy [166]. Similarly, pronounced complex IV defects were shown in both cardiac and skeletal muscle of patients with KSS and cardiomyopathy [167].

While an increasing incidence of cardiac mtDNA deletions has been reported in patients with DCM, scarce data are available regarding either the tissue specificity or correlation of the extent of cardiac mtDNA deletions with skeletal muscle deletions in the same patient. In isolated cases of KSS with cardiomyopathy, both skeletal muscle and heart were shown to harbor high levels of mtDNA deletions [168]. Also, multiple mtDNA deletions and mtDNA depletion have been detected in skeletal muscle of patients with cardiomyopathy [169]. The forementioned effects of AZT on mtDNA levels, respiratory complex activities, and bioenergetic phenotype were found in both heart and skeletal muscle from human and animal models.

Many of the cardiac cellular changes as well as the mitochondrial abnormalities often revealed during HF appear to be present in skeletal muscle. There is evidence that alterations in energy metabolism including decreased mitochondrial ATP production as well as altered transfer of energy through the phosphotransfer kinases occur in both cardiac and skeletal muscles and suggest a generalized metabolic myopathy in HF [170]. While more evidence confirming these findings is warranted, evaluation of skeletal muscle mitochondrial function can be informative in the overall diagnostic and prognostic evaluation of patients with HF. Determining what other parts of the HF signaling-pathway are truly cardiac specific and which might be also operative in skeletal muscle awaits further studies. Such studies might shed light about the relationship between the signaling pathways and mitochondrial energetics.

## Future prospects

The use of transgenic mice with defined mutations to study their impact and relationship to HF has been very informative. However, at present there still remains a gap in information about the physiological, biochemical, and molecular events in normal mouse heart. What is needed is a rigorous standardization of quantitative measurements relevant to mitochondrial bioenergetics, structure, and function in both cardiac and skeletal muscle. This should include an evaluation of the levels of mitochondrial enzyme activities, mtDNA, ATP, ADP, and NADH, as well as a comprehensive investigation of mitochondrial changes (including mtDNA deletions) as a function of age. Particular focus should be directed to the activity levels and content of complex V, mt-CK, and ANT, given the degree to which they appear affected in HF. Such information should provide the requisite database to investigate and compare the direct effects of introducing mutant genes in animal model (e.g., mouse) to test for pathogenic mutations that effect both mitochondria and cardiac function. Further refinement will also be needed to overcome the aforementioned technical hurdle that presently exists in introducing and testing specific mtDNA mutations and their pathogenic effects in a whole-animal model as well as more precise monitoring of cellular and molecular events in the myocardium in a less invasive manner than endomyocardial biopsy.

The need for new treatments for HF is obvious, and currently a number of new drugs are under development, including modulators of myocardial remodeling. Future strategies will also include antiapoptotic drugs and gene therapy. Undoubtedly, mitochondria have a particular aureole that is attracting cardiologists and students at large, and this interest will continue for a long time to come. Further research may bring, in the near future, a full understanding of the temporal order of changes in mitochondrial structure and function, as well as the organelle contribution to the pathophysiological events occurring in HF. These advances will facilitate a rational use of mitochondrial-targeted therapies.

# References

1. Kaasik A, Veksler V, Boehm E, Novotova M, Minajeva A, Ventura-Clapier R (2001) Energetic crosstalk between organelles: Architectural integration of energy production and utilization. Circ Res 89:153–9

2. James AM, Sheard PW, Wei YH, Murphy MP (1999) Decreased ATP synthesis is phenotypically expressed during increased energy demand in fibroblasts containing mitochondrial tRNA mutations. Eur J Biochem 259:462–9

3. Marín-García J, Goldenthal MJ, Pierpont ME, Ananthakrishnan R (1995) Impaired mitochondrial function in idiopathic dilated cardiomyopathy: Biochemical and molecular analysis. J Cardiac Fail 1:285–92

4. Marín-García J, Goldenthal MJ, Ananthakrishnan R, Pierpont ME, Fricker FJ, Lipshultz SE, Perez-Atayde A (1996) Mitochondrial

function in children with idiopathic dilated cardiomyopathy. J Inher Metab Dis 19:309–12

5.  Rustin P, Lebidois J, Chretien D, Bourgeron T, Piechaud JF, Rotig A, Munnich A, Sidi D (1994) Endomyocardial biopsies for early detection of mitochondrial disorders in hypertrophic cardiomyopathies. J Pediatr 124:224–8

6.  Buchwald A, Till H, Unterberg C, Oberschmidt R, Figulla HR,Wiegand V (1990) Alterations of the mitochondrial respiratory chain in human dilated cardiomyopathy. Eur Heart J 11:509–16

7.  Zeviani M, Mariotti C, Antozzi C, Fratta GM, Rustin P, Prelle A (1995) OXPHOS defects and mitochondrial DNA mutations in cardiomyopathy. Muscle Nerve 3:S170–4

8.  Marín-García J, Ananthakrishnan R, Goldenthal MJ, Filiano JJ, Perez-Atayde A (1997) Cardiac mitochondrial dysfunction and DNA depletion in children with hypertrophic cardiomyopathy. J Inherit Metab Dis 20:674–80

9.  Marín-García J, Goldenthal MJ, Pierpont EM, Ananthakrishnan R, Perez-Atayde A (1999) Is age a contributory factor of mitochondrial bioenergetic decline and DNA defects in idiopathic dilated cardiomyopathy? Cardiovasc Pathol 8:217–22

10.  Scheubel RJ, Tostlebe M, Simm A, Rohrbach S, Prondzinsky R, Gellerich FN, Silber RE, Holtz J (2002) Dysfunction of mitochondrial respiratory chain complex I in human failing myocardium is not due to disturbed mitochondrial gene expression. J Am Coll Cardiol 40: 2174–81

11.  Tanaka M, Ino H, Ohno K, Hattori K, Sato W, Ozawa T, Tanaka T, Itoyama S (1990) Mitochondrial mutation in fatal infantile cardiomyopathy. Lancet 336:1452

12.  Taniike M, Fukushima H, Yanagihara I, Tsukamoto H, Tanaka J, Fujimura H, Nagai T, Sano T, Yamaoka K, Inui K (1992) Mitochondrial tRNAIle mutation in fatal cardiomyopathy. Biochem Biophys Res Commun 186:47–53

13.  Silvestri G, Santorelli FM, Shanske S, Whitley CB, Schimmenti LA, Smith SA, DiMauro S (1994) A new mtDNA mutation in the tRNALEU(UUR) gene associated with maternally inherited cardiomyopathy. Hum Mutat 3:37–43

14.  Santorelli FM, Mak SC, Vazquez-Acevedo M, Gonzalez-Astiazaran A, Ridaura-Sanz C, Gonzalez-Halphen D, DiMauro S (1995) A novel mtDNA point mutation associated with mitochondrial encephalocardiomyopathy. Biochem Biophys Res Commun 216: 835–40

15.  Santorelli FM, Mak SC, El-Schahawi M, Casali C, Shanske S, Baram TZ, Madrid RE, DiMauro S (1996) Maternally inherited cardiomyopathy and hearing loss associated with a novel mutation in mitochondrial tRNALys gene (G8363). Am J Hum Genet 58:933–9

16.  Merante F, Tein I, Benson L, Robinson BH (1994) Maternally inherited cardiomyopathy due to a novel T-to-C transition at nt 9997 in the mitochondrial tRNAGly gene. Am J Hum Genet 55:437–46

17.  Zeviani M, Gellera C, Antozzi C, Rimoldi M, Morandi L, Villani F, Tiranti V, DiDonato S (1991) Maternally inherited myopathy and cardiomyopathy: Association with mutation in mitochondrial DNA tRNALeu. Lancet 338:143–47

18.  Casali C, Santorelli FM, D'Amati G, Bernucci P, DeBiase L, DiMauro S (1995) A novel mtDNA point mutation in maternally inherited cardiomyopathy. Biochem Biophys Res Commun 213: 588–93

19.  Anan R, Nakagawa M, Miyata M, Higuchi I, Nakao S, Suehara M, Osame M, Tanaka H (1995) Cardiac involvement in mitochondrial diseases: A study of 17 patients with mitochondrial DNA defects. Circulation 91:955–61

20.  Terasaki F, Tanaka M, Kawamura K, Kanzaki Y, Okabe M, Hayashi T, Shimomura H, Ito T, Suwa M, Gong JS, Zhang J, Kitaura Y (2001) A case of cardiomyopathy showing progression from the hypertrophic to the dilated form: Association of Mt8348A→G mutation in the mitochondrial tRNA(Lys) gene with severe ultra-structural alterations of mitochondria in cardiomyocytes. Jpn Circ J 65:691–4

21.  Akita Y, Koga Y, Iwanaga R, Wada N, Tsubone J, Fukuda S, Nakamura Y, Kato H (2000) Fatal hypertrophic cardiomyopathy associated with an A8296G mutation in the mitochondrial tRNA(Lys) gene. Hum Mutat 15:382

22.  Corona P, Lamantea E, Greco M, Carrara F, Agostino A, Guidetti D, Dotti MT, Mariotti C, Zeviani M  (2002) Novel heteroplasmic mtDNA mutation in a family with heterogeneous clinical presentations. Ann Neurol 51:118–22

23.  Karadimas C, Tanji K, Geremek M, Chronopoulou P, Vu T, Krishna S, Sue CM, Shanske S, Bonilla E, DiMauro S, Lipson M, Bachman R (2001) A5814G mutation in mtDNA can cause mitochondrial myopathy and cardiomyopathy. J Child Neurol 16:531–3

24.  Menotti F, Brega A, Diegoli M, Grasso M, Modena MG, Arbustini E (2004) A novel mtDNA point mutation in tRNA(Val) is

associated with hypertrophic cardiomyopathy and MELAS. Ital Heart J 5:460–5

25. McFarland R, Clark KM, Morris AA, Taylor RW, Macphail S, Lightowlers RN, Turnbull DM (2002) Multiple neonatal deaths due to a homoplasmic mitochondrial DNA mutation. Nat Genet 30:145–6

26. Grasso M, Diegoli M, Brega A, Campana C, Tavazzi L, Arbustini E (2001) The mitochondrial DNA mutation T12297C affects a highly conserved nucleotide of tRNA(Leu(CUN)) and is associated with dilated cardiomyopathy. Eur J Hum Genet 9:311–5

27. Merante F, Myint T, Tein I, Benson L, Robinson BH (1996) An additional mitochondrial tRNA(Ile) point mutation (A-to-G at nucleotide 4295) causing hypertrophic cardiomyopathy. Hum Mutat 8:216–22

28. Schon EA, Bonilla E, DiMauro S (1997) Mitochondrial DNA mutations and pathogenesis. J Bioenerg Biomembr 29:131–49

29. Santorelli FM, Tanji K, Manta P, Casali C, Krishna S, Hays AP, Mancini DM, DiMauro S, Hirano M (1999) Maternally inherited cardiomyopathy: An atypical presentation of the mtDNA 12S rRNA gene A1555G mutation. Am J Hum Genet 64:295–300

30. Hsieh RH, Li JY, Pang CY, Wei YH (2001) A novel mutation in the mitochondrial 16S rRNA gene in a patient with MELAS syndrome, diabetes mellitus, hyperthyroidism and cardiomyopathy. J Biomed Sci 8:328–35

31. Li YY, Maisch B, Rose ML, Hengstenberg C (1997) Point mutations in mitochondrial DNA of patients with dilated cardiomyopathy. J Mol Cell Cardiol 29:2699–709

32. Ozawa T, Katsumata K, Hayakawa M, Tanaka M, Sugiyama S, Tanaka T, Itoyama S, Nunoda S, Sekiguchi M (1995) Genotype and phenotype of severe mitochondrial cardiomyopathy: A recipient of heart transplantation and the genetic control. Biochem Biophys Res Commun 207:613–9

33. Arbustini E, Diegoli M, Fasani R, Grasso M, Morbini P, Banchieri N, Bellini O, Dal Bello B, Pilotto A, Magrini G, Campana C, Fortina P, Gavazzi A, Narula J, Vigano M (1998) Mitochondrial DNA mutations and mitochondrial abnormalities in dilated cardiomyopathy. Am J Pathol 153:1501–10

34. Marín-García J, Goldenthal MJ, Ananthakrishnan R, Pierpont ME (2000) The complete sequence of mtDNA genes in idiopathic dilated cardiomyopathy shows novel missense and tRNA mutations. J Card Fail 6:321–9

35.  Taylor RW, Giordano C, Davidson MM, d'Amati G, Bain H, Hayes CM, Leonard H, Barron MJ, Casali C, Santorelli FM, Hirano M, Lightowlers RN, DiMauro S, Turnbull DM (2003) A homoplasmic mitochondrial transfer ribonucleic acid mutation as a cause of maternally inherited hypertrophic cardiomyopathy. J Am Coll Cardiol 41:1786–96
36.  Carelli V, Giordano C, d'Amati G (2003) Pathogenic expression of homoplasmic mtDNA mutations needs a complex nuclear mitochondrial interaction. Trends Genet 19:257–62
37.  Chomyn A, Meola G, Bresolin N, Lai ST, Scarlato G, Attardi G (1991) *In vitro* genetic transfer of protein synthesis and respiration defects to mitochondrial DNA-less cells with myopathy patient mitochondria. Mol Cell Biol 11:2236–44
38.  Mariotti C, Tiranti V, Carrara F, Dallapiccola B, DiDonato S, Zeviani M (1994) Defective respiratory capacity and mitochondrial protein synthesis in transformant cybrids harboring the tRNA (Leu(UUR) mutation associated with maternally inherited myopathy and cardiomyopathy. J Clin Invest 93:1102–7
39.  Raha S, Merante F, Shoubridge E, Myint AT, Tein I, Benson L, Johns T, Robinson BH (1999) Repopulation of rho0 cells with mitochondria from a patient with a mitochondrial DNA point mutation in tRNA^GLY results in respiratory chain dysfunction. Hum Mutat 13:245–54
40.  Hayashi JI, Ohta S, Kikuchi A, Takemitsu M, Goto YI, Nonaka I (1991) Introduction of disease-related mitochondrial DNA deletions into HeLa cells lacking mitochondrial DNA results in mitochondria dysfunction. Proc Natl Acad Sci USA 88:10614–8
41.  Pastores GM, Santorelli FM, Shanske S, Gelb BD, Fyfe B, Wolfe D, Willner JP (1994) Leigh syndrome and hypertrophic cardiomyopathy in an infant with a mitochondrial point mutation (T8993G). Am J Med Genet 50:265–71
42.  Shoffner JM, Wallace DC (1992) Heart disease and mitochondrial DNA mutations. Heart Dis Stroke 1:235–41
43.  Marín-García J, Goldenthal MJ (2000) Mitochondrial biogenesis defects and neuromuscular disorders. Pediatr Neurol 22:122–9
44.  Silvestri G, Bertini E, Servidei S, Rana M, Zachara E, Ricci E, Tonali P (1997) Maternally inherited cardiomyopathy: A new phenotype associated with the A to G at nt 3243 in mitochondrial DNA. Muscle Nerve 20:221–5

45. Marín-García J, Ananthakrishnan R, Goldenthal MJ, Pierpont ME (2000) Biochemical and molecular basis for mitochondrial cardiomyopathy in neonates and children. J Inherit Metab Dis 23:625–33

46. Marín-García J, Ananthakrishnan R, Gonzalvo A, Goldenthal MJ (1995) Novel mutations in mitochondrial cytochrome b in fatal post partum cardiomyopathy. J Inherit Metab Dis 18:77–8

47. Andreu AL, Checcarelli N, Iwata S, Shanske S, DiMauro S (2000) A missense mutation in the mitochondrial cytochrome b gene in a revisited case with histiocytoid cardiomyopathy. Pediatr Res 48: 311–4

48. Valnot I, Kassis J, Chretien D, de Lonlay P, Parfait B, Munnich A, Kachaner J, Rustin P, Rotig A (1999) A mitochondrial cytochrome b mutation but no mutations of nuclearly encoded subunits in ubiquinol cytochrome c reductase (complex III) deficiency. Hum Genet 104:460–6

49. Hattori Y, Nakajima K, Eizawa T, Ehara T, Koyama M, Hirai T, Fukuda Y, Kinoshita M (2003) Heteroplasmic mitochondrial DNA 3310 mutation in NADH dehydrogenase subunit 1 associated with type 2 diabetes, hypertrophic cardiomyopathy, and mental retardation in a single patient. Diabetes Care 26:952–3

50. Zeviani M, Moraes CT, DiMauro S, Nakase H, Bonilla E, Schon EA, Rowland LP (1988) Deletions of mitochondrial DNA in Kearns-Sayre syndrome. Neurology 38:1339–46

51. Suomalainen A, Kaukonen J, Amati P, Timonen R, Haltia M, Weissenbach J, Zeviani M, Somer H, Peltonen L (1995) An autosomal locus predisposing to deletions of mitochondrial DNA. Nat Genet 9:146–51

52. Bohlega S, Tanji K, Santorelli FM, Hirano M, al-Jishi A, DiMauro S (1996) Multiple mitochondrial DNA deletions associated with auto-somal recessive ophthalmoplegia and severe cardiomyopathy. Neurology 46:1329–34

53. Suomalainen A, Paetau A, Leinonen H, Majander A, Peltonen L, Somer H (1992) Inherited idiopathic dilated cardiomyopathy with multiple deletions of mitochondrial DNA. Lancet 340:1319–20

54. Marín-García J, Goldenthal MJ, Ananthakrishnan R, Pierpont M, Fricker FJ, Lipshultz SE, Perez-Atayde A (1996) Specific mitochondrial DNA deletions in idiopathic dilated cardiomyopathy. Cardiovasc Res 31:306–14

55. Li YY, Hengstenberg C, Maisch B (1995) Whole  mitochondrial

genome amplification reveals basal level multiple deletions in mt-DNA of patients with dilated cardiomyopathy. Biochem Biophys Res Commun 210:211–8

56. Corral-Debrinski M, Stepien G, Shoffner JM, Lott MT, Kanter K, Wallace DC (1991) Hypoxemia is associated with mitochondrial DNA damage and gene induction: Implications for cardiac disease. J Am Med Assoc 266:1812–6

57. Esposito LA, Melov S, Panov A, Cottrell BA, Wallace DC (1999) Mitochondrial disease in mouse results in increased oxidative stress. Proc Natl Acad Sci USA 96:4820–5

58. Kaukonen J, Juselius JK, Tiranti V, Kyttala A, Zeviani M, Comi GP, Keranen S, Peltonen L, Suomalainen A (2000) Role of adenine nucleotide translocator 1 in mtDNA maintenance. Science 289:782–5

59. Tomomi I, Hiroyuki T, Shunji H, Dongchon K, Nobuhiro S, Kei-ichiro N, Hideo U, Naotaka H, Akira T (2001) Mitochondrial DNA damage and dysfunction associated with oxidative stress in failing hearts after myocardial infarction. Circ Res 88:529–35

60. Li YY, Chen D, Watkins SC, Feldman AM (2001) Mitochondrial abnormalities in tumor necrosis factor-alpha-induced heart failure are associated with impaired DNA repair activity. Circulation 104:2492–7

61. Lewis W, Dalakas MC (1995) Mitochondrial toxicity of antiviral drugs. Nat Med 1:417–22

62. Herskowitz A, Willoughby SB, Baughman KL, Schulman SP, Bartlett JD (1992) Cardiomyopathy associated with antiretroviral therapy in patients with HIV infection: A report of 6 cases. Ann Intern Med 116:311–3

63. Marín-García J, Ananthakrishnan R, Goldenthal MJ (1998) Hypertrophic cardiomyopathy with mitochondrial DNA depletion and respiratory enzyme defects. Pediatr Cardiol 19:266–8

64. Poulton J, Sewry C, Potter CG, Bougeron T, Chretien D, Wijburg FA, Morten KJ, Brown G (1995) Variation in mitochondrial DNA levels in muscle from normal controls: Is depletion of mtDNA in patients with mitochondrial myopathy a distinct clinical syndrome? J Inher Metab Dis 18:4–20

65. Poulton J, Morten K, Freeman-Emmerson C, Potter C, Sewry C, Dubowitz V, Kidd H, Stephenson J, Whitehouse W, Hansen FJ (1994) Deficiency of the human mitochondrial transcription factor h-mtTFA in infantile mitochondrial myopathy is associated with mtDNA depletion. Hum Mol Genet 3:1763–9

66.  Huizing M, Iacobazzi V, Ijlst L, Savelkoul P, Ruitenbeek W, van den Heuvel L, Indiveri C, Smeitink J, Trijbels F, Wanders R, Palmieri F (1997) Cloning of the human carnitine-acylcarnitine carrier cDNA and identification of the molecular defect in a patient. Am J Hum Genet 61:1239–45

67.  Babcock M, de Silva D, Oaks R, Davis-Kaplan S, Jiralerspong S, Montermini L, Pandolfo M, Kaplan J (1997) Regulation of mitochondrial iron accumulation by Yfh1p, a putative homolog of frataxin. Science 276:1709–12

68.  Campuzano V, Montermini L, Molto MD, Pianese L, Cossee M, Cavalcanti F, Monros E, Rodius F, Duclos F, Monticelli A (1996) Friedreich's ataxia: Autosomal recessive disease caused by an intronic GAA triplet repeat expansion. Science 271:1423–7

69.  Lodi R, Rajagopalan B, Blamire AM, Cooper JM, Davies CH, Bradley JL, Styles P, Schapira AH (2001) Cardiac energetics are abnormal in Friedreich ataxia patients in the absence of cardiac dysfunction and hypertrophy: An *in vivo* 31P magnetic resonance spectroscopy study. Cardiovasc Res 52:111–9

70.  Benit P, Beugnot R, Chretien D, Giurgea I, De Lonlay-Debeney P, Issartel JP, Corral-Debrinski M, Kerscher S, Rustin P, Rotig A, Munnich A (2003) Mutant NDUFV2 subunit of mitochondrial complex I causes early onset hypertrophic cardiomyopathy and encephalopathy. Hum Mutat 21:582–6

71.  Loeffen J, Elpeleg O, Smeitink J, Smeets R, Stockler-Ipsiroglu S, Mandel H, Sengers R, Trijbels F, van den Heuvel L (2001) Mutations in the complex I NDUFS2 gene of patients with cardiomyopathy and encephalomyopathy. Ann Neurol 49:195–201

72.  Papadopoulou LC, Sue CM, Davidson MM, Tanji K, Nishino I, Sadlock JE, Krishna S, Walker W, Selby J, Glerum DM, Coster RV, Lyon G, Scalais E, Lebel R, Kaplan P, Shanske S, De Vivo DC, Bonilla E, Hirano M, DiMauro S, Schon EA (1999) Fatal infantile cardioencephalomyopathy with COX deficiency and mutations in $SCO_2$, a COX assembly gene. Nat Genet 23:333–7

73.  Antonicka H, Leary SC, Guercin GH, Agar JN, Horvath R, Kennaway NG, Harding CO, Jaksch M, Shoubridge EA (2003) Mutations in COX10 result in a defect in mitochondrial heme A biosynthesis and account for multiple, early-onset clinical phenotypes associated with isolated COX deficiency. Hum Mol Genet 12:2693–702

74.  Kelly DP, Strauss AW (1994) Inherited cardiomyopathies. N Engl J Med 330:913–9

75. Strauss AW, Powell CK, Hale DE, Anderson MM, Ahuja A, Brackett JC, Sims HF. (1995) Molecular basis of human mitochondrial very-long-chain acyl CoA dehydrogenase deficiency causing cardiomyopathy and sudden death in childhood. Proc Natl Acad Sci USA 92:10496–500

76. Rocchiccioli F, Wanders RJ, Aubourg P, Vianey-Liaud C, Ijlst L, Fabre M, Cartier N, Bougneres PF (1990) Deficiency of long-chain 3-hydroxylacyl CoA dehydrogenase: A cause of lethal myopathy and cardiomyopathy in early childhood. Pediatr Res 28:657–62

77. Taroni F, Verderio E, Fiorucci S, Cavadini P, Finocchiaro G, Uziel G, Lamantea E, Gellera C, DiDonato S (1992) Molecular characterization of inherited carnitine palmitoyltransferase II deficiency. Proc Natl Acad Sci USA 89:8429–33

78. D'Adamo P, Fassone L, Gedeon A, Janssen EA, Bione S, Bolhuis PA, Barth PG, Wilson M, Haan E, Orstavik KH, Patton MA, Green AJ, Zammarchi E, Donati MA, Toniolo D (1997) The X-linked gene G4.5 is responsible for different infantile dilated cardiomyopathies. Am J Hum Genet 61:862–67

79. Schlame M, Kelley RI, Feigenbaum A, Towbin JA, Heerdt PM, Schieble T, Wanders RJ, DiMauro S, Blanck TJ (2003) Phospholipid abnormalities in children with Barth syndrome. J Am Coll Cardiol 42: 1994–9

80. Vreken P, Valianpour F, Nijtmans LG, Grivell LA, Plecko B, Wanders RJ, Barth PG (2000) Defective remodeling of cardiolipin and phosphatidylglycerol in Barth syndrome. Biochem Biophys Res Commun 279:378–82

81. Graham BH, Waymire KG, Cottrell B, Trounce IA, MacGregor GR, Wallace DC (1997) A mouse model for mitochondrial myopathy and cardiomyopathy resulting from a deficiency in heart/muscle isoform of the adenine nucleotide translocator. Nat Genet 16:226–34

82. Li Y, Huang TT, Carlson EJ, Melov S, Ursell PC, Olson JL, Noble LJ, Yoshimura MP, Berger C, Chan PH (1995) Dilated cardiomyopathy and neonatal lethality in mutant mice lacking manganese superoxide dismutase. Nat Genet 11:376–81

83. Wallace DC (2002) Animal models for mitochondrial disease. Methods Mol Biol 197:3–54

84. Ibdah JA, Paul H, Zhao Y, B nford S, Salleng K, Cline M, Matern D, Bennett MJ, Rinaldo P, Strauss AW (2001) Lack of mitochondrial trifunctional protein in mice causes neonatal hypoglycemia and sudden death. J Clin Invest 107:1403–9

85. Wang J, Wilhelmsson H, Graff C, Li H, Oldfors A, Rustin P, Bruning JC, Kahn CR, Clayton DA, Barsh GS, Thoren P, Larsson NG (1999) Dilated cardiomyopathy and atrioventricular conduction blocks induced by heart-specific inactivation of mitochondrial gene expression. Nat Genet 21:133–7

86. Puccio H, Simon D, Cossee M, Criqui-Filipe P, Tiziano F, Melki J, Hindelang C, Matyas R, Rustin P, Koenig M (2001) Mouse models for Friedreich ataxia exhibit cardiomyopathy, sensory nerve defect and Fe-S enzyme deficiency followed by intramitochondrial iron deposits. Nat Genet 27:181–6

87. Ingwall JS (2004) Transgenesis and cardiac energetics: new insights into cardiac metabolism. J Mol Cell Cardiol 37:613–23

88. Li H, Wilhelmsson H, Hanson A, Thoren P, Duffy J, Rustin P, Larsson N (2000) Genetic modification of survival in tissue-specific knockout mice with mitochondrial cardiomyopathy. Proc Natl Acad Sci USA 97:3467–72

89. Radford NB, Wan B, Richman A, Szczepaniak LS, Li JL, Li K, Pfeiffer K, Schagger H, Garry DJ, Moreadith RW (2002) Cardiac dysfunction in mice lacking cytochrome-c oxidase subunit VIaH. Am J Physiol Heart Circ Physiol 282:H726–33

90. Finck BN, Lehman JJ, Leone TC, Welch MJ, Bennett MJ, Kovacs A, Han X, Gross RW, Kozak R, Lopaschuk GD, Kelly DP (2002) The cardiac phenotype induced by PPARalpha overexpression mimics that caused by diabetes mellitus. J Clin Invest 109:121–30

91. Lehman JJ, Barger PM, Kovacs A, Saffitz JE, Medeiros DM, Kelly DP (2000) Peroxisome proliferator-activated receptor gamma coactivator-1 promotes cardiac mitochondrial biogenesis. J Clin Invest 106:847–56

92. Li YY, Chen D, Watkins SC, Feldman AM (2001) Mitochondrial abnormalities in tumor necrosis factor-alpha-induced heart failure are associated with impaired DNA repair activity. Circulation 104:2492–7

93. Sayen MR, Gustafsson AB, Sussman MA, Molkentin JD, Gottlieb RA (2003) Calcineurin transgenic mice have mitochondrial dysfunction and elevated superoxide production. Am J Physiol Cell Physiol 284:C562–70

94. Melov S, Schneider JA, Day BJ, Hinerfeld D, Coskun P, Mirra SS, Crapo JD, Wallace DC (1998) A novel neurological phenotype in mice lacking mitochondrial manganese superoxide dismutase. Nat Genet 18:159–63

95. Kajstura J, Zhang X, Liu Y, Szoke E, Cheng W, Olivetti G, Hintze TH, Anversa P (1995) The cellular basis of pacing-induced dilated cardiomyopathy: Myocyte cell loss and myocyte cellular reactive hypertrophy. Circulation 92:2306–17

96. Moe GW, Armstrong P (1999) Pacing-induced heart failure: a model to study the mechanism of disease progression and novel therapy in heart failure. Cardiovasc Res 42:591–9

97. O'Brien PJ, Moe GW, Nowack LM, Grima EA, Armstrong PW (1994) Sarcoplasmic reticulum Ca-release channel and ATP-synthesis activities are early myocardial markers of heart failure produced by rapid ventricular pacing in dogs. Can J Physiol Pharmacol 72: 999–1006

98. O'Brien PJ, Ianuzzo CD, Moe GW, Stopps TP, Armstrong PW (1990) Rapid ventricular pacing of dogs to heart failure: Biochemical and physiological studies. Can J Physiol Pharmacol 68:34–39

99. Marín-García J, Goldenthal MJ, Moe GW (2001) Abnormal cardiac and skeletal muscle mitochondrial function in pacing-induced cardiac failure. Cardiovasc Res 52:103–10

100. McCutcheon LJ, Cory CR, Nowack L, Shen H, Mirsalami M,Lahucky R, Kovac L, O'Grady M, Horne R, O'Brien PJ (1992) Respiratory chain defect of myocardial mitochondria in idiopathic dilated cardiomyopathy of Doberman pinscher dogs. Can J Physiol Pharmacol 70:1529–33

101. Kapelko VI, Kupriyanov VV, Novikova NA, Lakomkin VL, Steinschneider AYa, Severina MYu, Veksler VI, Saks VA (1988) The cardiac contractile failure induced by chronic creatine and phosphocreatine deficiency. J Mol Cell Cardiol 20:465–79

102. Kalsi KK, Smolenski RT, Pritchard RD, Khaghani A, Seymour AM, Yacoub MH (1999) Energetics and function of the human heart with dilated or hypertrophic cardiomyopathy. Eur J Clin Invest 29:469–77

103. De Sousa E, Veksler V, Minajeva A, Kaasik A, Mateo P, Mayoux E, Hoerter J, Bigard X, Serrurier B, Ventura-Clapier R (1999) Subcellular creatine kinase alterations: Implications in heart failure. Circ Res 85:68–76

104. Zhang J, Toher C, Erhard M, Zhang Y, Ugurbil K, Bache RJ, Lange T, Homans DC (1997) Relationship between myocardial bioenergetic and left ventricular function in hearts with volume-overload hypertrophy. Circulation 96:334–43

105. Janati-Idrissi R, Besson B, Laplace M, Bui MH (1995) In situ mitochondrial function in volume-overload and pressure-overload induced cardiac hypertrophy in rats. Basic Res Cardiol 90:305–13

106. Bache RJ, Zhang J, Murakami Y, Zhang Y, Cho YK, Merkle H, Gong G, From AH, Ugurbil K (1999) Myocardial oxygenation at high workstates in hearts with left ventricular hypertrophy. Cardiovasc Res 42:616–26

107. Balaban RS (1990) Regulation of oxidative phosphorylation in the mammalian cell. Am J Physiol 258:C377–89

108. Zhang J, Wilke N, Wang Y, Zhang Y, Wang C, Eijgelshoven MH, Cho YK, Murakami Y, Ugurbil K, Bache RJ, From AH (1996) Functional and bioenergetic consequences of postinfarction left ventricular remodelling in a new porcine model. Circulation 94:1089–100

109. Ning XH, Zhang J, Liu J, Ye Y, Chen SH, From AH, Bache RJ, Portman MA (2000) Signalling and expression for mitochondrial membrane proteins during left ventricular remodeling and contractile failure after myocardial infarction. J Am Coll Cardiol 36:282–7

110. Colucci WS (1997) Molecular and cellular mechanisms of myocardial failure. Am J Cardiol 80:15L–25L

111. Mittman C, Eschenhagen T, Scholz H (1998) Cellular and mole-molecular aspects of contractile dysfunction in heart failure. Cardiovasc Res 39:267–75

112. Hunter JJ, Chien KR (1999) Signalling pathways for cardiac hypertrophy and failure. N Engl J Med 341:1276–83

113. Anan R, Greve G, Thierfelder L, Watkins H, McKenna WJ, Solomon S, Vecchio C, Shono H, Nakao S, Tanaka H (1994) Prognostic implications of novel beta cardiac myosin heavy chain gene mutations that cause familial hypertrophic cardiomyopathy. J Clin Invest 93:280–5

114. Watkins H, McKenna WJ, Thierfelder L, Suk HJ, Anan R, O'Donoghue A, Spirito P, Matsumori A, Moravec CS, Seidman JG (1995) Mutations in the genes for cardiac troponin T and alpha-tropomyosin in hypertrophic cardiomyopathy. N Engl J Med 332:1058–64

115. Thierfelder L, Watkins H, MacRae C, Lamas R, McKenna W, Vosberg HP, Seidman JG, Seidman CE (1994) Alpha-tropomyosin and cardiac troponin T mutations cause familial hypertrophic cardiomyopathy: a disease of the sarcomere. Cell 77:701-12

116. Yu B, French JA, Carrier L, Jeremy RW, McTaggart DR, Nicholson MR, Hambly B, Semsarian C, Richmond DR, Schwartz K,

Trent RJ (1998) Molecular pathology of familial hypertrophic cardiomyopathy caused by mutations in the cardiac myosin binding protein C gene. J Med Genet 35:205–10

117. Olson TM, Michels VV, Thibodeau SN, Tai YS, Keating MT (1998) Actin mutations in dilated cardiomyopathy, a heritable form of heart failure. Science 280:750–2

118. Nigro V, Okazaki Y, Belsito A, Piluso G, Matsuda Y, Politano L, Nigro G, Ventura C, Abbondanza C, Molinari AM, Acampora D, Nishimura M, Hayashizaki Y, Puca GA (1997) Identification of the Syrian hamster cardiomyopathy gene. Hum Mol Genet 6:601–7

119. Towbin JA, Hejtmancik JF, Brink P, Gelb B, Zhu XM, Chamberlain JS, McCabe ER, Swift M (1993) An X-linked cardiomyopathy: Molecular genetic evidence of linkage to Duchenne muscular dystrophy gene at the Xp21. Circulation 87:1854–65

120. Dalakas MC, Park KY, Semino-Mora C, Lee HS, Sivakumar K, Goldfarb LG (2000) Desmin myopathy, a skeletal myopathy with cardiomyopathy caused by mutations in the desmin gene. N Engl J Med 342:770–80

121. Wang X, Osinska H, Gerdes AM, Robbins J (2002) Desmin filaments and cardiac disease: Establishing causality. J Card Fail 8: S287–92

122. Weisleder N, Taffet GE, Capetanaki Y (2004) Bcl-2 overexpression corrects mitochondrial defects and ameliorates inherited desmin null cardiomyopathy. Proc Natl Acad Sci USA 101:769–74

123. Fananapazir L, Dalakas MC, Cyran F, Cohn G, Epstein ND (1993) Missense mutations in the beta-myosin heavy-chain gene cause central core disease in hypertrophic cardiomyopathy. Proc Natl Acad Sci USA 90:3993–7

124. Thompson CH, Kemp GJ, Taylor DJ, Conway M, Rajagopalan B, O'Donoghue A, Styles P, McKenna WJ, Radda GK (1997) Abnormal skeletal muscle bioenergetics in familial hypertrophic cardiomyopathy. Heart 78:177–81

125. Arbustini E, Fasani R, Morbini P, Diegoli M, Grasso M, Dal Bello B, Marangoni E, Banfi P, Banchieri N, Bellini O, Comi G, Narula J, Campana C, Gavazzi A, Danesino C, Vigano M (1998) Coexistence of mitochondrial DNA and beta myosin heavy chain mutations in hypertrophic cardiomyopathy with late congestive heart failure. Heart 80:548–58

126. Ashrafian H, Redwood C, Blair E, Watkins H (2003) Hypertrophic cardiomyopathy: A paradigm for myocardial energy depletion. Trends Genet 19:263–8

127. Tardiff JC, Hewett TE, Palmer BM, Olsson C, Factor SM, Moore RL, Robbins J, Leinwand LA (1999) Cardiac troponin T mutations result in allele-specific phenotypes in a mouse model for hypertrophic cardiomyopathy. J Clin Invest 104:469–81

128. Lucas DT, Aryal P, Szweda LI, Koch WJ, Leinwand LA (2003) Alterations in mitochondrial function in a mouse model of hypertrophic cardiomyopathy. Am J Physiol Heart Circ Physiol 284:H575–83

129. Blair E, Redwood C, Ashrafian H, Oliveira M, Broxholme J, Kerr B, Salmon A, Ostman-Smith I, Watkins H (2001) Mutations in the gamma (2) subunit of AMP-activated protein kinase cause familial hypertrophic cardiomyopathy: Evidence for the central role of energy compromise in disease pathogenesis. Hum Mol Genet 10:1215–20

130. Carling D (2004) The AMP-activated protein kinase cascade: A unifying system for energy control. Trends Biochem Sci 29:18–24

131. Sakamoto A, Ono K, Abe M, Jasmin G, Eki T, Murakami Y, Masaki T, Toyo-oka T, Hanaoka F (1997) Both hypertrophic and dilated cardiomyopathies are caused by mutation of the same gene, delta-sarcoglycan, in hamster: An animal model of disrupted dystrophin-associated glycoprotein complex. Proc Natl Acad Sci USA 94:13873–8

132. Hoppel CL, Tandler B, Parland W, Turkaly JS, Albers LD (1982) Hamster cardiomyopathy: A defect in oxidative phosphorylation in the cardiac interfibrillar mitochondria. J Biol Chem 257:1540–8

133. Minieri M, Zingarelli M, Shubeita H, Vecchini A, Binaglia L, Carotenuto F, Fantini C, Fiaccavento R, Masuelli L, Coletti A, Simonelli L, Modesti A, Di Nardo P (2003) Related Identification of a new missense mutation in mtDNA of hereditary hypertrophic, but not dilated cardiomyopathic hamsters. Mol Cell Biochem 252:73–81

134. Szabo J, Nosztray K, Takacs I, Szegi J (1979) Thyroxin-induced cardiomegaly: Assessment of nucleic acid, protein content and myosin ATPase of rat heart. Acta Physiol Acad Sci Hung 54:69–79

135. Zak R, Rabinowitz M, Rajamanickam C, Merten S, Kwiatkowska-Patzer B (1980) Mitochondrial proliferation in cardiac hypertrophy. Basic Res Cardiol 75:171–8

136. Wiesner RJ, Aschenbrenner V, Ruegg JC, Zak R (1994) Coordi-

nation of nuclear and mitochondrial gene expression during the development of cardiac hypertrophy in rats. Am J Physiol 267:C229–35

137. Tanaka T, Morita H, Koide H, Kawamura K, Takatsu T (1985) Biochemical and morphological study of cardiac hypertrophy. Effect of thyroxin on enzyme activities in the rat myocardium. Basic Res Cardiol 80:165–74

138. Nelson BD, Luciakova K, Li R, Betina S (1995) The role of thyroid hormone and promoter diversity in the regulation of nuclear encoded mitochondrial proteins. Biochim Biophys Acta 1271:85–91

139. Goldenthal MJ, Weiss H, Marín-García J (2004) Bioenergetic remodeling of heart mitochondria by thyroid hormone. Mol Cell Biochem 265:97–106

140. Studer R, Reinecke H, Bilger J (1994) Gene expression of the cardiac $Na^+$-$Ca^{++}$ exchanger in end stage human heart failure. Circ Res 75:443–53

141. Takahashi T, Allen PD, Lacro RV, Marks AR, Dennis AR, Schoen FJ, Grossman W, Marsh JD, Izumo S (1992) Expression of dihydropyridine receptor (Ca2+ channel) and calsequestrin genes in the myocardium of patients with end-stage heart failure. J Clin Invest 90:927–35

142. Takahashi T, Allen P, Izumo S (1992) Expression of A-, B-, and C-type natriuretic peptide genes in failing and developing human ventricles. Correlation with expression of the Ca2+-ATPase gene. Circ Res 71:9–17

143. Linck B, Boknik P, Eschenhagen T, Muller FU, Neumann J, Nose M, Jones LR, Schmitz W, Scholz H. (1996) Messenger RNA expression and immunological quantification of phospholamban and SR-Ca ATPase in failing and nonfailing human heart. Cardiovasc Res 31:625–32

144. Gibbs C (1999) Respiratory control in normal and hypertrophic hearts. Cardiovasc Res 42:567-70

145. McCormack JG, Halestrap AP, Denton RM (1990) Role of calcium ions in regulation of mammalian intramitochondrial metabolism. Physiol Rev 70:391–425

146. Harris DA, Das AM (1991) Control of mitochondrial ATP synthesis in heart. Biochem J 280:561–73

147. Territo PR, Mootha VK, French SA, Balaban RS (2000) Ca2+ activation of heart mitochondrial phosphorylation: Role of the $F_0$/$F_1$-ATPase. Am J Physiol Cell Physiol 278:C423–35

148. Takaki M, Zhao DD, Zhao LY, Araki J, Mori M, Suga H (1995) Suppression of myocardial mitochondrial respiratory function in acute failing hearts made by a short term Ca2+ free, high Ca2+ coronary perfusion. J Mol Cell Cardiol 27:2009–13

149. Narula J, Haider N, Virmani R, DiSalvo TG, Kolodgie FD, Hajjar RJ, Schmidt U, Semigran MJ, Dec GW, Khaw BA (1996) Apoptosis in myocytes in end-stage heart failure. N Engl J Med 335: 1182–89

150. Olivetti G, Abbi R, Quaini F, Kajstura J, Cheng W, Nitahara JA, Quaini E, Di Loreto C, Beltrami CA, Krajewski S, Reed JC, Anversa P (1997) Apoptosis in the failing heart. N Engl J Med 336:1131–41

151. Regula KM, Ens K, Kirshenbaum LA (2003) Mitochondria-assisted cell suicide: A license to kill. J Mol Cell Cardiol 35:559–67

152. Czerski L, Nunez G (2004) Apoptosome formation and caspase activation: Is it different in the heart? J Mol Cell Cardiol 37:643–52

153. Narula J, Pandey P, Arbustini E, Haider N, Narula N, Kolodgie FD, Dal Bello B, Semigran MJ, Bielsa-Masdeu A, Dec GW, Israels S, Ballester M, Virmani R, Saxena S, Kharbanda S (1999) Apoptosis in heart failure: Release of cytochrome c from mitochondria and activation of caspase-3 in human cardiomyopathy. Proc Natl Acad Sci USA 96:8144–9

154. Zhang D, Mott JL, Farrar P, Ryerse JS, Chang SW, Stevens M, Denniger G, Zassenhaus HP (2003) Mitochondrial DNA mutations activate the mitochondrial apoptotic pathway and cause dilated cardiomyopathy. Cardiovasc Res 57:147–57

155. Bialik S, Cryns VL, Drincic A, Miyata S, Wollowick AL, Srinivasan A, Kitsis RN (1999) The mitochondrial apoptotic pathway is activated by serum and glucose deprivation in cardiac myocytes. Circ Res 85:403–14

156. Malhotra R, Brosius FC (1999) Glucose uptake and glycolysis reduce hypoxia-induced apoptosis in cultured neonatal rat cardiac myocytes. J Biol Chem 274:12567–75

157. Kang PM, Haunstetter A, Aoki H, Usheva A, Izumo S (2000) Morphological and molecular characterization of adult cardiomyocyte apoptosis during hypoxia and reoxygenation. Circ Res 87:118–25

158. Suzuki K, Murtuza B, Sammut IA, Latif N, Jayakumar J, Smolenski RT, Kaneda Y, Sawa Y, Matsuda H, Yacoub MH (2002) Heat shock protein 72 enhances manganese superoxide dismutase activity during myocardial ischemia-reperfusion injury, associated with mitochondrial protection and apoptosis reduction. Circulation 106:I270–6

159. Wiener DH, Fink LI, Maris J, Jones RA, Chance B, Wilson JR (1986) Abnormal skeletal muscle bioenergetics during exercise in patients with heart failure: role of reduced blood flow. Circulation 73: 1127–36

160. Duboc D, Jehenson P, Tamby JF, Payen JF, Syrota A, Guerin F (1991) Abnormalities of the skeletal muscle in hypertrophic cardiomyopathy: Spectroscopy using phosphorus-31 nuclear magnetic resonance. Arch Mal Coeur Vaiss 84:185–8

161. Caforio AL, Rossi B, Risaliti R, Siciliano G, Marchetti A, Angelini C, Crea F, Mariani M, Muratorio A (1989) Type 1 fiber abnormalities in skeletal muscle of patients with hypertrophic and dilated cardiomyopathy. J Am Coll Cardiol 14:1464–73

162. Adams V, Jiang H, Yu J, Mobius-Winkler S, Fiehn E, Linke A, Weigl C, Schuler G, Hambrecht R (1999) Apoptosis in skeletal myocytes of patients with chronic heart failure is associated with exercise intolerance. J Am Coll Cardiol 33:959–65

163. Vescovo G, Zennaro R, Sandri M, Carraro U, Leprotti C, Ceconi C, Ambrosio GB, Dalla Libera L (1998) Apoptosis of skeletal muscle myofibers and interstitial cells in experimental heart failure. J Mol Cell Cardiol 30:2449–59

164. Issacs H, Muncke G (1975) Idiopathic cardiomyopathy and skeletal muscle abnormality. Am Heart J 90:767–73

165. Hubner G, Grantzow R (1983) Mitochondrial cardiomyopathy with involvement of skeletal muscle. Virchow's Arch A Pathol Anat Histopathol 399:115–25

166. Marín-García J, Ananthakrishnan R, Goldenthal MJ, Filiano J, Perez-Atayde A (1999) Mitochondrial dysfunction in skeletal muscle of children with cardiomyopathy. Pediatrics 103:456–9

167. Muller-Hocker J, Johannes A, Droste M, Kadenbach B, Pongratz D, Hubner G (1986) Fatal mitochondrial cardiomyopathy in Kearns-Sayre syndrome with deficiency of cytochrome c oxidase in cardiac and skeletal muscle: An enzyme histochemical-ultraimmunocytochemical-fine structural study in longterm frozen autopsy tissue. Virchow's Arch B 52:353–67

168. Anan R, Nakagawa M, Higuchi I, Nakao S, Nomoto K, Tanaka H (1992) Deletion of mitochondrial DNA in the endomyocardial biopsy sample from a patient with Kearns-Sayre syndrome. Eur Heart J 13:1718–9

169. Marín-García J, Goldenthal JM (2002) Understanding theimpact

of mitochondrial defects in cardiovascular disease: A review. J Card Fail 8:347–61

170. Ventura-Clapier R, Garnier A, Veksler V (2004) Energy metabolism in heart failure. J Physiol 555:1–13

# Chapter 7

# Fatty Acid and Glucose Metabolism in Cardiac Disease

## Overview

Fatty acid and glucose metabolism have been extensively studied in the heart; however, information regarding the role(s) that mitochondria play in this metabolism and in the pathogenesis and progression of cardiac disease is rather limited. In this chapter, our understanding of the mechanisms, diagnosis, and treatment of metabolic defects occurring in human cardiac disorders and the experimental findings observed in animal models are discussed.

## Introduction

Fatty acids and associated lipids play an important role in cardiomyocyte structure and function. In the postnatal and adult mammalian heart, fatty acid β oxidation is the preferred pathway for the energy required for normal cardiac function. Glucose metabolism, which provides the bulk of ATP during prenatal growth, contributes significantly to the ATP production in the adult heart (up to 30% of myocardial ATP can be generated by glucose oxidation). In myocardial ischemia and hypertrophy, profound changes in both glucose and fatty acid metabolism occur, with glucose metabolism taking on greater importance. In addition, specific abnormalities in myocardial FAO metabolism, caused by either inherited or acquired physiological stresses, and in cardiac glucose utilization caused by chronic insulin deficiency or resistance may result in arrhythmias, cardiomyopathy, and HF.

In this chapter, the molecular and cellular basis of fatty acid, lipid, and glucose metabolic defects that can lead to cardiac disease are presented. In this context, the focus is on the molecular and biochemical events that can lead to myocardial hypertrophy, cardiomyopathy, and HF. Since there is a vast literature on acquired and inherited lipid disorders (e.g., cholesterol, the apolipoproteins, and HDL/ LDL), coronary artery disease, and stroke, these subjects are not included.

# Role of fatty acids and their metabolism in the normal cardiomyocyte: Structural and regulatory roles in cardiac cell membranes

Fatty acids play an integral role in the structure and function of the cardiac cell plasma and mitochondrial membranes. Their influence on the fluidity and stability of membrane structure markedly impacts on membrane functions such as transport of ions and substrates and electrophysiology intrinsic to cardiac function and excitability. In addition to their multiple structural and functional roles within the cardiac cell membrane, fatty acids and associated lipids are also regulatory molecules acting as second messengers in cell signaling, as effectors in apoptotic cell death, and in responses to oxidative and ischemic damage.

## *Fatty acid transporters and glucose carriers*

Entry of fatty acids into the cardiomyocyte is mediated by several proteins, including plasma membrane-associated fatty acid binding proteins (FABPs) and a myocardial-specific integral membrane transporter (fatty acid translocase or FAT/CD36), a homologue of human CD36.The nonenzymatic FABP also serves as a facilitator of intracellular transport of relatively insoluble long-chain fatty acids to sites of metabolic utilization (e.g., mitochondria). In mammals, the FABP content in skeletal, and cardiac muscle is related to the FAO capacity of the tissue [1]. FAT/CD36 is present in an intracellular compartment from which it can be translocated to the plasma membrane within minutes of stimulation by either muscle contraction or insulin treatment, leading to elevated myocardial uptake of long-chain fatty acids. In a rodent model of type 1 diabetes, fatty acid uptake into the heart and skeletal muscle is also elevated by increasing the expression of both FAT/CD36 and FABP [2].

Prior to their transport into mitochondria, fatty acids must be activated in the cytoplasm. This activation process requires ATP, CoA-SH, and is catalyzed by fatty acyl-CoA synthetases, associated with either the endoplasmic reticulum or the outer membrane of the mitochondria. At least 3 different acyl-CoA synthetase enzymes have been described whose specificities depend on fatty acid chain length.

For the β oxidation pathway to proceed, the fatty acyl-CoA has to be transported across the inner mitochondrial membrane. Long-chain fatty acyl-CoA molecules cannot pass directly across the inner mitochondrial membrane and need to be transported as carnitine esters, whereas short-chain and medium-chain fatty acids can be easily transported without the assistance of carnitine. The transport of long-chain fatty acyl-CoA into the mitochondria depicted in Figure 7.1 is accomplished via an acylcarnitine intermediate, which itself is generated by the action of carnitine palmitoyltransferase I (CPT-I), an enzyme residing in the inner face of the outer mitochondrial membrane. The resulting acylcarnitine molecule is subsequently transported into the mitochondria by the carnitine translocase, a transmembrane protein residing in the inner membrane that delivers acylcarnitine in exchange for free carnitine from the mitochondrial matrix. CPT-II located within the inner mitochondrial membrane catalyzes the regeneration of the fatty acyl-CoA molecule, with the acyl group transferred back to CoA from carnitine. Once inside the mitochondrion, the fatty acid-CoA is a substrate for the FAO machinery.

The uptake of fatty acids by heart mitochondria is regulated by the levels of the metabolite malonyl-CoA, which functions as a potent allosteric inhibitor of CPT-I. Malonyl-CoA is synthesized by the enzyme acetyl-CoA carboxylase (ACC) from cytoplasmic acetyl-CoA. The enzyme malonyl-CoA decarboxylase (MCD) is involved in the regulation of malonyl-CoA turnover. Levels of malonyl-CoA are affected by changes in acetyl-CoA levels or by modulation of the ACC and MCD activities. ACC activity is allosterically regulated by citrate and by kinase-mediated phosphorylation. In the ischemic heart, AMP-activated protein kinase (AMPK) promotes the phosphorylation and inhibition of ACC as well as activation of MCD, resulting in lower myocardial malonyl-CoA levels and increasing FAO [3].

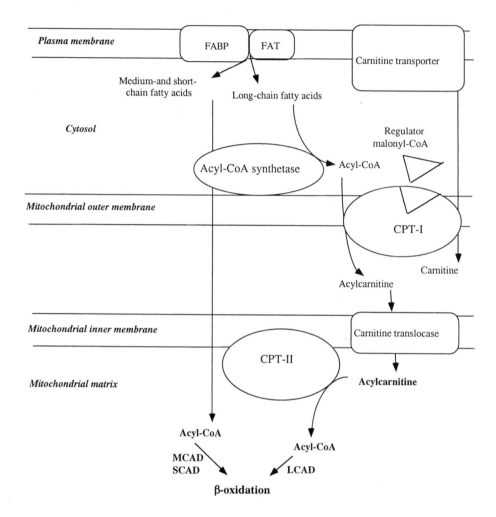

**Figure 7.1. Mitochondrial fatty acid import and oxidation.** *Fatty acid and carnitine after entry into the cardiomyocyte are transported into the mitochondria for oxidation. FABP, fatty acid binding protein; FAT, fatty acid translocase; CPT-I, carnitine palmitoyltransferase I; CPT-II, carnitine palmitoyltransferase II; MCAD, medium-chain acyl-CoA dehydrogenase; SCAD, short-chain acyl-CoA dehydrogenase; LCAD, long-chain acyl-CoA dehydrogenase.*

The level of cytoplasmic acetyl-CoA increases either as a function of decreased TCA cycle activity, reflecting lowered metabolic demand, or as a result of increased PDH activity. Therefore, malonyl-CoA production linked to altered metabolic demand or utilization of carbohydrate resources can in turn impact on either the down- or up-regulation of fatty acid import into mitochondria and myocardial FAO.

As in all other cells, the entry of glucose into cardiac myocytes is facilitated by members of the GLUT family of facilitative glucose transporters [4]. The GLUT1 transporter, which is localized on the plasma membrane under basal conditions, is thought to be the primary mediator of basal glucose uptake in the heart [5]. Its myocardial expression is stably increased within hours of ischemia or induction of hypertrophy. The most abundant glucose transporter in the heart is the insulin-responsive GLUT4 transporter. Insulin mediates the translocation of GLUT4 to the plasma membrane from a pool of intracellular vesicles and represents a critical control point by which the net flux of glucose is regulated. A variety of stimuli including hypoxia, ischemia, and cardiac work overload can induce this trans-location, thereby increasing glucose uptake and glycolytic metabolism. Defects in the ability of insulin to regulate GLUT4 translocation can lead to insulin resistance and non-insulin-dependent type 2 diabetes. HF in patients with diabetic cardiomyopathy results in a marked downregulation of myocardial GLUT transporters, limiting both glucose uptake and oxidation and contributing to the heart's inability to generate much needed ATP [6]. In diabetic cardiomyopathy, decreased glucose utilization results in an almost exclusive utilization of fatty acids as the myocardial energy source [7–8].

Fetal expression of myocardial GLUT4 is present throughout embryonic development, albeit at low levels, while GLUT1 is highly expressed in the prenatal heart [9]. At birth, the expression of genes that control myocardial glucose transport and oxidation is down-regulated. In the adult heart, GLUT4 becomes the main glucose transporter, although GLUT1 is expressed at a considerable level. The regulation of myocardial glucose transporter levels is primarily exerted transcriptionally [10].

## *Bioenergetics of FAO*

The mitochondrial fatty acid β oxidation pathway contains 4 reaction steps, including acyl-CoA dehydrogenases (short-chain, SCAD, medium-chain, MCAD, long-chain, LCAD, and very long-chain, VLCAD), short-chain enoyl-CoA hydratase, 3-hydroxyacyl-CoA dehydrogenase, and 3-ketoacyl-CoA thiolase as shown in Figure 7.2.

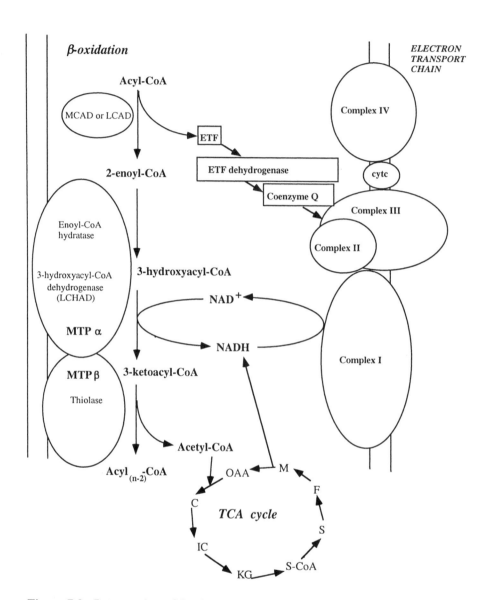

**Figure 7.2. Intersection of 3 mitochondrial bioenergetic pathways: Fatty acid β -oxidation, OXPHOS, and TCA cycle.** *ETF, electron transfer flavoprotein; cytc, cytochrome c; MTP, mitochondrial trifunctional protein; MCAD, medium-chain acyl-CoA dehydrogenase; LCAD, long-chain acyl-CoA dehydrogenase; LCHAD, long-chain 3-hydroxylacyl-CoA dehydrogenase; OAA, oxaloacetate; M, malate; C, citrate; F, fumarate; IC, isocitrate; KG, ketoglutarate; S, succinate; S-CoA, succinyl-CoA.*

In the initial acyl-CoA dehydrogenase reaction, VLCAD and LCAD are responsible for the enzymatic dehydrogenation of long-chain C8 to C22 fatty acids (e.g., palmitate and linoleic acids), with VLCAD having greater activity with the longer-chain substrates (e.g., C22 and C24 acyl-CoA esters). MCAD is active with the C4 to C12 straight-chain fatty acids (e.g., decanoic acid) and SCAD primarily is active with C2 to C4 fatty acids (e.g., butyryl-CoA). The remaining enzymatic reactions of FAO are performed by a highly organized single enzymatic complex known as the *mitochondrial trifunctional protein* (MTP), associated with the mitochondrial inner membrane. Recently, a different set of enzymes, localized in the mitochondrial matrix, has been reported to be responsible for the β-oxidation of medium- and short-chain fatty acids is [11–12].

The process of FAO is termed *β-oxidation* since it involves the sequential removal of 2-carbon units by oxidation at the β-carbon position of the fatty acyl-CoA molecule. Each round of β-oxidation produces NADH, $FADH_2$, and acetyl-CoA. Acetyl-CoA, the end product of each round of β-oxidation, enters the TCA cycle, where it is further oxidized to $CO_2$ with the concomitant generation of NADH, $FADH_2$, and ATP. The NADH and $FADH_2$ generated during FAO and acetyl-CoA oxidation in the TCA cycle, will subsequently enter the respiratory pathway for the production of ATP. Consequently, the oxidation of fatty acids yields more energy per carbon atom than does the oxidation of carbohydrates. However, while fatty acids produce more ATP during complete aerobic oxidation than glucose, this occurs at the expense of a higher rate of oxygen consumption. The supply of oxygen can be an important determinant of myocardial fuel utilization.

When circulating glucose and insulin levels are high, as occurs in the postprandial state, glucose is a primary contributor to cardiac energy metabolism [13]. During the fasting state, free fatty acids become the dominant fuel. With increased FAO, glucose oxidation is inhibited; during oxygen deprivation and anoxia, the inhibition of glucose utilization is removed, and glycolysis is accelerated. A significant increase in carbohydrate oxidation also occurs in the adult heart in response to an acute increase in cardiac work. Since increase in glucose uptake is delayed in this cardiac response, the increase in glucose oxidation is initiated by rapid glycogen breakdown [14].

## Cellular location of FAO and glucose oxidation

Both peroxisomes and mitochondria have multiple enzymes involved in fatty acid β-oxidation. The peroxisomal enzymes include palmitoyl -CoA oxidase, L-functional protein, and 3-ketoacyl oxidase, which are all inducible enzymes acting on straight-chain substrates. In addition, peroxisomes contain branched-chain acyl-CoA oxidase, D-functional protein, and sterol-carrier protein X, which are noninducible and primarily use branched-chain substrates. The inducible enzymes increase in response to the peroxisomal proliferating activating receptor (PPAR) resulting in increased peroxisomal biogenesis (see below).

It is important to note that while specific deficiencies in the mitochondrial-located enzymes involved in FAO may result in cardiomyopathy (as discussed below), defects in peroxisomal FAO enzymes primarily result in neurological pathology, including seizures, hypotonia, and psychomotor retardation. Cardiac abnormalities have been rarely described in peroxisomal deficiencies. This is also true of diseases involving general peroxisomal biogenesis abnormalities such as Zellweger syndrome and neonatal adrenoleukodystrophy, where there is little or no cardiac involvement. PPAR plays a pivotal role in both mitochondrial FAO and mitochondrial biogenesis, not only in normal cardiac growth and development but also in HF. This suggests an important interrelationship between the two cellular compartments and further underscores the mitochondrial compartment as a critical effector of cardiac homeostasis. The commonality of biogenesis and potential feedback between these two cellular organelles needs further elucidation in both normal growth and development and in cardiac disease (both FAO and mitochondrial OXPHOS disorders).

After entering the plasma membrane, glucose is oxidized by the glycolytic enzymes located primarily in the cytosol but often in association with specific organelles. Glyceraldehyde-3-phosphate dehydrogenase and pyruvate kinase bind to sarcolemmal and sarcoplasmic reticulum membranes. Both the first enzyme in the glycolytic pathway (i.e., hexokinase) and the last enzyme (i.e., PDH) are associated with the mitochondria. Hexokinase binds at the outer membrane to peripheral protein complexes such as the PT pore, while PDH (which determines the fate of the glycolytic product pyruvate) is entirely located within the mitochondrial matrix.

## *The effect of disorders of fatty acid and glucose metabolism on cardiac structure/function*

In cardiac failure following cardiac hypertrophy, there is a major switch in myocardial bioenergetic substrate used—from fatty acid to glucose. A key component and marker of the switch is the coordinate down-regulation of FAO enzymes and mRNA levels (>40%) in the human left ventricle [15]. This switch is thought to represent a reversal to a fetal energy substrate preference pattern of glucose oxidation in the heart. During the development of cardiac hypertrophy, a fetal metabolic gene program is initiated via the complicity of transcription factors that bind to regulatory elements, reducing gene expression of FAO enzymes (e.g., MCAD and CPT-I β). Although the molecular mechanisms mediating this down-regulation are not fully understood, the participation of several nuclear receptors, intermediate metabolites, and transcription factors (e.g., SP1 and PPAR) has been implicated in the programmatic change in myocardial gene expression (see further discussion below) [16].

The hypertrophied and failing heart becomes increasingly dependent on glucose as energy substrate. However, in the failing heart, it is unlikely that increased anaerobic glycolysis can compensate in ATP production for the decline in FAO, together with the diminished levels of high-energy phosphates resulting from declining phosphocreatine content, diminished creatine kinase activity, and mitochondrial OXPHOS dysfunction. Moreover, despite the rise in glycolysis, the rate of mitochondrial-localized pyruvate oxidation does not keep up with the increased pyruvate levels [17]. This has led to the conclusion that the failing heart is energetically, severely compromised [18].

The effects of diabetes and hyperglycemia on cardiac structure and function are also profound. Insulin deficiency or resistance are associated with LV hypertrophy and cardiomyopathy. Myocardial glucose uptake and utilization are affected with deficits in insulin signaling leading to an increased reliance of the heart on FAO for energy generation. This contributes to an increased accumulation of lipid intermediates, elevated cellular acidosis, decreased cardiac efficiency, and contractile dysfunction [19]. Moreover, hyperglycemia and diabetes affect cardiac mitochondria function directly. In animals treated with streptozocin to induce diabetes, cardiac mitochondria show pronounced swelling, increased damage, and targeting by lysosomes [20]. Mitochondria from a variety of diabetic animal models show diminished respiratory control as well as increased oxidative stress [21–22]. These changes in cardiac structure and function are reversed with insulin administration. Conversely, the activity of the PPAR-α gene regulatory pathway is increased in the diabetic heart, which relies primarily on FAO for energy production, providing further stimulus for the excessive FA import and oxidation underlying the cardiac remodeling of the diabetic heart.

Specific heritable (inborn) deficiencies in fatty acid and glucose metabolism are associated with cardiomyopathy and cardiac failure. Table 7.1 presents a list of disorders affecting fatty acid metabolism, which can result in cardiomyopathy or HF, with their characterized genetic loci. Heritable defects in mitochondrial acyl-CoA dehydrogenase have been described in cardiomyopathy and HF [23]. In general, defects in the oxidation of long-chain fatty acids are more likely to cause cardiomyopathy than defects in medium-chain or short-chain fatty acids. Specific defects in enzymes involved in short-chain, long-chain, and very long-chain fatty acids have been identified [24–27], and the genetic defects are described further in more detail in the molecular section below.

Although severe cardiomyopathy is unusual in patients exhibiting MCAD deficiency, sudden death in children is a common outcome, and its pathogenetic mechanism is presently undetermined.

Defects in malonyl-CoA decarboxylase due to mutations in MCD can also lead to cardiomyopathy and neonatal death [28]. HCM results from specific mutations in the regulatory subunit of AMPK, a critical bioenergetic sensor that activitates FAO by adjusting malonyl-CoA levels and increasing glucose uptake, particularly during chronic low-energy states, such as those that occur in cardiac hypertrophy and failure [29].

Carnitine deficiency has been frequently associated with severe cardiomyopathy. Mutations in proteins that participate in carnitine transport and metabolism may cause either DCM or HCM as a recessive trait [30–31]. One of the genetic loci affected in carnitine associated cardiac involvement encodes the plasma-membrane localized carrier that transports carnitine into the cell; its deficiency has been described

**Table 7.1. Fatty acid metabolism disorders in cardiac failure**

| Fatty Acid Metabolism Disorders | Affected Loci |
|---|---|
| CPT-II deficiency | ICV |
| Barth syndrome | G4.5 |
| SCAD deficiency | SCAD |
| MTP deficiency | MTPα subunit |
| (includes LCHAD defect) | MTPβ subunit |
| VLCAD deficiency | VLCAD |
| CPT-I deficiency | L-CPT-I |
| Carnitine transport | OCTN2 |
| Carnitine translocase deficiency | CACT |
| MCAD deficiency | MCAD |
| ETF deficiency | ETFα |
| ETF dehydrogenase deficiency | ETF-DH |
| FAT deficiency | CD36 |

as primary carnitine deficiency [32]. This transport deficiency is due to specific defects in the gene OCTN2 encoding the plasma-membrane localized organic cation/carnitine transporter [33].

The carnitine deficiency due to defects at this locus and its resultant pathology, which can prove lethal in childhood, have been recently shown to be dramatically reversed by intake of high-dose oral carnitine supplementation [34]. Defects in a second locus, the mitochondrial membrane localized carnitine-acylcarnitine translocase, also lead to an autosomal recessive carnitine deficiency, cardiomyopathy, and cardiac failure [35]. Carnitine supplementation has been shown to be an effective therapy in some cases [36].

Although generally not found in association with cardiomyopathy or cardiac failure, new evidence suggests that CPT-I deficiency can result in cardiac involvement [37]. In contrast, there is consensus that deficiencies in CPT-II (specifically infantile CPT-II deficiency), an autosomal recessive disorder, is associated with cardiac damage and sudden death [38].

## *Secondary effects on mitochondrial fatty acid β-oxidation: Relationship to mitochondrial respiration and OXPHOS*

The utilization of fatty acids as an energy source requires the functional operation of the mitochondrial ETC and OXPHOS. The NADH feeds into the ETC at complex I, and electrons are transferred from acyl-CoA dehydrogenases via the electron-transfer flavoprotein (ETF), ETF dehydrogenase, and ubiquinone (or coenzyme Q) to complex III as depicted in Figure 7.2 [39]. Affected individuals with deficiencies in the ETF pathway display impaired FAO and abnormal intramitochondrial accumulation of fatty acids and glutaric acid and may develop a fatal cardiomyopathy [39–40]. Similarly, patients with defects in respiratory complexes (e.g., complexes I and IV) will frequently develop cardiomyopathy and HF, largely as a result of impaired energy production [41]. However, the extent of the effects on cardiac FAO and on lipid accumulation in patients with defined respiratory activity defects and with defective coenzyme Q levels has not yet been fully assessed.

## Fatty acid metabolism defects and their association with cardiomyopathy and arrhythmias

### *Cardiomyopathy*

With the exception of defects in the MTP that affect long-chain L-3 hydroxylacyl-CoA activity and are associated with DCM [42], most of the disturbances in fatty acid metabolism are found in patients with HCM, and many of the reported mutations in fatty acid β oxidation pathway result in HCM rather than DCM [43].

The X-linked disorder Barth syndrome typically is characterized by DCM, skeletal myopathy, neutropenia, and increased levels of 3-methylglutaconic aciduria, with onset often occurring in infancy. Arrhythmias and HF are frequently present. The protein tafazzin encoded by the G4.5 gene is mutated and responsible for Barth syndrome with associated cardiomyopathy [44–45]. While the biochemical function of the tafazzin protein has not yet been determined, structural analysis suggests that tafazzin belongs to a family of acyltransferases involved in phospholipid synthesis [46]. Fatty acid composition of several phospholipids —including phospha tidylcholine, phosphatidylethanolamine, and cardiolipin— was altered in hearts of Barth patients [47]. Cardiolipin levels are also affected in other tissues including cultured fibroblasts [48]. Abnormal cardiolipin levels may prove useful as a diagnostic marker in patients with Barth syndrome.

## *Arrhythmias and conduction defects*

Conduction defects and cardiac arrhythmias frequently occur in patients with certain FAO defects [49]. Specifically, these electrocardiographic abnormalities were present in patients with deficiencies in CPT-II, carnitine translocase, and MTP enzyme acti-vities. On the other hand, cardiac arrhythmias were notably absent in patients with deficiencies in CPT-I, the primary carnitine carrier and MCAD. These findings support the notion that the accumulation of arrhythmogenic intermediary metabolites of fatty acids (e.g., long-chain acylcarnitines) may be responsible for arrhythmias and potentially contributory to HF and sudden death. This is also consis-tent with findings that long-chain acylcarnitines accumulate with defects in CPT-II, carnitine translocase, and MTP, whereas MCAD, CPT-I, and carnitine carrier defects do not result in the accumulation of these intermediates.

Amphiphilic long-chain acylcarnitines possess detergent-like prop-erties, can extensively modify membrane proteins and lipids, and have a variety of toxic effects on the electrophysiological function of the cardiac membranes including ion transport ($Na^+$, $Ca^{++}$) and impaired gap junction activity. This is further supported by the demonstration that patients with cardiomyopathy, due to inborn defects in carnitine translocase, have an increased incidence of cardiac arrhythmias [50]. Moreover, the accumulation of long-chain fatty acid intermediates (e.g., acylcarnitine) has been implicated in the genesis of ventricular
cardial ischemia [51]. Selective blocking of
the accumulation of potentially toxic long-
⟩xia/ischemia, thereby reducing the risk of
⟩ance and membrane disruption [52]. Studies
: of action of these toxic long-chain inter-
omyocytes (e.g., at the level of the plasma
matrix, or inner membrane) may prove to
the development of new therapies.

## Fatty acids, glucose, and cardiac apoptosis

The phospholipid cardiolipin is a component of the inner membrane associated with the mitochondrial PT pore (and its constituent protein ANT). Cardiolipin mediates the targeting of the proapoptotic protein tBid to mitochondria, implicating cardiolipin in the pathway for cytochrome *c* release [53]. It may also play a role in membrane permeability and proton conductance, as well as in the functioning of cytochrome *c* oxidase.

During ischemia, oxidation of the saturated fatty acid palmitate is associated with diminished myocyte function [54]. Saturated long-chain fatty acid substrates such as palmitate (but not monounsaturated fatty acids such as oleate) readily induce apoptosis in rat neonatal cardiomyocytes [55–56]. As an early feature of palmitate-induced cardiomyocyte apoptosis, palmitate diminishes the content of the mitochondrial cardiolipin by causing a marked reduction in cardiolipin synthesis. Decreased levels of cardiolipin synthesis and cytochrome *c* release have been reported to be temporally correlated suggesting that cardiolipin modulates the association of cytochrome *c* with the mitochondrial inner membrane [57].

Palmitate also decreases the oxidative metabolism of fatty acids and respiratory complex III activity, and has been associated with an increase in the intracellular second messenger ceramide [54].

Recent data have shown that the ceramide apoptotic pathway, which involves ROS production, is distinct from the palmitate-induced pathway, which involves neither ROS production nor oxidative stress [58–59]. The modulations in FAO metabolism (e.g., CPT-I activity decline) and complex III activity in fatty acid-induced apoptosis have been shown to be downstream occurring well after cytochrome *c* release [54, 60–61].

Glucose and glucose uptake can play an important role in modulating myocardial apoptosis. Glucose uptake in cardiomyocytes reduces hypoxia-induced apoptosis [62]. Overexpression of GLUT1, to promote increased glucose uptake, also blocked the progression of apoptosis in hypoxia-treated cardiomyocytes [63]. A protective apoptotic role of glucose is further supported by studies in glucose deprivation promoted myocardial apoptosis. Insuli tration attenuates cardiac ischemia-reperfusion induced activation of Akt-mediated cell-survival signaling [64 to normal myocardial glucose uptake and signali cell survival pathways (as discussed further in Chapter 10), there is evidence that defective glucose uptake and hyperglycemia, as found in diabetic cardiomyopathy, can lead to increased myocardial apoptosis. Hyperglycemia induces myocyte apoptosis, cytochrome $c$ release, and high levels of ROS in cardiomyocytes in culture as well as in a mouse model of diabetes produced by streptozocin treatment [66].

## Abnormalities in mtDNA and their association with both diabetes and cardiomyopathy

As noted earlier in this chapter, diabetes can often present with cardiomyopathy. Specific mtDNA mutations in association with both diabetes and cardiomyopathy are increasingly reported. Diabetes has been found in patients with large rearrangements (e.g., deletions) in mtDNA or in association with specific point mutations [67–68]. These point mutations have been found in tRNAs, including sites previously associated with MELAS (e.g., nt 3243) and MERRF (e.g., nt 8344), in structural genes (e.g., ND1 at nt 3310), and in 16s rRNA [69–71]. In addition, mitochondria are primary target of oxidative damage in the diabetic heart [72], which could lead to increased generation of mtDNA mutations at specific hotspots. However, the causal relationship between diabetes and mtDNA mutation remains unclear.

## Molecular players in FAO-related cardiac diseases; modulation of gene expression

### MCAD

MCAD deficiency is autosomally recessive and associated with sudden death and severe cardiac arrhythmias [73]. Over 90% of cases of MCAD deficiency are associated with a homozygous mutation at nt 985 (A985G). This mutation directs a glutamate replacement of lysine at residue 304 in the mature MCAD subunit, causing impairment of tetramer assembly and increased protein instability [74].

MCAD deficiency is the most frequent inborn metabolic disorder in populations of northwestern European origin [75].

At the gene level, 3 of the 7 reported non-A985G mutations found in MCAD deficiency localize to exon 11. At the protein level, the mutant residues cluster in helix H of the MCAD protein and are proposed to have their primary effect on the correct folding and assembly of the tetrameric MCAD enzyme structure. The amino acid residues effected are: M301T, S311R, and K304E [76].

## *VLCAD*

Pediatric cardiomyopathy is the most common clinical phenotype of VLCAD deficiency. A severe form of infantile cardiomyopathy is found in over 67% of cases, often resulting in sudden death [20].

VLCAD deficiency is characterized by a significant reduction of VLCAD mRNA and decreased levels and/or absence of VLCAD enzyme activity. Mutation analysis of the VLCAD gene revealed a large number of different mutant loci (21 in 19 patients) with few repeated mutations [77]. Distinguishing between truly pathogenic mutations and polymorphic variations remains to be done.

## *CPT-II*

The infantile form of CPT-II deficiency has frequent cardiac involvement and is associated with specific CPT-II mutations in contrast to the adult form of CPT-II deficiency that does not present with cardiac involvement. Infantile CPT-II deficiency has been associated with several mutations including a homozygous mutation at A2399C causing a Tyr→Ser substititution at residue 628. This mutation produces a marked decrease in CPT-II activity in fibroblasts [78]. Another mutation has been reported at C1992T predicting an Arg→Cys substitution at residue 631, which is associated with drastic reduction of CPT-II catalytic activity [79].

## *MTP*

MTP, an enzyme of β oxidation of long-chain fatty acids, is a multi-enzyme complex composed of 4 molecules of the α-subunit (encoded by HADHA) that contains both the enoyl-CoA hydratase and 3-

hydroxyacyl-CoA dehydrogenase domains, and 4 molecules of the β-subunit (encoded by HADHB) containing the 3-ketoacyl-CoA thiolase domain [80].

MTP deficiency has been classified into two different biochemical phenotypes. In one, both α and β subunits are present and only the 3-hydroxyacyl-CoA dehydrogenase (LCHAD) activity is effected. The most common mutation associated with MTP deficiency (G1528C) is associated with this phenotype. In the other, there is an absence of both subunits, and the complete lack of all 3 enzymatic activities of MTP. Mutations have been localized to the 5' donor splicing site of the β subunit gene, which can result in the entire loss of an exon in the mRNA (exon 3) and are associated with the second phenotype. Although there is some overlap between the clinical features found in each molecular/biochemical phenotype, patients with neonatal cardiomyopathy display the second biochemical phenotype only. Analysis of 2 children who died of HF and acidosis revealed that they were homozygous for a novel missense mutation G976C in the gene encoding the MTP β subunit [81]. This mutation caused the loss of all 3 MTP activities and near complete loss of the protein, as assayed by Western immunoblot analysis. The classification of MTP phenotypes has been recently expanded. Patients with a lethal form of cardiomyopathy harboring either α or β subunit mutations exhibit reduced activity levels of all 3 MTP activities, indicating that mutations in either subunit can contribute similarly to MTP complex instability [82]. Both DNA and enzymatic testing can be performed in fetal screening of this often devastating disease [83].

## *PPAR*

Members of the superfamily of nuclear gene receptors, the peroxisomal proliferating activating receptors (PPARs) have been identified as playing a key role in the transcriptional regulation of genes involved in intracellular lipid and energy metabolism including FAO enzymes [84–85]. Three isoforms of the PPAR subfamily (α, β and γ) are enriched in tissues that are dependent on lipid utilization for energy metabolism (e.g., heart, liver, brown adipose tissue as well as in all critical vascular cells) and have been implicated in the rapid mobilization of bioenergetic stores in response to physiological stresses.

By acting on DNA response elements, as heterodimers with the nuclear retinoid X receptor (RXR), PPAR acts as a transcriptional activator stimulating the expression of a constellation of genes encoding enzymes involved in both peroxisome and mitochondrial FAO (e.g., mitochondrial MCAD, CPT-I, and peroxisomal acyl-CoA oxidase). PPAR activity is dependent on the presence of a variety of activating ligands (e.g., prostaglandins, eicosanoids, and long-chain unsaturated fatty acids) and interacting proteins (i.e., coactivators and corepressors). The PPAR-ligand complex binds to a DNA response element in the promoter region of specific genes activating transcription [86]. The activity of PPAR-$\alpha$ is a critical determinant of myocardial energy production and can serve to match cardiac lipid delivery to oxidative capacity [87]. Cardiac metabolic gene expression is activated by PPAR-$\alpha$ regulation during postnatal development, during short-term starvation and in response to exercise training. One marker of PPAR activation is up-regulated MCAD expression.

Conversely, pressure-overload hypertrophy results in deactivation of PPAR-$\alpha$ with lower FAO enzyme expression, abnormal cardiac lipid homoeostasis, and reduced energy production [88]. The negative regulation of PPAR-$\alpha$ is mediated at the transcriptional level during ventricular overload in mice. In addition, PPAR activity is altered at the posttranscriptional level, via the extracellular signal-regulated MAP kinase pathway. Ventricular overload therefore results in hypertrophied myocytes with intracellular fat accumulation (in response to oleate loading). At this time, the role of PPAR in the activation of the fetal gene program, occurring during hypertrophy and HF, has not yet been fully delineated.

PPAR plays a pivotal role in mediating the effect of hypoxia on cardiomyocyte mitochondrial FAO resulting in diminished CPT-I $\beta$ mRNA levels. This is accomplished via PPAR transcriptional regulation (due to reduced binding of PPAR-$\alpha$), and its obligate partner, retinoid X receptor $\alpha$ (RXR-$\alpha$) to a DNA response element residing within the CPT-I $\beta$ promoter [89]. The cardiac phenotype of mice with overexpression of PPAR-$\alpha$ strikingly mimics the metabolic phenotype of diabetic cardiomyopathy, with increased myocardial FAO and decreased levels of glucose uptake and oxidation [90].

Although PPAR-γ specific agonists have cardioprotective effects in response to ischemia, the levels of PPAR-γ are barely detectable in the heart, even in isolated myocytes exposed to PPAR-γ agonists or FA ligands, arguing against a direct role for PPAR-γ in cardiac lipid metabolism [91]. In contrast, the less characterized myocardial PPAR-β isoform is similar in abundance to PPAR-α, fatty acid inducible, and promotes myocardial PPAR target gene expression. To precisely define the specific endogenous ligands used by these different PPARs, their specific coactivators and the full set of targeted genes for each receptor isoforms further research is needed. Eventually, this information may allow a finely tuned pharmacological modulation of cardiac metabolism.

## Peroxisome proliferator-activated receptor γ coactivator (PGC-1α)

PGC-1α has been identified as a regulator of mitochondrial respiratory function in tissues specialized for thermogenesis (e.g., brown adipose tissue and skeletal muscle) [92]. PGC-1α gene expression is induced in the mouse heart after birth and in response to short-term fasting, conditions known to increase cardiac mitochondrial energy production. Expression of PGC-1α in cardiac myocytes has been reported to induce nuclear and mitochondrial gene expression involved in multiple mitochondrial bioenergetic pathways, increased mitochondrial biogenesis, and respiration. Cardiac-specific overexpression of PGC-1α in transgenic mice resulted in uncontrolled mitochondrial proliferation in cardiac myocytes, leading to loss of sarcomeric structure and DCM. These results identify PGC-1α as a critical regulatory molecule in controlling myocardial mitochondrial number and function in response to energy demands [93].

PGC-1α also has been implicated in mediating the increased expression of mtTFA, involved in the control of both mtDNA transcription and replication, and NRF-1, which regulates the expression of a number of nuclear genes involved in OXPHOS including subunits of cytochrome *c* oxidase and ATP synthase [94].

PGC-1α overexpression in the myocardium can display strikingly developmental-specific differences. For instance, in the neonatal myocardium, PGC-1α overexpression leads to increased size and number of mitochondria, concurrent with the increased gene expression associated with mitochondrial biogenesis. In the adult mouse, PGC-1α overexpression produces a moderate increase in mitochondrial number, abnormal organelle structure, and eventually cardiomyopathy with increased ventricular mass and dilatation [95]. Cessation of PGC-1α expression reverses over time the cardiac phenotype.

## Animal models of defective fatty acid metabolism and cardiac failure

A number of animal models have been useful in our understanding of the initiation, severity, and progression of the cardiac phenotypes associated with specific abnormalities in fatty acid and glucose metabolism. Transgenic mice lacking PPAR-α display a cardiac phenotype of increased myocyte lipid accumulation [96]. Mice lacking MTP α and β subunits alleles show necrosis and acute degradation of the cardiac myocytes. They also accumulate long-chain fatty acid metabolites, have low birth weight, and develop neonatal hypoglycemia, with sudden death occurring between 6 and 36 hr after birth [97].

To test the hypothesis that disturbance in myocardial fatty acid uptake and utilization leads to the accumulation of cardiotoxic lipid species and to establish a mouse model of metabolic cardiomyopathy, transgenic mouse lines that overexpress long-chain acyl-CoA synthetase in the heart were generated. These mice showed cardiac-restricted expression of the transgene and marked cardiac myocyte triglyceride accumulation. Lipid accumulation was associated with initial cardiac hypertrophy, followed by the development of left-ventricular dysfunction and premature death [98].

The role of RXR-α in HF has been examined in transgenic mice as well. RXR-α null mutant mice display ocular and cardiac malformations and liver developmental delay and die from HF in early embryo life. A large percentage (over 50%) of the downstream target genes, identified by subtractive hybridization, encode proteins involved in fatty acid metabolism and electron transport, suggesting energy deficiency in the null RXR-α embryos. ATP content and MCAD mRNA were significantly lower in RXR-α mutant hearts compared to wild-type mice. These findings suggest that defects in intermediary metabolism may be a causative factor in the RXR-$\alpha$ -/- phenotype, an embryonic form of DCM [99].

Our understanding of the roles that mitochondrial gene expression and function play in defining cardiac metabolism has also been greatly enhanced by transgenic studies. The previously discussed studies with PGC-1$\alpha$ overexpression suggest that increased mitochondrial function and biogenesis may be fine in the neonatal heart but may result in cardiomyopathy in the adult. Disturbing mitochondrial bioenergetic function by creating null mutations in ANT1 can also lead to mitochondrial proliferation with dysfunctional mitochondria and cardiomyopathy [100]. Similarly, null mutations in mtTFA in mouse cause progressive cardiac dysfunction with depleted mtDNA and an associated decline in OXPHOS ATP production [101]. An early feature in the progression of this cardiac mitochondrial dysfunction is the activation of a fetal metabolic gene-expression program characterized by the decreased expression of FAO genes and increased expression of glycolytic genes [102]. The switch in the programming of cardiac metabolism was followed by increased myocardial mitochondrial biogenesis, which could not compensate in ATP production but rather contributes to the progression of heart failure, probably in a way similar to the PCG-1$\alpha$ overexpression in the adult heart.


## Advances in diagnostics and treatment of fatty acid/cardiac disease

At the biochemical level, the diagnostic evaluation of fatty acid defects and determination of carnitine levels are easily performed. Rapid and correct diagnosis (including newborn screening using a noninvasive, highly sensitive methodology profiling acylcarnitines, via tandem mass spectrometry, on blood spot collected on a Guthrie card) is critical since dramatic recovery from or prevention of arrhythmias and cardiac failure have been demonstrated in these disorders (e.g., VLCAD deficiency) [103]. As previously discussed, the use of carnitine supplementation in patients with carnitine deficiency may be of significant benefit in the prevention and treatment of potentially lethal disorders. The use of genetic analysis is also available, although the presence of nonrepeating mutations makes this analysis rather problematic.

The use of targeted dietary supplements and the pharmacological treatment of FAO and metabolic cardiac disorders are discussed in Chapter 11. In addition, gene therapy for some of the fatty acid disturbances of cardiac function and structure to decrease long-chain fatty acid intermediates and redirect metabolic programs holds great promise and is discussed in Chapter 11.

# References

1.   Glatz JF, Storch J (2001) Unraveling the significance of cellular fatty acid binding-protein. Curr Opin Lipidol 12:267–74

2.   Bonen A, Campbell SE, Benton CR, Chabowski A, Coort SL, Han XX, Koonen DP, Glatz JF, Luiken JJ (2004) Regulation of fatty acid transport by fatty acid translocase/CD36. Proc Nutr Soc 63:245–9

3.   Hopkins TA, Dyck JR, Lopaschuk GD (2003) AMP-activated protein kinase regulation of fatty acid oxidation in the ischaemic heart. Biochem Soc Trans 31:207–12

4.   Abel ED (2004) Glucose transport in the heart. Front Biosci 9:201–15

5.   Flier JS, Mueckler MM, Usher P, Lodish HF (1987) Elevated levels of glucose transport and transporter messenger RNA are induced by ras or src oncogenes. Science 235:1492–5

6.   Razeghi P, Young ME, Ying J, Depre C, Uray IP, Kolesar J, Shipley GL, Moravec CS, Davies PJ, Frazier OH, Taegtmeyer H (2002) Downregulation of metabolic gene expression in failing human heart before and after mechanical unloading. Cardiology 97:203–9

7.   Razeghi P, Young ME, Cockrill TC, Frazier OH, Taegtmeyer H (2002) Downregulation of myocardial myocyte enhancer factor 2C and myocyte enhancer factor 2C-regulated gene expression in diabetic patients with nonischemic heart failure. Circulation 106:407–11

8.   Stanley WC, Lopaschuk GD, McCormack JG (1997) Regulation of energy substrate metabolism in the diabetic heart. Cardiovasc Res 34:25–33

9. Vannucci SJ, Rutherford T, Wilkie MB, Simpson IA, Lauder JM (2000) Prenatal expression of the GLUT4 glucose transporter in the mouse. Dev Neurosci 22:274–82

10. Santalucia T, Boheler KR, Brand NJ, Sahye U, Fandos C, Vinals F, Ferre J, Testar X, Palacin M, Zorzano A (1999) Factors involved in GLUT-1 glucose transporter gene transcription in cardiac muscle. J Biol Chem 274:17626–34

11. Liang X, Le W, Zhang D, Schulz H (2001) Impact of the intramitochondrial enzyme organization on fatty acid organization. Biochem Soc Trans 29:279–82

12. Jackson S, Schaefer J, Middleton B, Turnbull DM (1995) Characterization of a novel enzyme of human fatty acid beta-oxidation: A matrix-associated, mitochondrial 2-enoyl CoA hydratase. Biochem Biophys Res Commun 214:247–53

13. Opie LH, Sack MN (2002) Metabolic plasticity and the promotion of cardiac protection in ischemia and ischemic preconditioning. J Mol Cell Cardiol 34:1077–89

14. Goodwin GW, Taegtmeyer H (2000) Improved energy homeostasis of the heart in the metabolic state of exercise. Am J Physiol Heart Circ Physiol 279:H1490–501

15. Sack MN, Rader TA, Park S, Bastin J, McCune SA, Kelly DP (1996) Fatty acid oxidation enzyme gene expression is downregulated in the failing heart. Circulation 94:2837–42

16. Kanda H, Nohara R, Hasegawa K, Kishimoto C, Sasayama S (2000) A nuclear complex containing PPARa/RXR is markedly downregulated in the hypertrophied rat left ventricular myocardium with normal systolic function. Heart Vessels 15:191–6

17. Leong HS, Brownsey RW, Kulpa JE, Allard MF (2003) Glycolysis and pyruvate oxidation in cardiac hypertrophy: Why so unbalanced? Comp Biochem Physiol A Mol Integr Physiol 135:499–513

18. van Bilsen M, Smeets PJ, Gilde AJ, van der Vusse GJ (2004) Metabolic remodelling of the failing heart: The cardiac burn-out syndrome? Cardiovasc Res 61:218–26

19. Avogaro A, Vigili de Kreutzenberg S, Negut C, Tiengo A, Scognamiglio R (2004) Diabetic cardiomyopathy: A metabolic perspective. Am J Cardiol 93:13A–16A

20. Seager MJ, Singal PK, Orchard R, Pierce GN, Dhalla NS (1984) Cardiac cell damage: A primary myocardial disease in streptozotocin-induced chronic diabetes. Br J Exp Pathol 65:613–23

21. Mokhtar N, Lavoie JP, Rousseau-Migneron S, Nadeau A (1993) Physical training reverses defect in mitochondrial energy production in heart of chronically diabetic rats. Diabetes 42:682–7

22. Tomita M, Mukae S, Geshi E, Umetsu K, Nakatani M, Katagiri T (1996) Mitochondrial respiratory impairment in streptozotocin induced diabetic rat heart. Jpn Circ J 60:673–82

23. Kelly DP, Strauss AW (1994) Inherited cardiomyopathies. New Engl J Med 330:913–9

24. Hale DE, Batshaw ML, Coates PM, Frerman FE, Goodman SI, Singh I, Stanley CA (1985) Long-chain acyl coenzyme A dehydrogenase deficiency: An inherited cause of nonketotic hypoglycemia. Pediatr Res 19:666–71

25. Rocchiccioli F, Wanders RJ, Aubourg P, Vianey-Liaud C, Ijlst L, Fabre M, Cartier N, Bougneres PF (1990) Deficiency of long-chain 3-hydroxyacyl-CoA dehydrogenase: A cause of lethal myopathy and cardiomyopathy in early childhood. Pediatr Res 28:657–62

26. Strauss AW, Powell CK, Hale DE, Anderson MM, Ahuja A, Brackett JC, Sims HF (1995) Molecular basis of human mitochondrial very-long-chain acyl-CoA dehydrogenase deficiency causing cardiomyopathy and sudden death in childhood. Proc Natl Acad Sci USA 92:10496–500

27. Tein I, Haslam RH, Rhead WJ, Bennett MJ, Becker LE, Vockley J (1999) Short-chain acyl-CoA dehydrogenase deficiency: A cause of ophthalmoplegia and multicore myopathy. Neurology 52:366–72

28. Surendran S, Sacksteder KA, Gould SJ, Coldwell JG, Rady PL, Tyring SK, Matalon R (2001) Malonyl CoA decarboxylase deficiency: C to T transition in intron 2 of the MCD gene. J Neurosci Res 65:591–4

29. Oliveira SM, Ehtisham J, Redwood CS, Ostman-Smith I, Blair EM, Watkins H (2003) Mutation analysis of AMP-activated protein kinase subunits in inherited cardiomyopathies: Implications for kinase function and disease pathogenesis. J Mol Cell Cardiol 35:1251–5

30. Roe CR, Ding JH. In: Scriver C, et al. ed. Metabolic and Molecular Basis of Inherited Disease. Vol. 2: McGraw-Hill 2001:2297–326

31. Engel AG, Angelini C (1973) Carnitine deficiency of human skeletal muscle with associated lipid storage myopathy: A new syndrome. Science 179:899–902

32. Stanley CA, Treem WR, Hale DE, Coates PM (1990) A genetic defect in carnitine transport causing primary carnitine deficiency. Prog Clin Biol Res 321:457–64

33. Nezu J, Tamai I, Oku A, Ohashi R, Yabuuchi H, Hashimoto N, Nikaido H, Sai Y, Koizumi A, Shoji Y, Takada G, Matsuishi T, Yoshino M, Kato H, Ohura T, Tsujimoto G, Hayakawa J, Shimane M, Tsuji A (1999) Primary systemic carnitine deficiency is caused by mutations in a gene encoding sodium ion-dependent carnitine transporter. Nat Genet 21:91–4

34. Tein I (2003) Carnitine transport: pathophysiology and metabolism of known molecular defects. J Inherit Metab Dis 26:147–69

35. Roschinger W, Muntau AC, Duran M, Dorland L, Ijlst L, Wanders RJ, Roscher AA (2000) Carnitine-acylcarnitine translocase deficiency: Metabolic consequences of an impaired mitochondrial carnitine cycle. Clin Chim Acta 298:55–68

36. Iacobazzi V, Pasquali M, Singh R, Matern D, Rinaldo P, Amat di San Filippo C, Palmieri F, Longo N (2004) Response to therapy in carnitine/acylcarnitine translocase (CACT) deficiency due to a novel missense mutation. Am J Med Genet 126A:150–5

37. Olpin SE, Allen J, Bonham JR, Clark S, Clayton PT, Calvin J, Downing M, Ives K, Jones S, Manning NJ, Pollitt RJ, Standing SJ, Tanner MS. (2001) Features of carnitine palmitoyltransferase type I deficiency. J Inherit Metab Dis 24:35–42

38. Demaugre F, Bonnefont JP, Colonna M, Cepanec C, Leroux JP, Saudubray JM (1991) Infantile form of carnitine palmitoyltransferase II deficiency with hepatomuscular symptoms and sudden death: Physiopathological approach to carnitine palmitoyltransferase II deficiencies. J Clin Invest 87:859–64

39. Salazar D, Zhang L, deGala GD, Frerman FE (1997) Expression and characterization of two pathogenic mutations in human electron transfer flavoprotein. J Biol Chem 272:26425–33

40. Gregersen N (1985) Riboflavin-responsive defects of beta-oxidation. J Inherit Metab Dis 8:65–9

41. Marín-García J, Goldenthal MJ, Moe GW (2001) Mitochondrial pathology in cardiac failure. Cardiovasc Res 49:17–26

42. Brackett JC, Sims HF, Rinaldo P, Shapiro S, Powell CK, Bennett MJ, Strauss AW (1995) Two alpha-subunit donor splice site mutations cause human trifunctional protein deficiency. J Clin Invest 95:2076–82

43. Schonberger J, Seidman CE (2001) Many roads lead to a broken heart: The genetics of dilated cardiomyopathy. Am J Hum Genet 69: 249–60

44. Bione S, D'Adamo P, Maestrini E, Gedeon AK, Bolhuis PA, Toniolo D (1996) A novel X-linked gene, G4.5 is responsible for Barth syndrome. Nat Genet 12:385–9

45. D'Adamo P, Fassone L, Gedeon A, Janssen EA, Bione S, Bolhuis PA, Barth PG, Wilson M, Haan E, Orstavik KH, Patton MA, Green AJ, Zammarchi E, Donati MA, Toniolo D (1997) The X-linked gene G4.5 is responsible for different infantile dilated cardiomyopathies. Am J Hum Genet 61:862–7

46. Neuwald AF (1997) Barth syndrome may be due to an acyltransferase deficiency. Curr Biol 7:R465–6

47. Schlame M, Kelley RI, Feigenbaum A, Towbin JA, Heerdt PM, Schieble T, Wanders RJ, DiMauro S, Blanck TJ (2003) Phospholipid abnormalities in children with Barth syndrome. J Am Coll Cardiol 42:1994–9

48. Vreken P, Valianpour F, Nijtmans LG, Grivell LA, Plecko B, Wanders RJ, Barth PG (2000) Defective remodeling of cardiolipin and phosphatidyl-glycerol in Barth syndrome. Biochem Biophys Res Commun 279:378–82

49. Bonnet D, Martin D, De Lonlay P, Villain E, Jouvet P, Rabier D, Brivet M, Saudubray JM (1999) Arrhythmias and conduction defects as presenting symptoms of fatty acid oxidation disorders in children. Circulation 100:2248–53

50. Stanley CA, Hale DE, Berry DT, Deleeuw S, Boxer J, Bonnefont JP. (1992) A deficiency of carnitine-acylcarnitine translocase in the inner mitochondrial membrane. New Engl J Med 327:19–23

51. Corr PB, Creer MH, Yamada KA, Saffitz JE, Sobel BE (1989) Prophylaxis of early ventricular fibrillation by inhibition of acylcarnitine accumulation. J. Clin. Invest 83:927–36

52. Tripp ME (1989) Developmental cardiac metabolism in health and disease. Pediatr Cardiol 10:150–8

53. Lutter M, Fang M, Luo X, Nishijima M, Xie X, Wang X (2000) Cardiolipin provides specificity for targeting of tBid to mitochondria. Nat Cell Biol 2:754–61

54. Hickson-Bick DL, Buja ML, McMillin JB (2000) Palmitate-mediated alterations in the fatty acid metabolism of rat neonatal cardiac myocytes. J Mol Cell Cardiol 32:511–19

55. De Vries JE, Vork MM, Roemen TH, de Jong YF, Cleutjens JP, van der Vusse GJ, van Bilsen M (1997) Saturated but not monounsaturated fatty acids induce apoptotic cell death in neonatal rat ventricular myocytes. J Lipid Res 38:1384–94

56. Sparagna GC, Hickson-Bick DL, Buja LM, McMillin JB (2001) Fatty acid-induced apoptosis in neonatal cardiomyocytes: Redox signaling. Antioxid Redox Signal 3:71–9

57. Ostrander DB, Sparagna GC, Amoscato AA, McMillin JB, Dowhan W (2001) Decreased cardiolipin synthesis corresponds with cytochrome c release in palmitate-induced cardiomyocyte apoptosis. J Biol Chem 276:38061–67

58. Kong JY, Rabkin SW (2003) Mitochondrial effects with ceramide-induced cardiac apoptosis are different from those of palmitate. Arch Biochem Biophys 412:196–206

59. Hickson-Bick DL, Sparagna GC, Buja LM, McMillin JB (2002) Palmitate-induced apoptosis in neonatal cardiomyocytes is not dependent on the generation of ROS. Am J Physiol Heart Circ Physiol 282:H656–64

60. Sparagna GC, Hickson-Bick DL, Buja LM, McMillin JB (2000) A metabolic role for mitochondria in palmitate-induced cardiac myocyte apoptosis. Am J Physiol Heart Circ Physiol 279:H2124–32

61. Sparagna GC, Hickson-Bick DL (1999) Cardiac fatty acid metabolism and the induction of apoptosis. Am J Med Sci 318:15–21

62. Malhotra R, Brosius FC (1999) Glucose uptake and glycolysis reduce hypoxia-induced apoptosis in cultured neonatal rat cardiac myocytes. J Biol Chem 274:12567–75

63. Lin Z, Weinberg JM, Malhotra R, Merritt SE, Holzman LB, Brosius FC (2000) GLUT-1 reduces hypoxia-induced apoptosis and JNK pathway activation. Am J Physiol Endocrinol Metab 278:E958–66

64. Fujio Y, Nguyen T, Wencker D, Kitsis RN, Walsh K (2000) Akt promotes survival of cardiomyocytes in vitro and protects against ischemia-reperfusion injury in mouse heart. Circulation 101:660–7

65. Aikawa R, Nawano M, Gu Y, Katagiri H, Asano T, Zhu W, Nagai R, Komuro I (2000) Insulin prevents cardiomyocytes from oxidative stress-induced apoptosis through activation of PI3 kinase/Akt. Circulation 102:2873–9

66. Cai L, Li W, Wang G, Guo L, Jiang Y, Kang YJ (2002) Hyperglycemia-induced apoptosis in mouse myocardium: Mitochondrial cytochrome c-mediated caspase-3 activation pathway. Diabetes 51:1938–48

67. Rotig A, Bonnefont JP, Munnich A (1996) Mitochondrial diabetes mellitus. Diabetes Metab 22:291–8

68. Maassen JA, 'T Hart LM, Van Essen E, Heine RJ, Nijpels G, Jahangir Tafrechi RS, Raap AK, Janssen GM, Lemkes HH (2004)

Mitochondrial diabetes: Molecular mechanisms and clinical presentation. Diabetes 53:S103–9

69. Hattori Y, Nakajima K, Eizawa T, Ehara T, Koyama M, Hirai T, Fukuda Y, Kinoshita M (2003) Heteroplasmic mitochondrial DNA 3310 mutation in NADH dehydrogenase subunit 1 associated with type 2 diabetes, hypertrophic cardiomyopathy, and mental retardation in a single patient. Diabetes Care 26:952–3

70. Suzuki S, Oka Y, Kadowaki T, Kanatsuka A, Kuzuya T, Kobayashi M, Sanke T, Seino Y, Nanjo K (2003) Clinical features of diabetes mellitus with the mitochondrial DNA 3243 (A-G) mutation in Japanese: Maternal inheritance and mitochondria-related complications. Diabetes Res Clin Pract 59:207–17

71. Hsieh RH, Li JY, Pang CY, Wei YH (2001) A novel mutation in the mitochondrial 16S rRNA gene in a patient with MELAS syndrome, diabetes mellitus, hyperthyroidism and cardiomyopathy. J Biomed Sci 8:328–35

72. Shen X, Zheng S, Thongboonkerd V, Xu M, Pierce Jr WM, Klein JB, Epstein PN (2004) Cardiac mitochondrial damage and biogenesis in a chronic model of type I diabetes. Am J Physiol Endocrinol Metab 287:E896–905

73. Feillet F, Steinmann G, Vianey-Saban C, de Chillou C, Sadoul N, Lefebvre E, Vidailhet M, Bollaert PE (2003) Adult presentation of MCAD deficiency revealed by coma and severe arrythmias. Intensive Care Med 29:1594–7

74. Kelly DP, Hale DE, Rutledge SL, Ogden ML, Whelan AJ, Zhang Z, Strauss AW. (1992) Molecular basis of inherited medium chain acyl-CoA dehydrogenase deficiency causing sudden child death. J Inherit Metab Dis 15:171–80

75. Tanaka K, Yokota I, Coates PM (1992) Mutations in the medium chain acyl-CoA dehydrogenase (MCAD) gene. Hum Mutat 1:271–9

76. Andresen BS, Bross P, Jensen TG, Knudsen I, Winter V, Kolvraa S, Bolund L, Gregersen N (1995) Molecular diagnosis and characterization of medium-chain acyl-CoA dehydrogenase deficiency. Scand J Clin Lab Invest Suppl 220:9–25

77. Mathur A, Sims HF, Gopalakrishnan D, Gibson B, Rinaldo P, Vockley J, Hug G, Strauss AW (1999) Molecular heterogeneity in very-long-chain acyl-CoA dehydrogenase deficiency causing pediatric cardiomyopathy and sudden death. Circulation 99:1337–43

78. Bonnefont JP, Taroni F, Cavadini P, Cepanec C, Brivet M, Sau-

dubray JM, Leroux JP, Demaugre F (1996) Molecular analysis of carnitine palmitoyltransferase II deficiency with hepatocardiomuscular expression. Am J Hum Genet 58:971–8

79. Taroni F, Verderio E, Fiorucci S, Cavadini P, Finocchiaro G, Uziel G, Lamantea E, Gellera C, DiDonato S (1992) Molecular characterization of inherited carnitine palmitoyltransferase II deficiency. Proc Natl Acad Sci 89:8429–33

80. Orii KE, Aoyama T, Wakui K, Fukushima Y, Miyajima H, Yamaguchi S, Orii T, Kondo N, Hashimoto T (1997) Genomic and mutational analysis of the mitochondrial trifunctional protein beta-subunit (HADHB) gene in patients with trifunctional protein deficiency. Hum Mol Genet 6:1215–24

81. Schwab KO, Ensenauer R, Matern D, Uyanik G, Schnieders B, Wanders RA, Lehnert W (2003) Complete deficiency of mitochondrial trifunctional protein due to a novel mutation within the beta-subunit of the mitochondrial trifunctional protein gene leads to failure of long-chain fatty acid beta-oxidation with fatal outcome. Eur J Pediatr 162:90–5

82. Spiekerkoetter U, Khuchua Z, Yue Z, Bennett MJ, Strauss AW (2004) General mitochondrial trifunctional protein (TFP) deficiency as a result of either alpha- or beta-subunit mutations exhibits similar phenotypes because mutations in either subunit alter TFP complex expression and subunit turnover. Pediatr Res 55:190–6

83. Ibdah JA, Zhao Y, Viola J, Gibson B, Bennett MJ, Strauss AW (2001) Molecular prenatal diagnosis in families with fetal mitochondrial trifunctional protein mutations. J Pediatr 138:396–9

84. Barger PM, Kelly DP (2000) PPAR signaling in the control of cardiac energy metabolism. Trends Cardiovasc Med 10:238–45

85. Finck BN, Kelly DP (2002) Peroxisome proliferator-activated receptor alpha (PPARalpha) signaling in the gene regulatory control of energy metabolism in the normal and diseased heart. J Mol Cell Cardiol 34:1249–57

86. Gulick T, Cresci S, Caira T, Moore DD, Kelly DP (1994) The peroxisome proliferator activated receptor regulates mitochondrial fatty acid oxidative enzyme gene expression. Proc Natl Acad Sci USA 91:11012–16

87. Kelly DP (2003) PPARs of the heart: Three is a crowd. Circ Res 92:482–4

88. Barger PM, Brandt JM, Leone TC, Weinheimer CJ, Kelly DP (2000) Deactivation of peroxisome proliferator-activated receptor-alpha during cardiac hypertrophic growth. J Clin Invest 105:1723–30

89. Huss JM, Levy FH, Kelly DP (2001) Hypoxia inhibits the peroxisome proliferator-activated receptor alpha/retinoid X receptor gene regulatory pathway in cardiac myocytes: A mechanism for $O_2$-dependent modulation of mitochondrial fatty acid oxidation. J Biol Chem 276:27605–12

90. Finck BN, Lehman JJ, Leone TC, Welch MJ, Bennett MJ, Kovacs A, Han X, Gross RW, Kozak R, Lopaschuk GD, Kelly DP (2002) The cardiac phenotype induced by PPARalpha overexpression mimics that caused by diabetes mellitus. J Clin Invest 109:121–30

91. Gilde AJ, van der Lee KA, Willemsen PH, Chinetti G, van der Leij FR, van der Vusse GJ, Staels B, van Bilsen M (2003) Peroxisome proliferator-activated receptor (PPAR) alpha and PPARbeta/delta, but not PPARgamma, modulate the expression of genes involved in cardiac lipid metabolism. Circ Res 92:518–24

92. Wu Z, Puigserver P, Andersson U, Zhang C, Adelmant G, Mootha V, Troy A, Cinti S, Lowell B, Scarpulla RC, Spiegelman BM (1999) Mechanisms controlling mitochondrial biogenesis and respiration through the thermogenic coactivator PGC-1. Cell 98:115–24

93. Lehman JJ, Barger PM, Kovacs A, Saffitz JE, Medeiros DM,Kelly DP (2000) Peroxisome proliferator-activated receptor gamma coactivator-1 promotes cardiac mitochondrial biogenesis. J Clin Invest 106:847–56

94. Vega RB, Huss JM, Kelly DP (2000) The coactivator PGC-1 cooperates with peroxisome proliferator-activated receptor in transcriptional control of nuclear genes encoding mitochondrial fatty acid oxidation enzymes. Mol Cell Biol 20:1868–76

95. Russell LK, Mansfield CM, Lehman JJ, Kovacs A, Courtois M, Saffitz JE, Medeiros DM, Valencik ML, McDonald JA, Kelly DP (2004) Cardiac-specific induction of the transcriptional coactivator peroxisome proliferator-activated receptor gamma coactivator-1alpha promotes mitochondrial biogenesis and reversible cardiomyopathy in a developmental stage-dependent manner. Circ Res 94:525–33.

96. Djouadi F, Brandt JM, Weinheimer CJ, Leone TC, Gonzalez FJ, Kelly DP (1999) The role of the peroxisome proliferator-activated receptor alpha (PPAR a) in the control of cardiac lipid metabolism. Prostaglandins Leukot Essent Fatty Acids 60:339–43

97. Ibdah JA, Paul H, Zhao Y, B nford S, Salleng K, Cline M, Matern D, Bennett MJ, Rinaldo P, Strauss AW (2001) Lack of mitochondrial trifunctional protein in mice causes neonatal hypoglycemia and sudden death. J Clin Invest 107:1403–9

98. Chiu HC, Kovacs A, Ford D, Hsu FF, Garcia R, Herrero P, Saffitz JE, Schaffer JE (2001) A novel mouse model of lipotoxic cardiomyopathy. J Clin Invest 107:813–22

99. Ruiz-Lozano P, Smith SM, Perkins G, Kubalak SW, Boss GR, Sucov HM, Evans RM, Chien KR (1998) Energy deprivation and a deficiency in downstream metabolic target genes during the onset of embryonic heart failure in RXR alpha -/- embryos. Development 125:533–44

100. Graham BH, Waymire KG, Cottrell B, Trounce IA, MacGregor GR, Wallace DC (1997) A mouse model for mitochondrial myopathy and cardiomyopathy resulting from a deficiency in the heart/muscle isoform of the adenine nucleotide translocator. Nat Genet 16:226–34

101. Wang J, Wilhelmsson H, Graff C, Li H, Oldfors A, Rustin P, Bruning JC, Kahn CR, Clayton DA, Barsh GS, Thoren P, Larsson NG (1999) Dilated cardiomyopathy and atrioventricular conduction blocks induced by heart-specific inactivation of mitochondrial DNA gene expression. Nat Genet 21:133–7

102. Hansson A, Hance N, Dufour E, Rantanen A, Hultenby K, Clayton DA, Wibom R, Larsson NG (2004) A switch in metabolism precedes increased mitochondrial biogenesis in respiratory chain-deficient mouse hearts. Proc Natl Acad Sci USA 101:3136–41

103. Touma EH, Rashed MS, Vianey-Saban C, Sakr A, Divry P, Gregersen N, Andresen BS (2001) A severe genotype with favourable outcome in very long chain acyl-CoA dehydrogenase deficiency. Arch Dis Child 84:58–60

# Chapter 8

# Mitochondria in Pediatric Cardiology

## Overview

Abnormalities in cardiac mitochondrial respiratory enzyme function and mtDNA have been identified in an increasing number of children and infants with either DCM or HCM, giving rise to the entity known as *mitochondrial cardiomyopathy*. In addition, children with congenital heart defects (CHD) and in particular those in HF often present with defects in the structure and function of mitochondria. Awareness of the mitochondrial role in heart bioenergetics and of the potential association of CHD with gene mutations that may affect mitochondrial respiration and metabolism is important. The histochemical, biochemical, and molecular findings of mitochondrial cardiomyopathy, which will be helpful for its diagnosis in neonates and children, and the role that mitochondrial defects play in a number of congenital heart defects are presented in this chapter.

## MITOCHONDRIAL CARDIOMYOPATHY

## Introduction

Mitochondrial cardiomyopathy (MCM) can be defined as an OXPHOS disease characterized by abnormal cardiac mitochondria either in number, structure or function. By altering ETC function, specific pathogenic mtDNA mutations or depletion of mtDNA levels may also result in cardiomyopathy. MCM may present either a hypertrophic phenotype (characterized primarily by left ventricular or biventricular hypertrophy often accompanied by myofibril disarray) or a dilated phenotype (characterized by increased ventricular size and impaired ventricular function).

Many of the described mitochondrial cardiomyopathies occur in conjunction with primarily neurological disorders such as MELAS, MERRF, KSS, and Leigh syndromes and with the less characterized family of cardioneuropathies [1–3]. This association likely stems from the strong demand that neural (e.g., brain and ocular tissue) and cardiac tissue have for oxidative energy, as well as their extreme sensitivity to its deprivation. These disorders may present early in childhood, while others manifest themselves later (adult or adolescent onset). Mitochondrial abnormalities have also been reported in a number of cases of fatal infantile cardiomyopathy [4–7].

Biochemical analysis has demonstrated that specific defects in mitochondrial ETC and/or OXPHOS are the major loci of mitochondrial dysfunction in MCM [1–2]. Since the 5 multisubunit respiratory complexes (I to V) located in the mitochondrial inner membrane consist of over 70 different types of polypeptide components, a large number of potential sites for defects are present in the pathway for energy generation (Figure 8.1).

In MCM as well as in other OXPHOS diseases, single or multiple defects in each of the respiratory complex activities can be present [4, 8–10]. Some of these defects are attributable to defined changes in mtDNA, such as specific mutations in the mitochondrial protein synthesis apparatus (e.g., mitochondrial encoded tRNAs) [4] or mutations in structural protein-encoding genes [11–12]. However, in the majority of mitochondrial based cardiomyopathies, the primary site of defect has not yet been elucidated.

A pattern of maternal inheritance can be used to corroborate the presence of a mitochondrial-based pathology in a number of familial cardiomyopathies [4, 13–14]. However, mutations in nuclear genes may also be associated with MCM. For instance, a mutation in a nuclear gene involved in mtDNA replication has been implicated in an autosomally inherited cardiomyopathy characterized by the accumulation of multiple mtDNA deletions in the patient's brain and heart [15–16]. Mutations in 2 nuclear genes NDUFV2 and NDUFS2, encoding subunits of respiratory complex I, have been implicated in the development of early onset HCM [17–18].

Moreover, fatal infantile cardiomyopathy can result from the severe skeletal and cardiac muscle complex IV deficiency found in patients with mutations in the nuclear $SCO_2$ gene. This gene encodes the copper-binding protein involved in the assembly of COX subunits into a functional complex IV enzyme [19].

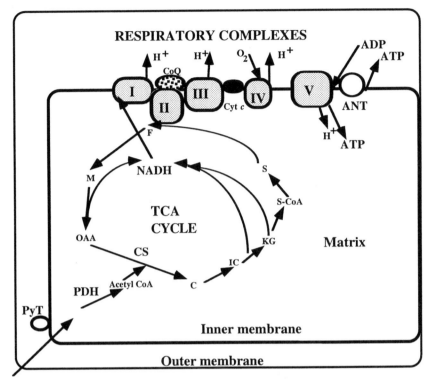

**Figure 8.1. Mitochondrial structure and major metabolic reactions involved in OXPHOS**. *The electron transport chain with respiratory complexes I to V is illustrated showing directional proton movement ($H^+$) as indicated. The electron carriers CoQ (coenzyme Q) and cytochrome c (Cyt c) are depicted with stippled circles. The TCA cycle is shown with several key metabolic intermediates identified: malate (M), oxaloacetic acid (OAA), citric acid (C), isocitrate (IC), α-ketoglutarate (KG), succinate (S), succinyl-CoA (S-CoA), fumarate (F), and NADH. Pyruvate transporters (PyT) and the ATP/ADP translocator (ANT) are indicated by the light circles. Other key enzymes shown are PDH (pyruvate dehydrogenase) and CS (citrate synthase). Also noted is the general organization of the mitochondrial compartments: inner and outer membranes and matrix.*

MCM can also occur in a sporadic fashion. Various agents that cause damage to the mitochondria can result in cardiomyopathy. Some of these agents may have nonspecific or multiple modes of action on both mitochondria and the cell (e.g., alcohol, adriamycin, and ischemia). The relationship of sporadic mtDNA damage to cardiomyopathy is of great interest since somatically generated mtDNA deletions increase during myocardial ischemia [20]. In addition, KSS, a neuromuscular disorder with atrioventricular conduction defects and cardiomyopathy, is commonly associated with abundant large-scale mtDNA deletions whose generation is thought to be spontaneous, since they are rarely detected in mothers or siblings. In contrast, a severe cardiomyopathy associated with multiple mtDNA deletions and progressive external ophthalmoplegia (PEO) is transmitted by an autosomally recessive nuclear gene defect [21]. This defect along with mutations in other nuclear genes such as Twinkle, ANT1, and POLγ presumably affects proteins involved in DNA maintenance, leading to the development of multiple mtDNA deletions and cardiac pathology. This unique etiology of cardiac pathology, involving both Mendelian transmission and mitochondrial cytopathy has been termed a "dual genome" disease [22].

As previously discussed, the molecular basis and pathogenic significance of mtDNA deletions in the cardiomyopathic heart in most clinical cases remains undefined. Among the agents that have been shown to result in specific mitochondrial damage and cardiomyopathy are adriamycin and zidovudine (AZT) [23–24].

## Diagnosis

Findings at the clinical, histochemical, biochemical, and molecular levels are used in the characterization of MCM. The highly variable clinical manifestations of MCM are indicative of both the heterogeneity of the disease as well as its frequent association with multisystemic disorder. Histochemical and morphological analysis to determine abnormality in mitochondria structure or number has proven informative in some cases but is not always specific. Biochemical analysis demonstrating reductions in specific respiratory enzymes activities is probably the most consistent assay for MCM. The biochemical analysis of the respiratory chain requires (in most cases) highly invasive endomyocardial biopsy, although enzyme analysis of biopsied skeletal muscle can be informative as noted in Chapter 6. Another important diagnostic tool in evaluating MCM is the analysis of specific molecular genetic changes such as mtDNA point mutations and deletions, increasingly identified in cardiomyopathies. The molecular genetic analysis of mtDNA mutations with blood, biopsied skeletal muscle, or cultured cells can also be informative. A definitive assessment of MCM should include both a molecular genetic and biochemical analysis combined with a comprehensive clinical and histochemical profile.

## Clinical signs

MCM has often been found in association with certain "soft" clinical signs in patients and maternal relatives including hearing loss, hypotonia, and migraine-like headaches. Manifestations of cardiac involvement include DCM, HCM, and ventricular dysrhythmias [25]. Lactic acidosis is commonly present, and many patients display generalized muscle weakness [26–27].

## Histological and electron microscopic (EM) analysis

Abnormalities in mitochondrial structure may be found including but not limited to distended cristae, electron dense and paracrystalline inclusions, and swollen or distended mitochondrial membranes. In addition to these abnormalities, giant mitochondria may also be present [28]. Increased number and aggregation of abnormal mitochondria are often detected in particular with cardiac hypertrophy. Ragged-red fibers (RRF) are often present in skeletal muscle as shown in Figure 8.2. RRF are associated with disorders of adult/adolescent onset [29], commonly present in disorders caused by defects in mitochondrial protein synthesis and rarely present in disorders associated with mitochondrial structural gene defects [30]. EM will allow assessment of mitochondria number and structural abnormalities (Figure 8.3).

Enzyme immunostaining has proved to be a useful adjunct in assessing the relative amounts of specific enzyme activity in muscle fibers and specific enzyme content (e.g., cytochrome $c$ oxidase) [31]. In addition, immunohistochemical studies of skeletal muscle biopsies of children with COX deficiencies have been used to distinguish between mtDNA and nuclear DNA specific defects, based on the levels of mtDNA-encoded subunits COXI and COXII relative to changes in nuclear DNA-encoded subunits COXIV and COXVA [32].

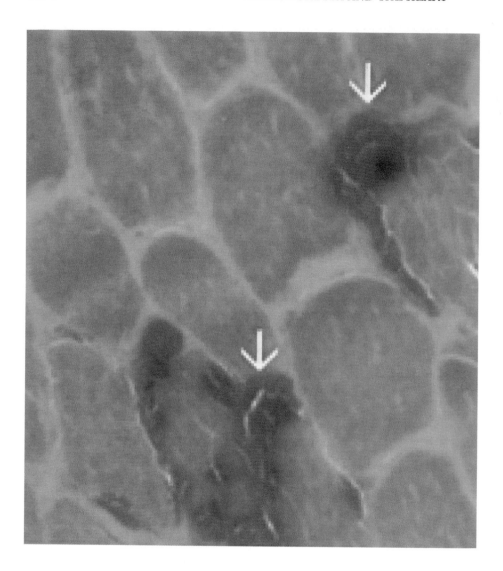

**Figure 8.2. Quadriceps femoris muscle biopsy.** *This biopsy shows fibers with basophilic sarcoplasmic masses, corresponding to ragged-red fibers (arrows) clearly identified with modified Gomori trichrome stain because these subsarcolemmal zones are irregular in shape and intensely red in color, whereas the normal myofibrils are green.*

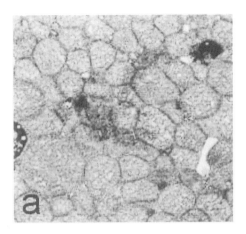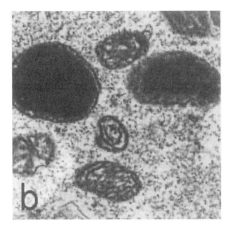

**Figure 8.3. Mitochondrial defects.** *( a) Increased mitochondrial number in cardiac muscle and ( b) giant mitochondria with electron-dense deposits in skeletal muscle of a child with mitochondrial cardiomyopathy*

## *Biochemical analysis*

Using either crude tissue homogenates or isolated mitochondria, the specific activity levels of each respiratory complex can be evaluated. Mitochondrial based diseases such as MELAS and MERRF most often exhibit deficiencies in complex I and complex IV activities [33–34]. Deficiencies in either complex V, complex IV, or PDH activities have been described in Leigh syndrome [12, 35–37]. Complex IV deficiency has also been described in isolated cases of pediatric cardiomyopathy [38–39] and is the most common recognized respiratory chain defect in childhood. Infants with histiocytoid cardiomyopathy —which is characterized by cardiomegaly, ventricular tachycardia, and frequently sudden death occurring within the first 2 years of life— harbor defects in respiratory enzyme activities including complexes III [40] and IV [41]. Moreover, in children with DCM, reduced levels of specific cardiac respiratory chain enzyme activities were frequently found that ranged from 35 to 70% of age-matched control values [42]. Reduced activity levels of complex III were most often observed although cases exhibiting reduced activities of complexes I, IV, and V were also noted. Other studies using biopsied cardiac tissue from children with HCM found reduced complex I and IV activities [43]. Why specific mtDNA-encoded enzymes are affected while others are unaffected is not known.

## MtDNA analysis

As previously noted, a number of mtDNA mutations have been reported to play a role in the pathogenesis of cardiomyopathies. Defects in mtDNA identified thus far include specific point mutations in mitochondrial tRNA genes and in several of the 13 protein-encoding mitochondrial structural genes.

Other mtDNA abnormalities include increased abundance of specific large-scale mtDNA deletions in cardiomyopathic tissues, although their pathogenic role remains to be established. Additional types of mtDNA rearrangement (including tandem duplications of sequence) and defective genetic loci (including mitochondrial ribosomal RNA genes) have also been reported [44–45].

Distinguishing pathogenic mutations from polymorphic variations in nucleotide sequence is not simple. Moreover, a number of mtDNA sequence changes previously characterized as polymorphic variants have been found to be associated with an increased incidence of cardiomyopathy; these include both homoplasmic and heteroplasmic modifications in the D-loop regulatory region (e.g., nt 16093, 16168, 16186, and 16189) [46–48].

## Mitochondrial tRNA mutations

Defects in mitochondrial tRNAs, which play a key role in protein synthesis, are involved in the genesis of multisystemic diseases with associated cardiomyopathy including MELAS [49], MERRF [50], and Leigh syndrome [51]. Children with cardiomyopathy have been screened for evidence of tRNA mutation using a variety of techniques such as single-strand conformation polymorphism (SSCP) analysis [52], restriction enzyme digestion [53], and automated DNA sequencing [54]. Point mutations in tRNA genes (e.g. $tRNA^{Leu}$, $tRNA^{Ile}$, $tRNA^{Val}$, $tRNA^{Lys}$, and $tRNA^{Gly}$) have been associated with HCM [55–60], a number of which are shown in Figure 8.4.

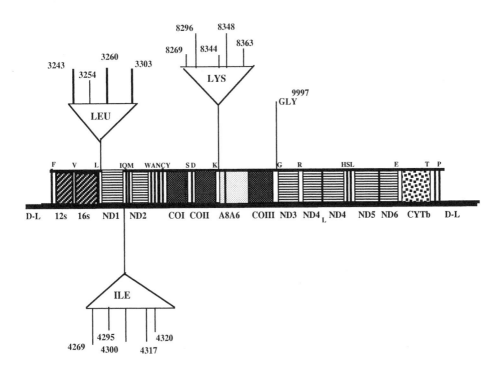

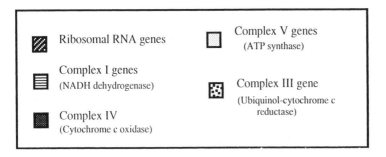

**Figure 8.4. Linear representation of the circular 16,569 basepair human mtDNA molecule.** *It shows the location of all 13 protein-encoding genes (ND1-ND6, COI- COIII, cytb, ATP6, and ATP8), 22 tRNAs identified by their cognate amino acid using single-letter code (F, V, L, I, Q, M, W, A, N, C, Y, S, D, K, G, R, H, S, L, E, T, P), the 2 rRNA genes (12S and 16S), and the noncoding D-loop region (D-L). Position of pathogenic mtDNA mutations in tRNA genes, including leu, lys, ile, and gly, are shown.*

Molecular data concerning the location of these mutations, biochemical findings concerning the enzymes affected, the inheritance pattern, the relative proportion of mutant relative to wild type alleles (heteroplasmy), and pertinent clinical findings are presented in Table 8.1. For certain mutations (e.g., 3243 in tRNA$^{Leu}$ and 8344 in tRNA$^{Lys}$) clinical manifestations are often delayed occurring primarily in adolescents or adults. However, although atypical, early presentation of cardiomyopathy has been reported in cases with mutation at nt 3243 [61] and recently in a case of fatal infantile histiocytoid cardiomyopathy with a sporadic nt 8344 mutation in heart and liver [41]. For other less frequent tRNA mutations, particularly those associated with fatal infantile cardiomyopathy (e.g., 4269 tRNA$^{Ile}$, 4317 tRNA$^{Ile}$, 4320 tRNA$^{Ile}$, and 3303 tRNA$^{Leu}$), given the limited number of cases reported thus far, it is presently unknown whether or not the clinical outcome will invariably be the same. The majority of the aforementioned studies detected tRNA mutations using mtDNA derived from biopsied skeletal muscle. In some instances, the amount of the mutant allele is high enough to be detected in blood as well [62]. However, more often, analysis of the patient's blood has provided limited information since hematopoietic cells may lose mtDNA mutations [1–2]. Moreover, different quantities of both normal and mutant alleles may be found in the patient (i.e., heteroplasmy), an intracellular mixture of wild-type and mutant genomes that may be different dependent on the tissue examined. This is in contrast with situations where only one allele or the other is found (i.e., homoplasmy). Only when the percentage of mutant tRNA genes increases above a certain tissue-specific threshold does protein synthesis become inhibited resulting in decreased activity levels of specific respiration enzymes and abnormal cellular phenotypes [1–3]. Young individuals (<20 years of age) appear to have higher thresholds requiring as much as 95% of mutant mtDNAs in order to express the disease phenotype.

Moderately and severely deleterious mtDNA mutations are likely to be heteroplasmic while mildly deleterious mtDNA mutations are homoplasmic [63]. For example, the 3303 tRNA$^{Leu}$ mutation was described as homoplasmic in the proband and a close relative both who died of fatal infantile cardiomyopathy; however, maternal relatives with milder symptoms were heteroplasmic for this allele [4].

**Table 8.1. tRNA mutations in mitochondrial cardiomyopathy**

| Gene | Site | Freq | HOM/ HET | Signs and Symptoms | Ref | Biochemical Findings |
|------|------|------|----------|--------------------|-----|----------------------|
| leu | 3243 A→G | NUM | HET | MELAS, RRF, HCM | [41] | Defects in I + IV activities and protein translation |
| leu | 3260 A→G | LIM | HET | Dypsnea, CM, tachycardia | [48] | I + IV defects |
| leu | 3303 C→T | LIM | HOM/ HET | FICM myopathy | [4] | Unknown |
| ile | 4300 A→G | LIM | HOM/ HET | Dyspnea, RRF, HCM | [14] | No defects in muscle or heart |
| ile | 4317 A→G | ND | ND | FICM | [5] | IV defect |
| ile | 4320 C→T | LIM | HET | FICM, seizures | [49] | No defects in OXPHOS |
| ile | 4269 A→G | LIM | HOM/ HET | Deafness, epilepsy, RRF HF at 18 yr, | [6] | IV defect |
| lys | 8344 A→G | NUM | HET | Leigh, MERRF, hist CM | [42] | I and IV defects |
| lys | 8296 A→G | LIM | HET | Fatal HCM | [66] | N.D. |
| lys | 8363 G→A | LIM | HET | Hearing loss, ataxia, HCM | [13, 43] | I, III + IV defects; high II activity |
| gly | 9997 T→C | LIM | HET | Arrhythmia, HCM | [47] | I, III + IV defects |

*Note*: Freq, frequency; LIM, limited; NUM, numerous; FICM, fatal infantile cardiomyopathy; Ref, references; HOM, homoplasmy; HET, heteroplasmy; RRF, ragged red fiber; hist CM, histiocytoid cardiomyopathy; HCM, hypertrophic cardiomyopathy; HF, heart failure; MELAS, mitochondrial myopathy, encephalopathy, lactic acidosis and strokelike episodes; MERRF, myoclonic epilepsy and ragged red fibers; N.D., not determined.

A homoplasmic mutation at 12192 in tRNA$^{His}$ has been reported in several patients with DCM [64]. A pathogenic mutation in tRNA$^{Ile}$ at nt 4300 was homoplasmic in all samples from several unrelated children affected with severe HCM as well as their maternal relatives [65]. Such findings suggest that caution is warranted in assessing pathogenicity as a function of heteroplasmy.

Detection of specific tRNA mutations has been made relatively simple by the use of restriction fragment digestion of PCR amplified products containing the gene sequence of interest. Defective mtDNA genes can be characterized by either a loss or a gain of a restriction enzyme site. For the analysis of sequence changes that do not alter natural restriction sites, a restriction site can been created using "mismatched" primers that will distinguish between the presence of the wild-type and mutant alleles [67]. All of the point mutations in tRNA noted in Table 8.1 have been analyzed by restriction digestion. This approach has made possible the detection of each of the defective alleles described above using minimal tissue, limited technology, and resources. Similar diagnostic tests can also be performed with genes (e.g., β-MHC and acyl-CoA dehydrogenase) in which a number of specific mutations have been identified that are associated with a poor clinical outcome in patients with HCM, as described in Chapters 6 and 7 [68–69]. These molecular genetic tests in combination with an analysis of pedigree/inheritance (e.g., an autosomal dominant pattern for β-MHC defects) can be used in excluding these defects, which are particularly common in cases of familial HCM [70–71], in the differential diagnosis of MCM.

As frequently found with nuclear gene mutations (e.g., β-MHC mutations) associated with HCM [72], the consensus experience with mtDNA mutations has been that each specific HCM-causing mutation tends to be relatively rare, challenging the view of common mutations and that most families have "private" or novel mutations; however, some pathogenic mtDNA mutations are more prevalent. Nevertheless, correlation of the clinical course and prognosis with the presence of specific mutant alleles (and with their overall proportion relative to wild type alleles) has proved highly informative in several cases.

Other mitochondrial tRNA mutations have been reported whose association with cardiomyopathy remain to be confirmed. For instance, a heteroplasmic mutation in tRNA$^{Pro}$ at 15990 converting the tRNA$^{Pro}$ anticodon to that of tRNA$^{Ser}$ was reported in a child with a myopathy characterized by progressive weakness of the extremities [73]. While mitochondrial respiratory complex activity levels in the patient's biopsied skeletal muscle were severely decreased, there was no evidence of cardiac involvement.

Mutations have also been found in the anticodon stem and loop of tRNA$^{Thr}$ at 15923 and 15924 in 2 unrelated cases of fatal infantile respiratory failure [74] and in tRNA$^{Thr}$ at 15928 in several cases of cardiomyopathy [75]. Although the pathogenicity of these mutations has been called into question, since the 15924 tRNA$^{Thr}$ and 15928 tRNA$^{Thr}$ mutations have been observed in control tissues [76], the mutant allele at nt 15924 has been confirmed in patients with cardiomyopathy rather than in normal subjects [77].

## *Mitochondrial structural gene mutations*

An important criteria in assessing pathogenicity of a specific mutant allele in a mtDNA protein-encoding gene relates to how conserved in evolution is the amino acid residue that is altered [63]. Albeit rarely present, point mutations in moderately and highly conserved amino acid residues associated with cardiomyopathy have been identified in many of the 13 mtDNA-encoded proteins including ATPase6, cyt*b*, COXI, COXII, ND3, ND5, and ND1 and are discussed in more detail below.

## *ATP synthase (ATPase6)*

Leigh syndrome is a rapidly progressive neurodegenerative childhood disease with variable clinical manifestations including seizures, ataxia, basal ganglia lesions, and muscle weakness that can be associated with HCM [12, 78]. A mutation in ATPase6 has been reported in several independent cases of Leigh syndrome with associated cardiomyopathy. The ATPase6 mutation is a T→G transversion at np 8993 converting a highly conserved hydrophobic leucine 156 to arginine [79–81]. In biochemical studies with cultured lymphocytes derived from patients with Leigh disease, a pronounced defect was noted in the proton channel of the H$^+$-translocating ATP synthase, thus inhibiting ATP generation from OXPHOS [80]. Abnormal activity of complex V was also found in the heart and skeletal muscle of an unrelated individual with Leigh cardiomyopathy containing the same mutation [35]. This mutation has been shown to present itself heteroplasmically in maternal relatives while the patient had >95%

mutant mtDNA in several tissues (e.g., heart, brain and skeletal muscle). The relative concentration of the mutant allele correlates with the clinical severity of the disease.

A severe phenotype ("true" Leigh syndrome) occurs with a higher percentage of mutant genomes; lesser amounts of the mutant allele are associated with milder symptoms often termed *NARP syndrome* (neurogenic muscle weakness, ataxia, and retinitis pigmentosa) [63]. A second heteroplasmic, maternally inherited mutation located at the same position 8993 (T→C) resulting in a leucine →proline change has also been reported [82]. Mutations at a variety of other genetic loci can also cause Leigh syndrome (e.g., point mutations at several sites including the mitochondrial $tRNA^{Lys}$ gene [51], nuclear genes encoding subunits of PDH [37], the flavoprotein subunit of complex II [83], and COX assembly factor $SCO_2$ [19]).

## Cytochrome b (cytb)

Several mutations in the cyt*b* gene have been identified in children with cardiomyopathy. The first, an A→G mutation at nt 14927 in cyt*b*, converting a highly conserved threonine to an alanine residue, was found in the cardiac mtDNA of a 1-year-old male with marked cardiomegaly who died of HF [11]. Second, a mutation at nt 15236 converting a highly conserved isoleucine to a valine at residue 164 has been described in 2 unrelated patients [84]; a 7-year-old female with familial DCM and a 19-year-old male presenting with HCM. Unfortunately, data concerning the extent of heteroplasmy, inheritance pattern, and respiratory enzyme activity analysis were not reported in these cases. The third cyt*b* mutation, a C→A at nt 15452 in cyt*b*, converted a leucine to an isoleucine at residue 236 [85]. This mutation was heteroplasmic, present in 7 of 33 cases of DCM screened and not found in controls (18 individuals), with 4 of the 7 mutant alleles detected in infants under 2 years of age.

In these patients, there was a striking reduction in cardiac complex III activity with levels ranging from 0 to 40% of the control value. Since this mutation does not result in changing a highly conserved amino acid residue, its presence in several cases of Leber's hereditary optic neuropathy (LHON) was previously considered nonpathogenic [86]. Nevertheless, to rigorously prove the pathogenicity of this mutation, its relationship to both the defective complex III activity and to the cellular phenotype will require the analysis of cybrids in which defective mitochondria containing the mutant gene are introduced into cultured cells by cell fusion [87].

In a child with COX deficiency displaying severe histiocytoid cardiomyopathy, a mutant allele in cyt*b* at nt 15498 was detected [88]. This mutation results in the replacement of a neutral amino acid (glycine) with an acidic amino acid (aspartic acid) at a highly conserved residue (251), altering the interactions of cyt*b* with other subunits, thereby affecting complex III assembly and proton transfer function [88–89]. Another study identified a cyt*b* mutation at nt 15243 in a patient with severe HCM and complex III deficiency. This mutation changes a highly conserved glycine to a glutamic acid residue situated within the cd2 helical region of cyt*b* in close proximity to the hinge region of the Rieske iron-sulfur protein and was found to profoundly alter the subunit interactions, conformation of the *bc1* complex, and complex III stability and activity [90–91]. A cyt*b* mutation at nt 15508 in a highly conserved aspartic acid with a glutamic acid residue was found in a female infant with DCM in association with marked complex III deficiency [75].

It is noteworthy that a relatively large number of pathogenic mutations in cyt*b* have been found in cardiomyopathic tissues. While a subset of these mutations represent either neutral amino acid substitutions or likely polymorphisms, it remains to be seen whether there is some additive or synergistic effect of these mutations on mitochondrial function. These findings also imply that cyt*b* represents a hitherto uncharacterized "hotspot" for mtDNA defects, some of which could play an important role in the pathogenesis of cardiomyopathy, adding it to a list that includes several mitochondrial tRNA genes (e.g., tRNA$^{Leu}$, tRNA$^{Ile}$, and tRNA$^{Lys}$) and ATPase6 [1–3].

## *Mutations in COX and ND subunits*

Obayashi and associates [11] found a mutation at COII at nt 7673 converting a highly conserved isoleucine to valine at residue 30 in a 1 year-old patient with cardiomegaly. Ozawa and associates [84] reported a mutation in COI at nt 6521 causing a change from highly conserved isoleucine to methionine at residue 206 in a 7-year-old female with DCM. However, lack of information concerning allele heteroplasmy and enzymatic data precluded a complete evaluation of these mutations' pathogenicity.

Several potentially pathogenic mutations in mtDNA genes encoding complex I subunits have been reported. One in ND5 at nt 13258 converted a highly conserved serine to a cysteine residue in a child with HCM [11] and a second mutation in ND1 at nt 3394 converting a highly conserved threonine to a histidine residue in a child with DCM [84]. Another mutation in ND1 at nt 3310 has been described in a case of HCM in conjunction with type 2 diabetes [92]. As with the COX mutations described above, no biochemical data were available. A severe reduction of complex I activity was found in association with a mutation in ND5 at nt 14069 resulting in a serine to leucine transition in a female of 14 years old with DCM [75].

## *MtDNA depletion*

As previously noted, mtDNA depletion in cardiac cells can also play a role in the pathogenesis of cardiomyopathy. Depletion of wild-type mtDNA has been found as a primary defect in several young patients with mitochondrial myopathy and respiratory enzyme defects [93–94] and has also been shown, in some cases, to be tissue-specific and autosomally transmitted [95–96]. Recently, several nuclear loci have been identified as likely responsible for mtDNA depletion. Autosomal recessive mutations in enzymes that play a role in mitochondrial nucleotide metabolism (e.g., thymidine kinase, thymidine phosphorylase, and deoxyguanosine kinase) have been identified in a subset of patients with mtDNA depletion and represent an example of the "dual genome" disorders. In addition, depletion of cardiac mtDNA levels can be specifically induced by AZT, which inhibits both the viral reverse transcriptase and mitochondrial DNA polymerase γ, abrogating mtDNA replication [23]. Moreover, a causative role for zidovudine in the development of cardiomyopathy in AZT-treated infants and children has been proposed [97]. The role of mtDNA depletion in cardiomyopathy remains to be demonstrated by the systematic and accurate estimation of total undeleted mitochondrial genomes and their relationship to cardiac respiratory enzyme defects.

## MITOCHONDRIA AND CONGENITAL HEART DEFECTS (CHD)

CHD, cardiomyopathy, and arrhythmias are common causes of mortality and morbidity in infants and children, in particular during the perinatal period. Single gene mutations have been implicated in the pathogenesis of CHD. These mutations are more common than previously thought and may be present in a number of genes involved in cardiac structure and function, including extracellular matrix proteins, metabolic enzymes and membrane transporters, fatty acid and mitochondrial biosynthesis, cardiac OXPHOS metabolism, sarcomeric structural and contractile proteins, as well as nuclear transcription factors, which control myocardial gene expression and developmental programming [98]. In addition, abnormalities in the structure and function of mitochondria have been found in a significant number of children with CHD and several subclasses of these mitochondrial defects will be discussed in this section.

## Structural and functional cardiac defects

Ultrastructural changes and abnormal mitochondrial number have been reported in a variety of CHD, including ventricular septal defect, patent ductus arteriosus (PDA), and right ventricular dysplasia [99–102]. In addition, DiGeorge/velo-cardio-facial syndrome, which can present with Tetralogy of Fallot results from a large chromosomal deletion ranging from 1.5 to 3 mB in chromosome 22 excising over 30 genes, some of which appear to be involved in mitochondrial function [103]. The loss of the gene for the mitochondrial citrate transporter was initially proposed as contributing to the distinct phenotype of this syndrome [104]. However, recent evidence implicated the deletion of the gene encoding the T-box transcription factor TBX1 in the cardio-vascular abnormalities present in velo-cardio-facial/DiGeorge syndrome [105].

It is well established that functional closure of PDA at birth is initiated by $O_2$-induced vasoconstriction. Mitochondrial ETC and generation of $H_2O_2$ are essential components of the $O_2$ sensing apparatus [106–107]. Mitochondrial-generated $H_2O_2$ has been demonstrated to function as a diffusible redox-mediator that can directly inhibit the activity of voltage-gated $K^+$ channels and thereby regulate the tone and patency of human ductus arteriosus *in vivo*. Modulation of this mitochondrial-based $O_2$ sensing apparatus may prove useful as a potential therapeutic target in treating this common congenital heart disease in preterm infants.

## Cardiac arrhythmias

The accumulation of intermediary metabolites of fatty acids, such as long-chain acylcarnitines, can result in severe cardiac arrhythmias and conduction defects in the neonate. Inborn errors of FAO (e.g., carnitine palmitoyltransferase II, mitochondrial trifunctional protein, and carnitine-acylcarnitine translocase deficiencies) have been reported in cases of unexplained sudden infant death or near misses and in infants with conduction defects or ventricular tachycardia [108]. In Wolff-Parkinson-White (WPW) syndrome, a disorder of preexcitation of the ventricle characterized by rapid and variable atrioventricular conduction, a subset of cases have been found to be caused by mutations in the regulatory subunit of AMPK, a key sensor and mediator in cellular energy metabolism [109].

## Other congenital cardiomyopathies with mitochondrial defects

Significant mitochondrial defects have been demonstrated in cases of FRDA with HCM and in the X-linked Barth syndrome with DCM. The mutant genes frataxin in FRDA and G4.5 in Barth syndrome have been mapped and fully characterized [110–111]. Also, as previously noted, a number of genetic defects in lipid metabolism and mitochondrial FAO can result in pediatric cardiomyopathy, including VLCAD, carnitine metabolism, and MTP defects [112]. Another type of congenital pediatric cardiomyopathy, left ventricular noncompaction (LVNC), has recently been found to have a frequent association with mitochondrial myopathy [113]. This disorder appears to be genetically heterogenous, linked to defects at a variety of genetic loci including X-linked G4.5. Autosomal dominant LVNC has recently been mapped to an unidentified gene at chromosome 11p15 [114]. Congenital HCM and defective OXPHOS in association with infantile cataracts and mitochondrial myopathy have been described in children with Sengers syndrome [115–116]. Although patients with Sengers syndrome exhibit a pronounced ANT protein deficiency in skeletal muscle and abnormal mitochondrial structure [115–117], the underlying genetic defect has not yet been determined. In addition, patients with Alpers syndrome display HCM with skeletal muscle RRF in association with reduced mitochondrial respiration, including COX deficiency and extensive mtDNA depletion [28, 118]. In addition, pronounced mtDNA polymerase γ deficiency [119] and specific lesions in the POLγ gene have been reported in patients with Alpers syndrome [120]. Wilson's disease, an autosomal recessive disorder of copper homeostasis, is characterized by abnormal accumulation of copper in several tissues and has been reported to display a range of cardiac abnormalities, including HCM, supraventricular tachycardia, and autonomic dysfunction [121–122]. The disease associated gene encodes a copper-transporting P-type ATPase, the WND protein. The excessive accumulation of copper is particularly toxic to mitochondria resulting in increased ROS formation, inhibition of mitochondrial dehydrogenases (e.g., PDH) and reduced mitochondrial OXPHOS activities [123–125].

## Congenital heart defects and mitochondrial respiration

Recent studies have further examined the effects of CHD on mitochondrial respiration and metabolism. NO binds to complex IV decreasing myocardial oxygen consumption; in HF this regulation is abrogated due to reduced levels of available NO. Myocardial NO-mediated regulation of mitochondrial respiration has been evaluated comparing patients with end-stage CHD and nonischemic cardiomyopathy [126]. Both eNOS antagonists (e.g., bradykinin, ramiprilat, and amlodipine) and NO donors (e.g., nitroglycerin and S-nitroso-N-acetylpenicillamine [SNAP]) caused a significantly smaller decrease in mitochondrial respiration in CHD hearts compared to cardiomyopathic hearts, suggesting abnormal NO-mediated mitochondrial regulation in CHD. In contrast, the abnormal regulation in the cardiomyopathic heart is related to reduced NO levels and can be reversed by NO donors or agonists.

Exercise tolerance is also compromised in patients with CHD [127]. Using $^{31}P$ nuclear magnetic spectroscopy, skeletal muscle metabolites were assessed in patients with CHD and age-matched healthy controls. In patients with CHD, resting muscle showed a significant elevation in cytosolic pH and in inorganic phosphate levels. However, exercised muscle had increased cytosolic acidification and increased phosphocreatine depletion, whose levels took significantly longer to recover, consistent with a decrease in oxidative ATP synthesis in the skeletal muscle of children with CHD.

## Conclusions

Defects in the structure and function of mitochondria have been found in an increasing number of cardiomyopathies, a subset of which have all the hallmarks of mitochondrial disease. While the molecular basis of the majority of these mitochondrial defects has not yet been established, mtDNA mutations (both point mutations and deletions) are increasingly being identified in MCM. To draw valid conclusions concerning their role in the pathophysiology of cardiomyopathy, these mutations should be (1) compared to previously established mtDNA sequences as well as to unaffected controls to exclude polymorphic variation (an updated database of common mtDNA polymorphisms is available at www.mitomap.org), (2) evaluated for levels of tissue-specificity and heteroplasmy, (3) assessed as to their inheritance pattern, (4) correlated with the presence of other mtDNA point mutations and deletions, and (5) correlated with OXPHOS enzymatic defects.

   Increased awareness and knowledge of MCM will enhance the prospects for developing both a finely tooled diagnostic methodology as well as a range of possible therapeutic modalities. Although no "magic bullet" is yet available to treat mitochondrial-based disorders, delineation of the specific molecular defect can allow treatment with metabolic intermediates (e.g., succinate), coenzymes, and vitamins serving as electron donors and transporters (e.g., vitamin K, thiamine, ascorbate, and riboflavin) to at least partially bypass the defect in OXPHOS and increase ATP production [128]. Coenzyme $Q_{10}$ and its analogue idebenone have been reported to have beneficial effects in the treatment of stroke-like episodes, lactic acidosis, and fatigability in MELAS, in the cardiac conduction disturbance associated with KSS, and in the management of other mitochondrial cardiomyopathies, including FRDA [128–131]. Alternative therapeutic approachs may also include the use of gene therapy to replace defective genes and override abnormal cardiac mitochondrial function and are discussed further in Chapter 11.

# References

1. Marín-García J, Goldenthal MJ (1994) Cardiomyopathy and abnormal mitochondrial function. Cardiovasc Res 28:456–63

2. DiMauro S, Hirano M (1998) Mitochondria and heart disease.Curr Opin Cardiol 13:190–7

3. Wallace DC (1992) Diseases of the mitochondrial DNA. Annu Rev Biochem 61:1175–212

4. Silvestri G, Santorelli FM, Shanske S, Whitley CB, Schimmenti LA, Smith SA, DiMauro S (1994) A new mtDNA mutation in the tRNA$^{Leu(UUR)}$ gene associated with maternally inherited cardiomyopathy. Hum Mutat 3:37–43

5. Tanaka M, Ino H, Ohno K, Hattori K, Sato W, Ozawa T, Itoyama S (1990) Mitochondrial mutation in fatal infantile cardiomyopathy. Lancet 336:1452

6. Taniike M, Fukushima H, Yanagihara I, Tsukamoto H, Tanaka J, Fujimura H, Nagai T, Sano T, Yamaoka K, Inui K, Okada S (1992) Mitochondrial tRNA$^{Ile}$ mutation in fatal cardiomyopathy. Biochem Biophys Res Commun 186:47–53

7. Marín-García J, Ananthakrishnan R, Carta M, Dubois R, Gu J, Goldenthal MJ (1994) Mitochondrial dysfunction in fatal infantile cardiomyopathy. J Inher Metab Dis 17:756–7

8. Marín-García J, Goldenthal MJ, Pierpont ME, Ananthakrishnan R (1995) Impaired mitochondrial function in idiopathic dilated cardiomyopathy: Biochemical and molecular analysis. J Cardiac Fail 1: 285–92

9. Marín-García J, Ananthakrishnan R, Goldenthal MJ, Filiano JJ, Perez-Atayde A (1997) Cardiac mitochondrial dysfunction and DNA depletion in children with hypertrophic cardiomyopathy. J Inherit Metab Dis 20:674–80

10. Marín-García J, Ananthakrishnan R, Goldenthal MJ, Pierpont ME

(2000) Biochemical and molecular basis for mitochondrial cardiomyopathy in neonates and children. J Inherit Metab Dis 23: 625–33

11. Obayashi T, Hattori K, Sugiyama S, Tanaka M, Tanaka T, Itoyama S., Deguchi H, Kawamura K, Koga Y, Toshima H, Takeda N, Nagano M, Ito T, Ozawa T (1992) Point mutations in mitochondrial DNA in patients with hypertrophic cardiomyopathy. Am Heart J 124: 1263–9

12. Pastores GM, Santorelli FM, Shanske S, Gelb BD, Fyfe B, Wolfe D, Willner JP (1994) Leigh syndrome and hypertrophic cardiomyopathy in an infant with a mitochondrial point mutation (T8993G). Amer J Med Genet 50:265–71

13. Santorelli FM, Mak S-C, El-Schahawi M, Casali C, Shanske S, Baram TZ, Madrid RE, DiMauro S (1996) Maternally inherited cardiomyopathy and hearing loss associated with a novel mutation in the mitochondrial tRNA$^{Lys}$ gene (G8363). Am J Hum Genet 58:933–9

14. Casali C, Santorelli FM, D'Amati G, Bernucci P, DeBiase L, DiMauro S (1995) A novel mtDNA point mutation in maternally inherited cardiomyopathy. Biochem Biophys Res Commun 213: 588–93

15. Suomalainen A, Kaukonen J, Amati P, Timonen R, Haltia M, Weissenbach J, Zeviani M, Somer H, Peltonen L (1995) An autosomal locus predisposing to deletions of mitochondrial DNA. Nature Genet 9:146–51

16. Zeviani M, Servidei S, Gellera C, Bertini E, DiMauro S, DiDonato S (1989) An autosomal dominant disporder with multiple deletions of mitochondrial DNA starting at the D loop region. Nature 339: 309–11

17. Benit P, Beugnot R, Chretien D, Giurgea I, De Lonlay-Debeney P, Issartel JP, Corral-Debrinski M, Kerscher S, Rustin P, Rotig A, Munnich A (2003) Mutant NDUFV2 subunit of mitochondrial complex I causes early onset hypertrophic cardiomyopathy and encephalopathy. Hum Mutat 21:582–6

18. Loeffen J, Elpeleg O, Smeitink J, Smeets R, Stockler-Ipsiroglu S, Mandel H, Sengers R, Trijbels F, van den Heuvel L (2001) Mutations in the complex I NDUFS2 gene of patients with cardiomyopathy and encephalomyopathy. Ann Neurol 49:195–201

19. Papadopoulou LC, Sue CM, Davidson MM, Tanji K, Nishino I, Sadlock JE, Krishna S, Walker W, Selby J, Glerum DM, Coster RV, Lyon G, Scalais E, Lebel R, Kaplan P, Shanske S, De Vivo DC,

Bonilla E, Hirano M, DiMauro S, Schon EA (1999) Fatal infantile cardioencephalomyopathy with COX deficiency and mutations in $SCO_2$, a COX assembly gene. Nat Genet 23:333–7

20. Marín-García J, Goldenthal MJ, Ananthakrishnan R, Mirvis D(1996) Specific mitochondrial DNA deletions in canine myocardial ischemia. Biochem Mol Biol Int 40:1057–65

21. Bohlega S, Tanji K, Santorelli FM, Hirano M, alJishi A, DiMauro S (1996) Multiple mitochondrial DNA deletions associated with autosomal recessive ophthalmoplegia and severe cardiomyopathy. Neurology 46:1329–34

22. Fosslien E (2003) Review: Mitochondrial medicine— cardiomyopathy caused by defective oxidative phosphorylation. Ann Clin Lab Sci 33:371–95

23. Lewis W, Dalakas MC (1995) Mitochondrial toxicity of antiviral drugs. Nature Med 1:417–22

24. Wallace KB (2003) Doxorubicin-induced cardiac mitochondrionopathy. Pharmacol Toxicol 93:105–15

25. Shoffner JM, Wallace DC (1992) Heart disease and mitochondrial DNA mutations. Heart Dis Stroke 1:235–41

26. Guenthard J, Wyler F, Fowler B, Baumgartner R (1995) Cardiomyopathy in respiratory chain disorders. Arch Dis Child 72:223–6

27. Lev D, Nissenkorn A, Leshinsky-Silver E, Sadeh M, Zeharia A, Garty BZ, Blieden L, Barash V, Lerman-Sagie T (2004) Clinical presentations of mitochondrial cardiomyopathies. Pediatr Cardiol 25:443–50

28. Holmgren D, Wahlander H, Eriksson BO, Oldfors A, Holme E, Tulinius M (2003) Cardiomyopathy in children with mitochondrial disease: Clinical course and cardiological findings. Eur Heart J 24: 280–8

29. Shoffner JM, Lott MT, Lezza AMS, Seibel P, Ballinger SW, Wallace DC (1990) Myoclonic epilepsy and ragged red fiber disease (MERRF) is associated with a mitochondrial DNA tRNA$^{Lys}$ mutation. Cell 61:931–7

30. Shoffner JM, Lott MT, Voljavec AS, Soueidan SA, Costigan DA, Wallace DC (1989) Spontaneous Kearns-Sayre chronic ophthalmoplegia plus syndrome associated with mitochondrial DNA deletion: a slip replication model and metabolic therapy. Proc Natl Acad Sci USA 86:7952–6

31. Tiranti V, Corona P, Greco M, Taanman JW, Carrara F, Lamantea E, Nijtmans L, Uziel G, Zeviani M (2000) A novel frame-

shift mutation of the mtDNA COIII gene leads to impaired assembly of cytochrome c oxidase in a patient affected by Leigh-like syndrome. Hum Mol Genet 9:2733–42

32. Rahman S, Lake BD, Taanman JW, Hanna MG, Cooper JM, Schapira AH, Leonard JV (2000) Cytochrome oxidase immunohistochemistry: Clues for genetic mechanisms. Brain 3:591–600

33. Morgan-Hughes JA, Sweeney MG, Cooper JM, Hammans SR, Brockington M, Schapira AH, Harding AE, Clark JB (1995) Mitochondrial DNA (mtDNA) diseases: Correlation of genotype to phenotype. Biochem Biophys Acta 1271:135–40

34. Moraes CT, Ricci E, Bonilla E, DiMauro S, Schon EA (1992) The mitochondrial tRNA(Leu(UUR)) mutation in mitochondrial encephalomyopathy, lactic acidosis, and strokelike episodes (MELAS): Genetic, biochemical, and morphological correlations in skeletal muscle. Am J Hum Genet 50:934–49

35. Marín-García J, Ananthakrishnan R, Korson M, Goldenthal MJ, Perez-Atayde A (1996) Cardiac mitochondrial dysfunction in Leigh syndrome. Pediatr Cardiol 17:387–9

36. DiMauro S, Servidei S, Zeviani M, DiRocco M, DeVivo DC, DiDonato S, Uziel G, Berry K, Hoganson G, Johnsen SD, Johnson PC (1987) Cytochrome c oxidase deficiency in Leigh syndrome. Ann Neurol 22:498–506

37. Matthews PM, Marchington DR, Squier M, Land J, Brown R, Brown GK (1993) Molecular genetic characterization of an X-linked form of Leigh's syndrome. Ann Neurol 33:652–5

38. Servidei S, Bertini E, Manfredi G, Dionnisi Vici C, Silvestri G, Ricci E, Burlina A, Tonali P (1993) Familial infantile myopathy and cardiomyopathy with deficiency of cytochrome c oxidase and mitochondrial adenosine triphosphate synthase. Ann Neurol 34:463–4

39. Zeviani M, Van Dyke DH, Servidei E, Bauserman SC, Bonilla E, Beaumont ET, Sharda J, VanderLaan K, DiMauro S (1986) Myopathy and fatal cardiopathy due to cytochrome c oxidase deficiency. Arch Neurol 43:1198–202

40. Papadimitriou A, Neustein HB, DiMauro S, Stanton R, Bresolin N (1984) Histiocytoid cardiomyopathy of infancy: Deficiency of reducible cytochrome b in heart mitochondria. Pediatr Res 18:1023–8

41. Vallance HD, Jeven G, Wallace DC, Brown M (2004) A case ofsporadic infantile histiocytoid cardiomyopathy caused by the

A8344G (MERRF) mitochondrial DNA mutation. Pediatr Cardiol 25:538–40

42. Marín-García J, Goldenthal MJ, Ananthakrishnan R, Pierpont M, Fricker FJ, Lipshultz SE, Perez-Atayde A (1996) Mitochondrial function in children with idiopathic dilated cardiomyopathy. J Inher Metab Dis 19:309–12

43. Rustin P, Lebidois J, Chretien D, Bourgeron T, Piechaud JF, Rotig A, Munnich A, Sidi D (1994) Endomyocardial biopsies for early detection of mitochondrial disorders in hypertrophic cardiomyopathies. J Pediatr 124:224–8

44. Santorelli FM, Tanji K, Manta P, Casali C, Krishna S, Hays AP, Mancini DM, DiMauro S, Hirano M (1999) Maternally inherited cardiomyopathy: An atypical presentation of the mtDNA 12S rRNA gene A1555G mutation. Am J Hum Genet 64:295–300

45. Hsieh RH, Li JY, Pang CY, Wei YH (2001) A novel mutation in the mitochondrial 16S rRNA gene in a patient with MELAS syndrome, diabetes mellitus, hyperthyroidism and cardiomyopathy. J Biomed Sci 8:328–35

46. Boles RG, Luna C, Ito M (2003) Severe reversible cardiomyopathy in four unrelated infants associated with mitochondrial DNA D-loop heteroplasmy. Pediatr Cardiol 24:484–7

47. Marín-García J, Zoubenko O, Goldenthal MJ (2002) Mutations in the cardiac mitochondrial DNA control region associated with cardiomyopathy and aging. J Card Fail 8:93–100

48. Khogali SS, Mayosi BM, Beattie JM, McKenna WJ, Watkins H, Poulton J (2001) A common mitochondrial DNA variant associated with susceptibility to dilated cardiomyopathy in two different populations. Lancet 357:1265–7

49. Goto Y, Nonaka I, Horai S (1990) A mutation in the tRNA$^{Leu(uur)}$ gene associated with the MELAS subgroup of mitochondrial encephalomyopathies. Nature 348:651–3

50. Silvestri G, Ciafaloni E, Santorelli FM, Shanske S, Servidei S, Graf WD, Sumi M, DiMauro S (1993) Clinical features associated with the A→ G transition at nucleotide 8344 of mtDNA ("MERRF" mutation). Neurology 43:1200–6

51. Graf WD, Marín-García J, Gao HG, Pizzo S, Naviaux RK, Markusic D, Barshop BA, Courchesne E, Haas RH (2000) Autism associated with the mitochondrial DNA G8363A transfer RNA(Lys) mutation. J Child Neurol 15:357–61

52.  Houshamond M, Larsson NG, Holme E, Oldfors A, Tulinius MH, Andersen O (1994) Automatic sequencing of mitochondrial tRNA genes in patients with mitochondrial encephalomyopathy. Biochem Biophys Acta 1226:49–55

53.  Suomalainen A, Ciafaloni E, Koga Y, Peltonen L, DiMauro S, Schon EA (1992) Use of single strand polymorphism analysis to detect point mutations in human mitochondrial DNA. J Neurol Sci 111:222–6

54.  Lauber J, Marsac C, Kadenbach B, Seibel P (1991) Mutations in mitochondrial tRNA genes: A frequent cause of neuromuscular diseases. Nucleic Acids Res 19:1393–7

55.  Merante F, Tein I, Benson L, Robinson BH (1994) Maternally inherited cardiomyopathy due to a novel T-to-C transition at nucleotide 9997 in the mitochondrial tRNA$^{Gly}$ gene. Am J Hum Genet 55: 437–46

56.  Zeviani M, Gellera C, Antozzi C, Rimoldi M, Morandi L, Villani F, Tiranti V, DiDonato S (1991) Maternally inherited myopathy and cardiomyopathy: Association with mutation in mitochondrial DNA tRNA$^{Leu}$. Lancet 338:143–7

57.  Santorelli FM, Mak S-C, Vazquez-Acevedo M, Gonzalez-Astiazaran A, Ridaura-Sanz C, Gonzalez-Halphen D, DiMauro S (1995) A novel mitochondrial DNA point mutation associated with mitochondrial encephalocardiomyopathy. Biochem Biophys Res Commun 216:835–40

58.  Zeviani M, Amati P, Bresolin N, Antozzi C, Piccolo G, Toscano A, DiDonato S (1991) Rapid detection of the A→G$^{8344}$ mutation of mtDNA in Italian families with myoclonus epilepsy and ragged-red fibers (MERRF). Am J Hum Genet 48:203–11

59.  Campos Y, Garcia A, del Hoyo P, Jara P, Martin MA, Rubio JC, Berbel A, Barbera JR, Ribacoba R, Astudillo A, Cabello A, Ricoy JR, Arenas J (2003) Two pathogenic mutations in the mitochondrial DNA tRNA$^{Leu(UUR)}$ gene (T3258C and A3280G) resulting in variable clinical phenotypes. Neuromuscul Disord 13:416–20

60.  Menotti F, Brega A, Diegoli M, Grasso M, Modena MG, Arbustini E (2004) A novel mtDNA point mutation in tRNA(Val) is associated with hypertrophic cardiomyopathy and MELAS. Ital Heart J 5:460–5

61.  Okhuijsen-Kroes EJ, Trijbels JM, Sengers RC, Mariman E, van den Heuvel LP, Wendel U, Koch G, Smeitink JA (2001) Infantile pre-

sentation of the mtDNA A3243G tRNA$^{Leu(UUR)}$ mutation. Neuropediatrics 32:183–90

62. Hammans SR, Sweeney MG, Brockington M, Morgan-Hughes JA, Harding AE (1991) Mitochondrial encephalopathies: Molecular genetic diagnosis from blood samples. Lancet 337:1311–3

63. Wallace DC (1994) Mitochondrial DNA sequence variation in human evolution and disease. Proc Natl Acad Sci USA 91:8739–46

64. Shin WS, Tanaka M, Suzuki J, Hemmi C, Toyo-oka T (2000) A novel homoplasmic mutation in mtDNA with a single evolutionary origin as a risk factor for cardiomyopathy. Am J Hum Genet 67: 1617–20

65. Taylor RW, Giordano C, Davidson MM, d'Amati G, Bain H, Hayes CM, Leonard H, Barron MJ, Casali C, Santorelli FM, Hirano M, Lightowlers RN, DiMauro S, Turnbull DM (2003) A homoplasmic mitochondrial transfer ribonucleic acid mutation as a cause of maternally inherited hypertrophic cardiomyopathy. J Am Coll Cardiol 41:1786–96

66. Akita Y, Koga Y, Iwanaga R, Wada N, Tsubone J, Fukuda S, Nakamura Y, Kato H (2000) Fatal hypertrophic cardiomyopathy associated with an A8296G mutation in the mitochondrial tRNA(Lys) gene. Hum Mutat 15:382

67. Seibel P, DeGoul N, Romero N, Marsac C, Kadenbach B (1990) Identification of point mutations by mispairing PCR as exemplified in MERRF disease. Biochem Biophys Res Commun 173:561–5

68. Roe CR, Coates PM (1989) Acyl CoA deficiencies. In: Scriver CR, Beaudet AL, Slys WS, Valle D, eds. The Metabolic Basis of Inherited Disease. 6th ed. NY: McGraw-Hill 889–914

69. Anan R, Greve G, Thierfelder L, Watkins H, McKenna WJ, Solomon S, Vecchio C, Shono H, Nakao S, Tanaka H, Mares A, Towbin JA, Spirito P, Roberts R, Seidman JG, Seidman CE (1994) Prognostic implications of novel ß cardiac myosin heavy chain gene mutations that cause familial hypertrophic cardiomyopathy. J Clin Invest 93: 280–5

70. Towbin J (1993) Molecular genetic aspects of cardiomyopathy. Biochem Med Metab Biol 49:285–320

71. Watkins H, Rosenzweig A. Hwang DS, Levi T, McKenna W, Seidman C, Seidman J (1992) Characteristics and prognostic implications of myosin missense mutations in familial hypertrophic cardiomyopathy. N Eng J Med 326:1108–14

72. Maron BJ, Moller JH, Seidman CE, Vincent GM, Dietz HC, Moss AJ, Sondheimer HM, Pyeritz RE, McGee G, Epstein AE (1998) Impact of laboratory molecular diagnosis on contemporary diagnostic criteria for genetically transmitted cardiovascular diseases: Hypertrophic cardiomyopathy, long-QT syndrome, and Marfan syndrome. Circulation 98:1460–71

73. Moraes CT, Ciacci F, Bonilla E, Ionasescu VV, Schon EA, DiMauro S (1993) A mitochondrial tRNA anticodon swap associated with a muscle disease. Nat Genet 4:284–8

74. Yoon KL, Aprille JR, Ernst SG (1991) Mitochondrial tRNA (Thr) mutation in fatal infantile respiratory enzyme deficiency. Biochem Biophys Res Commun 176:1112–6

75. Marín-García J, Goldenthal MJ, Ananthakrishnan R, Pierpont ME (2000) The complete sequence of mtDNA genes in idiopathic dilated cardiomyopathy shows novel missense and tRNA mutations. J Card Fail 6:321–9

76. Brown MD, Torroni A, Shoffner JM, Wallace DC (1992) Mitochondrial tRNA$^{Thr}$ mutations and lethal infantile mitochondrial myopathy. Am J Hum Genet 51:446–7

77. Ruppert V, Nolte D, Aschenbrenner T, Pankuweit S, Funck R, Maisch B (2004) Novel point mutations in the mitochondrial DNA detected in patients with dilated cardiomyopathy by screening the whole mitochondrial genome. Biochem Biophys Res Commun 318: 535–43

78. Rutledge JC, Haas JE, Monnat R, Milstein JM (1982) Hypertrophic cardiomyopathy is a component of subacute necrotizing encephalomyelopathy. J Pediatr 101:706–10

79. Tatuch Y, Christodolou J, Feigenbaum A, Clark JT, Wherret J, Smith C, Rudd N, Petrova-Benedict R, Robinson BH (1992) Heteroplasmic mitochondrial DNA mutation (T to G) at 8993 can cause Leigh disease when the percentage of abnormal mtDNA is high. Am J Hum Genet 50:852–8

80. Tatuch Y, Robinson BH (1993) The mitochondrial DNA mutation at 8993 associated with NARP slows the rate of ATP synthesis in isolated lymphoblast mitochondria. Biochem Biophys Res Commun 144:124–8

81. Tatuch Y, Pagon RA, Vlcek B, Roberts R, Korson M, Robinson BH (1994) The 8993 mtDNA mutation: Heteroplasmy and clinical presentation in three families. Eur J Hum Genet 2:35–43

82. Santorelli FM, Shanske S, Jain KD, Tick D, Schon EA, DiMauro S (1994) A T→C mutation at nt 8993 of mitochondrial DNA in a child with Leigh syndrome. Neurology 44:972–4

83. Bourgeron T, Rustin P, Chretien D, Birch-Machin M, Bourgeois M, Viegas-Pequignot E, Munnich A, Rotig A (1995) Mutation of a nuclear succinate dehydrogenase gene results in mitochondrial respiratory chain deficiency. Nat Genet 11:144–9

84. Ozawa T, Katsumata K, Hayakawa M, Tanaka M, Sugiyama S, Tanaka T, Itoyama S, Numoda S, Sekiguchi M (1995) Genotype and phenotype of severe mitochondrial cardiomyopathy: A recipient of heart transplantation and the genetic control. Biochem Biophys Res Commun 207:613–9

85. Marín-García J, Hu Y, Ananthakrishnan R, Pierpont ME, Pierpont GL, Goldenthal MJ (1996) A point mutation in the cytb gene of cardiac mtDNA associated with complex III deficiency in ischemic cardiomyopathy. Biochem Mol Biol Int 40:487–95

86. Brown MD, Voljavec AS, Lott MT, Torroni A, Yang CC, Wallace DC (1992) Mitochondrial DNA complex I and III mutations associated with Leber's hereditary optic neuropathy. Genetics 130: 163–73

87. Chomyn A, Meola G, Bresolin N, Lai ST, Scarlato G, Attardi G (1991) *In vitro* genetic transfer of protein synthesis and respiration defects to mitochondrial DNA-less cells with myopathy patient mitochondria. Mol Cell Biol 11:2236–44

88. Andreu AL, Checcarelli N, Iwata S, Shanske S, DiMauro (2000) A missense mutation in the mitochondrial cytochrome b gene in a revisited case with histiocytoid cardiomyopathy. Pediatr Res 48: 311–4

89. Saint-Georges Y, Bonnefoy N, di Rago JP, Chiron S, Dujardin G (2002) A pathogenic cytochrome b mutation reveals new interactions between subunits of the mitochondrial bc1 complex. J Biol Chem 277: 49397–402

90. Valnot I, Kassis J, Chretien D, de Lonlay P, Parfait B, Munnich A, Kachaner J, Rustin P, Rotig A (1999) A mitochondrial cytochrome b mutation but no mutations of nuclearly encoded subunits in ubiquinol cytochrome c reductase (complex III) deficiency. Hum Genet 104:460–6

91. Fisher N, Bourges I, Hill P, Brasseur G, Meunier B (2004) Disruption of the interaction between the Rieske iron-sulfur protein and

cytochrome b in the yeast bc1 complex owing to a human disease-associated mutation within cytochrome b. Eur J Biochem 271:1292–8

92. Hattori Y, Nakajima K, Eizawa T, Ehara T, Koyama M, Hirai T, Fukuda Y, Kinoshita M (2003) Heteroplasmic mitochondrial DNA 3310 mutation in NADH dehydrogenase subunit 1 associated with type 2 diabetes, hypertrophic cardiomyopathy, and mental retardation in a single patient. Diabetes Care 26:952–3

93. Moraes CT, Shanske S, Tritschler HJ, Aprille JR, Andreetta F, Bonilla E, Schon EA, DiMauro S (1991) mtDNA depletion with variable tissue expression: A novel genetic abnormality in mitochondrial diseases. Am J Hum Genet 48:492–501

94. Poulton J, Sewry C, Potter CG, Bougeron T, Chretien D, Wijberg FA, Morten KJ, Brown G (1995) Variation in mitochondrial DNA levels in muscle from normal controls: Is depletion of mtDNA in patients with mitochondrial myopathy a distinct clinical syndrome? J Inher Metab Dis 18:4–20

95. Zeviani M (1992) Nucleus-driven mutations of human mitochondrial DNA. J Inher Metab Dis 15:456–71

96. Zeviani M, Spinazzola A, Carelli V (2003) Nuclear genes in mitochondrial disorders. Curr Opin Genet Dev 13:262–70

97. Herskowitz A, Willoughby SB, Baughman KL, Schulman SP, Bartlett JD (1992) Cardiomyopathy associated with antiretroviral therapy in patients with HIV infection: A report of 6 cases. Ann Intern Med 116:311–3

98. Marino B, Digilio MC (2000) Congenital heart disease and genetic syndromes: Specific correlation between cardiac phenotype and genotype. Cardiovasc Pathol 9:303–15

99. Pham TD, Wit AL, Hordof AJ, Malm JR, Fenoglio JJ (1978) Right atrial ultrastructure in congenital heart disease. I. Comparison of ventricular septal defect and endocardial cushion defect. Am J Cardiol 42:973–82

100. Blankenship DC, Hug G, Balko G, van der Bel-Kann J, Coith RL, Engel PJ (1993) Hemodynamic and myocyte mitochondrial ultrastructural abnormalities in arrhythmogenic right ventricular dysplasia. Am Heart J 126:989–95

101. Sakashita I, Matsukawa T, Ando T, Asano K (1971) Morphological comparison of infundibular pulmonary stenosis and tetralogy of Fallot. Jpn Heart J 12:205–13

102. Dastur DK, Vevaina SC, Manghani DK (1989) Fine structure of A: autonomic nerve fibers and terminals in human myocardium and B: myocardial changes in congenital heart disease. Ultrastruct Pathol 13: 413–31

103. Strauss AW (1998) The molecular basis of congenital cardiac disease. Semin Thorac Cardiovasc Surg Pediatr Card Surg Annu 1: 179–88

104. Stoffel M, Karayiorgou M, Espinosa R, Beau MM (1996) The human mitochondrial citrate transporter gene (SLC20A3) maps to chromosome band 22q11 within a region implicated in DiGeorge syndrome, velo-cardio-facial syndrome and schizophrenia. Hum Genet 98:113–5

105. Merscher S, Funke B, Epstein JA, Heyer J, Puech A, Lu MM, Xavier RJ, Demay MB, Russell RG, Factor S, Tokooya K, Jore BS, Lopez M, Pandita RK, Lia M, Carrion D, Xu H, Schorle H, Kobler JB, Scambler P, Wynshaw-Boris A, Skoultchi AI, Morrow BE, Kucherlapati R (2001) TBX1 is responsible for cardiovascular defects in velo-cardio-facial/DiGeorge syndrome. Cell 104:619–29

106. Michelakis ED, Rebeyka I, Wu X, Nsair A, Thebaud B, Hashimoto K, Dyck JR, Haromy A, Harry G, Barr A, Archer SL (2002) $O_2$ sensing in the human ductus arteriosus: Regulation of voltage-gated K+ channels in smooth muscle cells by a mitochondrial redox sensor. Circ Res 91:478–86

107. Archer SL, Wu XC, Thebaud B, Moudgil R, Hashimoto K, Michelakis ED. $O_2$ sensing in the human ductus arteriosus: Redox-sensitive K+ channels are regulated by mitochondria-derived hydrogen peroxide. Biol Chem 385:205–16

108. Bonnet D, Martin D, Pascale De Lonlay, Villain E, Jouvet P, Rabier D, Brivet M, Saudubray JM (1999) Arrhythmias and conduction defects as presenting symptoms of fatty acid oxidation disorders in children. Circulation 100:2248–53

109. Gollob MH, Green MS, Tang AS, Gollob T, Karibe A, Ali Hassan AS, Ahmad F, Lozado R, Shah G, Fananapazir L, Bachinski LL, Roberts R, Hassan AS (2001) Identification of a gene responsible for familial Wolff-Parkinson-White syndrome. N Engl J Med 344:1823-31

110. Palau F (2001) Friedreich's ataxia and frataxin: Molecular genetics, evolution and pathogenesis. Int J Mol Med 7:581–9

111. Bolhuis PA, Hensels GW, Hulsebos TJ, Baas F, Barth PG (1991) Mapping of the locus for X-linked cardioskeletal myopathy

with neutropenia and abnormal mitochondria (Barth syndrome) to Xq28. Am J Hum Genet 48:481–5

112. Kelly DP, Strauss AW (1994) Inherited cardiomyopathies. N Eng J Med 330:913–9

113. Pignatelli RH, McMahon CJ, Dreyer WJ, Denfield SW, Price J, Belmont JW, Craigen WJ, Wu J, El Said H, Bezold LI, Clunie S, Fernbach S, Bowles NE, Towbin JA (2003) Clinical characterization of left ventricular noncompaction in children: A relatively common form of cardiomyopathy. Circulation 108:2672–8

114. Sasse-Klaassen S, Probst S, Gerull B, Oechslin E, Nürnberg P, Heuser A, Jenni R, Hennies HC, Thierfelder L (2004) Novel gene locus for autosomal dominant left ventricular noncompaction maps to chromosome 11p15. Circulation 109:2720–3

115. Sengers RC, Stadhouders AM, Jaspar HH, Trijbels JM, Daniels O (1976) Cardiomyopathy and short stature associated with mitochondrial and/or lipid storage myopathy of skeletal muscle. Neuropadiatrie 7:196–208

116. Morava E, Sengers R, Ter Laak H, Van Den Heuvel L, Janssen A, Trijbels F, Cruysberg H, Boelen C, Smeitink J (2004) Congenital hypertrophic cardiomyopathy, cataract, mitochondrial myopathy and defective oxidative phosphorylation in two siblings with Sengers-like syndrome. Eur J Pediatr 163:467–71

117. Jordens EZ, Palmieri L, Huizing M, van den Heuvel LP, Sengers RC, Dorner A, Ruitenbeek W, Trijbels FJ, Valsson J, Sigfusson G, Palmieri F, Smeitink JA (2002) Adenine nucleotide translocator 1 deficiency associated with Sengers syndrome. Ann Neurol 52:95–9

118. Rasmussen M, Sanengen T, Skullerud K, Kvittingen EA, Skjeldal OH (2000) Evidence that Alpers-Huttenlocher syndrome could be a mitochondrial disease. J Child Neurol 15:473–7

119. Naviaux RK, Nyhan WL, Barshop BA, Poulton J, Markusic D, Karpinski NC, Haas RH (1999) Mitochondrial DNA polymerase gamma deficiency and mtDNA depletion in a child with Alpers' syndrome. Ann Neurol 45:54–8

120. Naviaux RK, Nguyen KV (2004) POLG mutations associated with Alpers' syndrome and mitochondrial DNA depletion. Ann Neurol 55:706–12

121. Hlubocka Z, Marecek Z, Linhart A, Kejkova E, Pospisilova L, Martasek P, Aschermann M (2002) Cardiac involvement in Wilson disease. J Inherit Metab Dis 25:269–77

122. Kuan P (1987) Cardiac Wilson's disease. Chest 91:579-83

123. Gu M, Cooper JM, Butler P, Walker AP, Mistry PK, Dooley JS, Schapira AH (2000) Oxidative-phosphorylation defects in liver of patients with Wilson's disease. Lancet 356:469–74

124. Davie CA, Schapira AH (2002) Wilson disease. Int Rev Neurobiol 53:175–90

125. Sheline CT, Choi DW (2004) Cu2+ toxicity inhibition of mitochondrial dehydrogenases *in vitro* and *in vivo*. Ann Neurol 55: 645–53

126. Mital S, Loke KE, Chen JM, Mosca RS, Quaegebeur JM, Addonizio LJ, Hintze TH (2004) Mitochondrial respiratory abnormalities in patients with end-stage congenital heart disease. J Heart Lung Transplant 23:72–9

127. Adatia I, Kemp GJ, Taylor DJ, Radda GK, Rajagopalan B, Haworth SG (1993) Abnormalities in skeletal muscle metabolism in cyanotic patients with congenital heart disease: A $^{31}$P nuclear magnetic resonance spectroscopy study. Clin Sci (Lond) 85:105–9

128. Shoffner JM, Wallace DC (1994) Oxidative phosphorylation diseases and mitochondrial DNA mutations: Diagnosis and treatment. Annu Rev Nutr 14:535–68

129. Lerman-Sagie T, Rustin P, Lev D, Yanoov M, Leshinsky-Silver E, Sagie A, Ben-Gal T, Munnich A (2001) Dramatic improvement in mitochondrial cardiomyopathy following treatment with idebenone. J Inherit Metab Dis 24:28–34

130. Langsjuen P, Vadhanavikit S, Folkers K (1985) Response of patients in classes III and IV of cardiomyopathy to therapy in a blind and cross-over trial with coenzyme $Q_{10}$. Proc Natl Acad Sci USA 82: 4240–4

131. Geromel V, Darin N, Chretien D, Benit P, DeLonlay P, Rotig A, Munnich A, Rustin P (2002) Coenzyme Q(10) and idebenone in the therapy of respiratory chain diseases: Rationale and comparative benefits. Mol Genet Metab 77:21–30

# Chapter 9

# Mitochondria and the Aging Heart

## Overview

The mitochondrial theory of aging states that somatic mutations in mtDNA initiate a vicious cycle in which the organelle bioenergetic function is progressively compromised leading to tissue dysfunction, degeneration, and eventually death. As the human population ages and the average life span increases, so does the burden of cardiovascular disease. While risk factors such as lifestyle patterns, genetic traits, blood lipid levels, and diabetes can contribute to its development, advancing age unequivocally remains the most significant predictor of cardiac disease. Several parameters of left ventricular function may be affected with aging (including increased duration of systole, decreased sympathetic stimulation and increased left ventricle ejection time), while compliance decreases. In addition, changes in cardiac phenotype with diastolic dysfunction, reduced contractility, left ventricular hypertrophy, and heart failure all increase in incidence with age. Given the limited capacity that the heart has for regeneration, reversing or slowing the progression of these abnormalities poses a major challenge. Moreover, during aging a significant loss of cardiac myocytes occurs, probably related to programmed cell death (apoptosis). This loss in cardiomyocytes may be secondary to mitochondrial dysfunction caused by chronic exposure to oxidative radicals and damage to mtDNA and mitochondrial membranes. While mtDNA damage (point mutations and deletions) occurs with cardiac aging, mtDNA levels, although decreased mainly in liver and skeletal muscle, are for the most part preserved in the aging heart. In this chapter, the bioenergetic, biogenesis, and molecular changes occurring with aging in human and animal models are discussed, including our own experience with senescent rats and innovative therapies that may reverse the process.

## Introduction

Cellular manifestations of aging are most pronounced in postmitotic organs (e.g., brain and heart), and abnormalities in cardiomyocyte structure and function may be the definitive factors in the overall cardiac aging process. As the heart ages, myocytes undergo some degree of hypertrophy, and this may be accompanied by mitochondria-derived oxidative injury, contributing to the overall cellular aging process as well as to ischemia-induced tissue damage. While the aging heart suffers greater damage following an episode of ischemia and reperfusion than the young or adult heart, the occurrence and degree of aging-related defects in OXPHOS remain uncertain. Many of the aging-related defects have been found to be limited to interfibrillar mitochondria (e.g., COX activity and rate of OXPHOS were decreased), while the subsarcolemmal mitochondria remained unaffected [1]. The selective alteration of interfibrillar mitochondria during aging raises the possibility that the consequences of aging-induced mitochondrial dysfunction will be enhanced in specific subcellular regions of the senescent cardiomyocyte. In addition, in the aging heart during ischemia, ATP and tissue adenosine levels are reduced compared to adult controls [2]. However, the reduction of ATP content in early ischemia is unlikely to provide a mechanism for the increased damage observed following more prolonged periods of ischemia in the aging heart. The interaction of mitochondria and lysosomes in cellular homeostasis may also be of significance, since both organelles suffer the most remarkable age-related alterations in postmitotic cells [3]. Many mitochondria undergo enlargement and structural disorganization, while lysosomes responsible for mitochondrial turnover experience a loss of function. The rate of total mitochondrial protein turnover declines with age [4]. The coupled mitochondrial and lysosomal defects contribute to irreversible functional impairment and cell death. Similarly, mitochondrial interaction with other functional compartments of the cardiac cell (e.g., the ER for $Ca^{++}$ metabolism; peroxisomes for the interchange of antioxidant enzymes essential in the production and decomposition of $H_2O_2$) must be kept in check since defects in communication between these organelles may accelerate the aging process.

# Bioenergetics and gene expression in the aging heart

A thorough discussion of mitochondrial bioenergetics and the heart is presented in Chapter 2. Here it suffices to say that in the aging heart of a variety of animal models, including bovine, dog, and rat, as well as in humans, defects in the ETC and OXPHOS have been found [5–12] and the respiratory complexes primarily affected (I, III, IV, and V) have subunits encoded by both the nuclear and mitochondrial genomes. Studies with rat heart have found that the respiratory complexes of the interfibrillar population of mitochondria (particularly complexes III and IV) are more likely to be affected in aging than the sarcolemmal mitochondrial populations [10]. Other studies have shown that complex I, the respiratory enzyme with the largest complement of mtDNA-encoded subunits (i.e., 7 of the 13 mtDNA encoded proteins), appears to be the most affected with aging, and also becomes more strongly rate-limiting for electron transfer [11]. Complex I also plays a major role in the formation of superoxide radicals. A decline in complex I activity (with increased state 4 respiration) elevates ROS production during aging likely promoting the generation of prooxidant compounds, the modulation of the PT pore and mitochondrial membrane potential, and finally the induction of apoptosis. However, it is important to note that there is considerable disagreement in the literature concerning the extent or significance of mitochondrial ETC dysfunction in the aging heart. A recent study in humans found that mitochondrial respiratory enzymes maintained normal activities in the aging heart and concluded that defects in ETC cannot be considered the main cause of the increased oxidative damage associated with aging [13]. These conflicting results may be related to the difficulties involved in accessing fresh control cardiac tissues from humans for gauging enzymatic values, as well as from the different populations of mitochondria studied.

Age-related changes in mitochondrial adenine nucleotide metabolism may also underlie progressive decline in cardiac function. Reduced myocardial ANT activity has been reported in the aging rat heart [14], probably as a consequence of both a diminished pool of exchangeable adenine nucleotides (ADP + ATP) and lower ANT velocity. Membrane lipids of cardiac mitochondria from aged rat displayed a 43% higher cholesterol/phospholipid ratio and a significantly lower phosphatidylethanolamine/phosphatidylcholine ratio compared to the young rat. Moreover, older rats display a marked decline in levels of myocardial cardiolipin, the primarily inner-membrane localized phospholipid implicated in mediating the stability and enzymatic activities of respiratory complexes I and IV [15–17]. These findings suggest that changes in the lipid components of the mitochondrial inner membrane, in which the ANT and the respiratory complexes are embedded, may be contributory to the aging-related decrease in cardiac mitochondrial function.

## Mitochondrial function and gene expression in the aging heart

The mitochondrial theory of aging suggests that somatic mutations in mtDNA, induced by oxygen radicals, are the primary cause of energy decline (Figure 9.1). Also, ROS, considered as the pathogenic agent of many diseases and aging, are mainly the product of the mitochondrial respiratory chain. The free radical theory of aging and its particular targeting of mtDNA is supported by a large number of observations describing the limited mtDNA repair machine, the absence in mitochondria of histones and a chromatin structure, which serve to protect the nuclear genome from damage. With aging, increased level of ROS-induced changes in mtDNA, including base modifications and increased number of mtDNA deletions might be expected to cause increased errors or mutations in mtDNA-encoded enzyme subunits, resulting in impaired OXPHOS and defective ETC, which in turn creates more ROS.

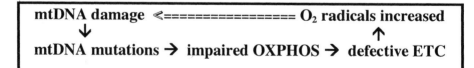

**Figure 9.1. Vicious cycle initiated by somatic mtDNA damage.** *Somatic mtDNA damage can lead to eventual injury in the aging heart.*

During aging, myocardial mitochondrial gene expression may be down-regulated [5, 18–20], although this view has been recently challenged [21–22]. The effect of senescence on mtDNA transcription has been studied with an *in organello* system using intact isolated rat heart mitochondria [23]. The electrophoretic patterns of mtDNA transcription products in young, adult, and senescent rats showed an age-related reduction in newly synthesized mitochondrial transcripts, as a consequence of a reduction in the synthesis rate. These results correlate with reduced enzyme activity levels of complexes I and IV, which are partially encoded by the mitochondrial genome, and with an age-related increase in the protein carbonyl content of the mitochondrial membranes, which has been observed in senescent mitochondria, suggesting an accumulation of mitochondrial oxidative damage.

Other studies using transcription profiling have not clarified the effect of age on myocardial mitochondrial transcription. One study (with the aging mouse model) found that aging cardiac myocytes have reduced mtDNA-encoded ETC expression and reduced levels of cardiac transcription factors [20], while another study with rat documented an increase in the myocardial expression of OXPHOS genes [22].

The potential role that nuclear gene expression of mitochondrial proteins plays needs to be further examined. Gene expression profiles in both the senescent mice and rat hearts indicated decreased cellular adaptation and protection against stress-induced injury, together with the development of contractile dysfunction. Moreover, there is definitive evidence that the aging process is associated with a genetic component and that the senescent phenotype, which is the endpoint of the aging process, may be due to changes in the expression of a limited number of genes that remain to be identified.

A large number of changes in mitochondrial structure and function has been reported with cardiac aging. Besides OXPHOS/ETC functions, it is evident that other aspects of the organelle function are affected during cardiac aging including the down-regulation of FAO metabolism, changes in mitochondrial $Ca^{++}$ transport and mitochondrial import of nuclear-encoded proteins [24–26]. There is considerably evidence that the structural components of the mitochondria are modified in the aging heart, including the phospholipid content of mitochondrial membranes, mitochondrial protein modification as well as the generation of extensive mtDNA damage [27–31]. These defects are likely to contribute to the progression of mitochondrial impairment and provide a contextual setting for the mitochondrial dysfunction developing in the aging heart. Decline in overall mitochondrial function during the aging process may lead to cellular energy deficits, especially in times of greater energy demand (e.g., exercise) and compromise vital ATP-dependent cellular processes, including detoxification, DNA repair, DNA replication, and osmotic balance. Mitochondrial decay may also lead to enhanced oxidant production rendering the cell more prone to oxidative insult. In addition, these mitochondrial alterations may be contributory elements in the increased susceptibility of the aging heart to ischemia-reperfusion damage, which also targets mitochondrial function [32]. Due to its reliance for energy on β-oxidation of fatty acids and the postmitotic nature of cardiac myocytes, which would allow for greater accumulation of mitochondrial mutations and deletions, the heart is especially susceptible to a dysfunctional mitochondria. Thus, maintenance of mitochondrial function is essential to preserve overall myocardial function.

## ROS in the aging heart

The production of ROS and oxidative stress is a function of both the inefficiency of the transfer of electrons through the respiratory chain and the overall level of antioxidant defenses in the cell [33]. Because ROS are the result of normal metabolic processes, the more active tissues, such as the heart, suffer the most damage. In addition, the bioenergetic dysfunction occurring with aging will further increase the accumulation of ROS. Among its many targets, ROS can reduce inner-membrane fluidity by attacking the polyunsaturated fatty acids and cardiolipin, which can substantially affect protein transport function and the ETC. There is also extensive evidence for increased ROS-mediated oxidative damage to a wide spectrum of myocardial lipids and proteins in the aging heart. Both myocardial mitochondrial and nuclear DNA damage may result in further accumulation of oxidative species. In particular, mtDNA damage accumulates due to its inefficient repair and its close proximity to the sources of ROS.

In the aging heart, the neutralization of ROS by both cytosolic and mitochondrial antioxidants such as superoxide dismutase (SOD), catalase (CA), glutathione peroxidase (GPx), and glutathione becomes of critical significance as presented in Figure 9.2. Markedly declining levels of ascorbate and reduced glutathione in interfibrillar (but not sarcolemmal) mitochondria have been found in the aging heart [34].

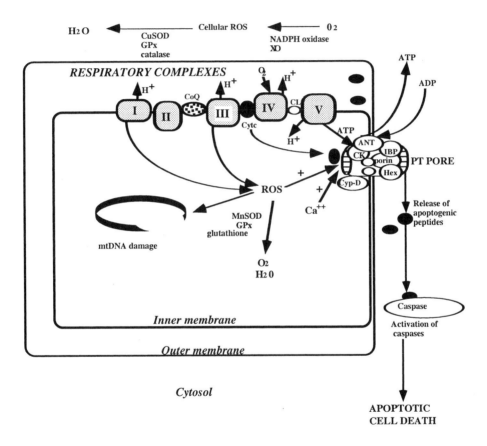

**Figure 9.2. Location of antioxidant enzymes and ROS generation in the aging heart.** *Shown are the cytosolic pathways of ROS generation involving NADPH oxidase and xanthine oxidase (XO), the cytosolic antioxidant enzymes copper SOD (CuSOD), glutathione peroxidase (GPx ), and catalase as well as the mitochondrial pathway of ROS generation (primarily through complexes I and III) and mitochondrial antioxidant response featuring MnSOD, GPx, and glutathione. Also depicted are the primary mitochondrial targets of ROS including the PT pore and mitochondrial apoptotic pathway and mtDNA.*

Several studies have reported elevated levels of myocardial glutathione peroxidase and reductase presumably as an adaptive mechanism to cope with increased ROS generation [35–36]. Most studies (with one exception [37]) have found no changes with aging in the myocardial activity levels of the antioxidant MnSOD [36, 38–39]. Mimetics of the antioxidant enzymes CA and SOD have been considered as a way of fighting back against the accumulation of ROS and therefore aging. However, we have to be prudent since this modality of therapy may also produce undesirable effects on the "good role" of ROS as signaling molecules.

As discussed in Chapter 4, ROS can induce myocardial apoptosis. During aging, there is a significant loss of postmitotic cells such as cardiac myocytes potentially triggered by the onset of mytochondrial dysfunction and ROS generation. For instance, *in vitro* studies of $H_2O_2$-treated cardiomyocytes show that increased mitochondrial oxidative stress and declining mitochondrial energy production lead to the activation of apoptotic pathways [40–41], but whether this also occurs in the aging heart *in vivo* is unclear. Although the role and extent of apoptosis in normal myocardial aging is presently under considerable debate, evidence of cardiomyocyte apoptosis has been corroborated by studies demonstrating the release of cytochrome *c* from the aging rat heart mitochondria and decreased levels of the antiapoptotic protein Bcl-2 while proapoptotic Bax remained unchanged [42]. Moreover, myocytes derived from the hearts of old mice displayed increased levels of markers of cell death and senescence, compared to myocytes from younger animals [43].

## Mitochondrial DNA damage in the aging heart

Mitochondria of postmitotic cells (e.g., cardiomyocytes) have a limited life span of a few weeks. Their replacement during normal turnover requires an intergenomic coordination between both the mitochondrial and the nuclear genome. Over the last decade, a significant number of mtDNA point mutations have been reported in humans above a certain age. Initially, increased levels of mutations at specific sites within the mtDNA D-loop control region were reported in skin fibroblasts and skeletal muscle of aging individuals [44]. More recently, Marín-García et al. [45], in their study on the incidence and location of myocardial D-loop mutations as a function of age, found no evidence of an age-related correlation in the accumulation of homoplasmic mutations in either patients with cardiomyopathy or in normal controls. Similarly, no age-related accumulation was found for heteroplasmic mutations in either the D-loop or cytochome *b* gene. This contrasts with age-dependent increases in mtDNA deletions found in human cardiac tissues from aging patients with and without cardiac disease [46]. Recently, research has focused on the role that pathogenic mtDNA mutations may have in programmed cell death in human, even though mtDNA damage and defective mitochondrial respiration may not be essential factors for the process of apoptosis to occur. The integrity of mtDNA may influence the rate of apoptosis during aging, most probably by regulating ROS production.

Experimental evidence reveals that for mtDNA mutations to have a phenotypic effect, they must be present in high proportion (often calculated at over 80%) compared to their wildtype counterparts. Given that mtDNA is a multicopy genome estimated at over 1,000 copies per cardiomyocyte, the occurrence of a somatic mutation in a single mtDNA molecule must have some replicative advantage to multiply (by clonal expansion) to become the predominant mtDNA molecule in a cell. Recent studies have shown that a high proportion of cells in the normal human heart (as well as other tissues) contain high levels of clonal mutant mtDNA derived from a single mtDNA molecule containing somatic mutations [47]. While such a selective replicative advantage has been demonstrated with *in vitro* studies of mtDNA deletions in human cells [48] and clonal expansion of mtDNA deletions have been found with *in vivo* human cardiomyocytes [49], this represents the first definitive evidence for clonal expansion of mtDNA point mutations. The cardiomyocyte phenotypes resulting from clonal expansions might be expected to include neutral phenotypes, hyporespiratory phenotypes (with less ROS production and reduced ATP production), or phenotypes with defective ETC, enhanced ROS generation and oxidative stress triggered apoptosis. Since the mechanism by which mutant mtDNAs are selectively replicated is not known, further research effort in this area may have great impact in our understanding of mitochondria's role in the aging myocardium [50].

Experimental observations in 6- and 27-month-old rats have shown an age-related reduction of mtDNA copy number in skeletal muscle and liver but not in the heart [5]. In human however, it is unclear if there is an aging-related decrease in mtDNA copy number. Recently, one study described no changes in the heart nor in skeletal muscle with age [51], while another found decreased levels of skeletal muscle mtDNA copy number in older healthy humans (65 to 75 years old) compared to young adults (20 to 30 years old) [52]. Nevertheless, it appears that the effects of aging on mitochondrial gene expression are tissue-specific and mtDNA levels are preserved in the aging heart muscle, presumably due to its continual aerobic activity. In this regard, it is noteworthy that no changes in the levels or activity of the mtTFA protein, implicated in mtDNA replication and transcription, have been demonstrated in the aging rat heart as compared to an age-related increase in liver and brain [53]. In our laboratory, we have found increased levels of heart mtDNA deletions in aging patients with idiopathic DCM compared to young patients [46]. In the older patient group, the age-related decline in ETC and the increased accumulation of mtDNA deletions may be the result of oxidative damage, which increase with aging [54]. Moreover, age appears to play a role in increasing the incidence of specific mtDNA deleletions (the common 5 and 7kb deletions) and in the development of multiple respiratory enzymes defects in patients with DCM but appears to be noncontributory to the severity or frequency of single enzyme activity defects.

Recently, the potential causative effects of point mutations and de-letions on aging have been addressed experimentally by creating homozygous knock-in mice that express a proof-reading-deficient version of Polγ, the nuclear-encoded catalytic subunit of mtDNA polymerase [55]. The knock-in mice developed a three-to fivefold in-crease in the levels of mtDNA point mutations, as well as an increased amount of deleted mtDNA. The increase in somatic mtDNA mutations was associated with reduced life span and the premature onset of aging-related phenotypes, including heart enlargement, thus providing a causative link between mtDNA mutations and aging. The accumulation of age-dependent point mutations and deletions in postmitotic tissues has also recently been demonstrated to be signifi-cantly elevated in individuals with mutations in the mitochondrial helicase Twinkle or in Polγ [56].

## Rat model of cardiac aging: Defects in ETC

In our institution, we have performed a comprehensive analysis of mitochondrial enzyme activities, mtDNA, and specific expression analysis of mitochondrial and nuclear genes in the heart of senescent Fischer rat (30 months of age) compared to young adults (4 months). Using hearts derived from Fischer rats allowed us to work with an isogenic background, in both young and older animals, as well as a consistency of parameters (e.g., diet and exercise) that are difficult to control with other species, including the human.

As depicted in Figure 9.3, the specific activity level of respiratory complex IV was significantly reduced (by 26%) in the 30-month-old heart compared to 4-month-old heart. Complex I activity declined by a similar amount in the senescent heart although the difference between age groups was not statistically significant. Complex V activity was markedly reduced (by 46%) in the senescent heart. Both complex II and CS (citrate synthase) activity levels were not significantly reduced in the senescent compared to the young adult heart.

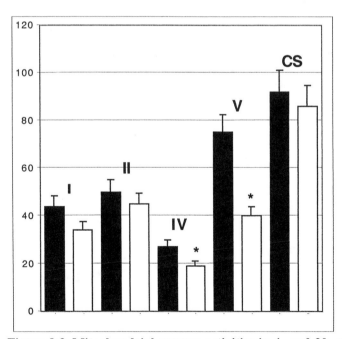

**Figure 9.3. Mitochondrial enzyme activities in 4- and 30- month-old rat hearts.** *Specific activity levels are shown for respiratory complexes I, II, IV and V, and citrate synthase (CS) in hearts from 4-(■) and 30-month-old rats(□). Values shown are in nm substrate/min/mg protein (except CS which is at 10 fold higher levels) and represent mean ±SE (n=6); \*, p < 0.05 relative to control.*

When enzyme activities were normalized relative to CS (often used as a gauge of overall mitochondrial content), the activity ratios obtained for complexes I, IV, and V (i.e., I/CS, IV/CS, and V/CS) as depicted in Figure 9.4 exhibited significant declines in the older age group. However, the activity ratio of complex II showed no significant change with age.

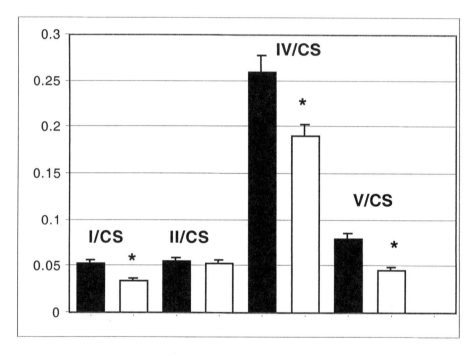

**Figure 9.4. Mitochondrial respiratory enzyme activity ratios in 4- and 30-month-old rat hearts.** *Activity ratios (i.e. specific activity of each respiratory enzyme normalized to CS activity) are shown for respiratory complex I (i.e. I/CS), II (II/CS), IV (IV/CS) and V (V/CS) in hearts from 4-(■) and 30-month (□)-old rats. Values shown represent mean $\pm$ SE (n=6); *, p < 0.05 relative to control.*

The mechanisms for mitochondrial enzymatic defects observed in myocardial aging may include posttranscriptional and translational regulation, the import of mitochondrial subunits as well as factors that can modulate the successful assembly, functioning, and activity of the subunits within the mitochondrial inner membrane.

## Gene expression

Gene expression in cardiac aging was evaluated by northern blots. A significant increase was found in the age-dependent expression levels of mtDNA encoded genes examined including 12S rRNA, cyt*b* and COI ranging from 1.3 to 1.6-fold in senescent as compared to young adult heart (Table 9.1). Transcript levels of myocardial nuclear transcription factors NF-κB are 1.5-fold up-regulated in senescent compared to young adult hearts. Expression of GPx, a mitochondrial-located stress response protein, was significantly up-regulated (1.4-fold) in the senescent heart. The housekeeping gene GAPDH showed no significant change with aging.

**Table 9.1. RNA analysis: Genes grouped by function**

| mtDNA genes | Ratio S/YA |
|---|---|
| cyt*b* | $1.31 \pm 0.08$* |
| COI | $1.60 \pm 0.09$* |
| 12S rRNA | $1.48 \pm 0.05$* |
| **Transcription factors** | |
| NF-κ B | $1.52 \pm 0.15$* |
| **Stress response** | |
| Glutathione peroxidase | $1.39 \pm 0.04$* |
| **Cytoplasmic genes** | |
| GAPDH | $1.04 \pm 0.013$ |

*Note:* S/YA = normalized transcript level in senescent heart /level in young adult heart;  Standard mean $\pm$ SEM;  * indicates $p < 0.05$.

## DNA copy number and damage analysis

To determine whether modulation in mtDNA copy number was involved in the altered levels of mitochondrial enzyme activities observed in the senescent heart, we determined mtDNA levels using quantitative competitive PCR. No significant change in mtDNA levels was detected in the 30-month-old as compared to 4-month-old hearts. However, significant mtDNA damage was found in the senescent heart as gauged by the attenuated amplification of progressively larger DNA fragments. Amplification of smaller 406 and 618 bp fragments displayed no significant difference in efficiency when comparing template DNA derived from young and older myocardium. However, larger fragments of 2193 and 3115 bp exhibited a marked decline in amplification efficiency with template DNA in older heart (Table 9.2).

**Table 9.2. Amplification efficiency of myocardial mtDNA fragments**

| Amplified Fragment Size | Senescent Adult (% Relative to Young Adult) |
|---|---|
| 406 bp | 97 |
| 618 bp | 89 |
| 2193 bp | 56* |
| 3115 bp | 43* |

*Note:* * $p < 0.05$.

## Comments

### *On mitochondrial dysfunction*

In the senescent heart, we found a moderate decrease in complex I and IV activities and a more significant decline in complex V activity. On the other hand, and in marked contrast to the significant decline in activities found in mtDNA encoded enzymes (e.g., complexes I, IV, and V), entirely nuclear-encoded mitochondrial enzymes (e.g., complex II and CS) exhibited no significant changes. These findings were very similar to those previously reported by our laboratory using 18-month-old rats compared to 2-month-old young adults [5].

The molecular basis for the marked decline in complex I, IV, and V activities during aging remains unclear. Immunoblot studies with specific antibodies directed against both nuclear-encoded (ATPγ and ATPα) and mitochondrial-encoded (ATP6) subunits have not detected either a qualitative or quantitative difference in these complex V subunits in senescent rats. Moreover, our data do not support the hypothesis that reduced levels of complexes I, IV, and V activities in aging occur as a function of altered mtDNA levels, which were unchanged. Transcript analysis of mtDNA-encoded subunits (COI and cyt*b*) failed to detect any significant reduction (but rather an increase) in the mtDNA transcription of these subunits, suggesting that decline in gene transcription is unlikely to provide the molecular basis for the enzymatic defects found in the senescent heart. This is in agreement with the findings of Barazonni and associates [22] but different than those reported by Gadaleta [18, 57]. In an entirely novel model of aging, the primate *Macaca fascicularis,* and utilizing proteomic analysis, Yan and associates reported a marked aging-mediated decline in the levels of myocardial proteins involved in glycolysis (e.g., pyruvate kinase, α−enolase,  and triosephosphate isomerase), glucose oxidation (e.g., PDH E1 β-subunit), and OXPHOS (ATP synthase α and β subunits and COXIV subunit).  The effect was gender-specific (i.e., present only in older males) [58].

## *On mitochondrial DNA damage*

The marked decline in mtDNA integrity in the senescent heart does not result in lower transcription of those genes, suggesting the presence of an adaptive mechanism to promote mitochondrial transcription in the presence of mitochondrial dysfunction and mtDNA damage. Such a mechanism has been described in patients with mitochondrial disease. It could be argued that the generation of mtDNA damage in the senescent heart may be secondary to increased ROS and mitochondrial enzymatic dysfunction. This hypothesis may be tested by overcoming the aging-mediated mitochondrial dysfunction and/or the generation of mitochondrial ROS and examining the extent of mtDNA damage. While overall levels of mtDNA were not changed, significant specific mtDNA nucleotide damage was prevalent in the senescent heart, as gauged by reduced PCR amplification of larger mtDNA fragments. This damage is likely a result of increased oxidative damage to mtDNA.

## *On gene expression of mitochondrial stress proteins and cellular programming*

Genes encoding mitochondrial stress proteins including both heat-shock and antioxidant response proteins such as HSP60 and GPx are up-regulated in the senescent heart. Increased levels of HSP60 protein have been reported in association with increased level of protein import into mitochondria [25], indicating that mitochondrial protein import is unlikely to be a primary cause of mitochondrial dysfunction.

A significant increase in myocardial mitochondrial GPx activity has been reported in the senescent heart [35–36]. Elevated GPx levels may be an important mechanism in coping with free radical damage, which increases in the senescent heart. In our study, the increased gene expression of GPx is a novel finding suggesting that a signaling mechanism for this transcriptional response needs to be identified.

Aging can induce and activate transcription factors affecting cellular programming. The transcription factor Nf-κB—which is involved in triggering a broad array of inflammatory, cytokine and stress proteins responses in myocardium—was increased in the senescent heart. The transcriptional stimulation of NF-κB is ROS-sensitive.

## *On mitochondrial PT pore*

It is known that the opening of the mitochondrial PT pore occurs as a landmark event of apoptosis and as a result of oxidative stress in cardiomyocytes; however, there is little information concerning the PT pore opening in the aging rat heart. We found increased $Ca^{++}$ sensitivity of the PT pore opening in the senescent heart compared to the young adult. Whether this inner membrane event contributes to the early mitochondrial dysfunction observed, serves as a by-product of the production of mitochondrial ROS, or is an intrinsic component of the myocardial apoptosis trigger during aging remains to be determined.

## Conclusions

Mitochondria are an important focal point in the events of myocardial aging process. Mitochondrial enzymatic dysfunction is unlikely to be a result of an aging-induced decline in mitochondrial transcription, mtDNA depletion, or defective mitochondrial biogenesis. The search for the mechanism of mitochondrial enzyme dysfunction should focus on the posttranslational modification of the component proteins, particularly mtDNA-encoded subunits. Comprehensive examination of all the peptide subunits involved in each aging-affected respiratory enzyme using blue native polyacrylamide gel electrophoresis (BN-PAGE) analysis (in which catalytic activities can be maintained) may be informative in distinguishing among the possible mechanisms for enzymatic dysfunction [59]. A strong mitochondrial stress response with increased gene expression of HSP60 and GPx, presumably secondary to elevated ROS production, occurs in the senescent heart, which may be mediated by the increased transcription of NF-κB. The role(s) of both aging-dependent mtDNA damage and increased sensitivity of the PT pore need to be further delineated both as indicators of oxidative damage and as potential stimuli or signaling events of downstream cellular transcriptional and apoptotic events in myocardial aging. The larger context of myocardial nuclear gene expression governing mitochondrial function needs to be considered and fully examined, given the relative scarcity of aging-regulation data presently available. A comprehensive analysis of mitochondrial events may be extremely useful in assessing both the individual pathway responses and the overall cardiac phenotype in aging.

## Potential approaches to reverse mitochondrial dysfunction in the aging heart

Although in Chapters 11 and 12 we address in detail where we are and where we are going in the treatment of the mitopathies of the aging heart and cardiovascular diseases at large, in this chapter we comment briefly on the recently suggested therapies for mitochondrial dysfunction secondary to ROS and defective FAO metabolism occurring in the aging heart.

To reverse the mitochondrial dysfuntion found in the aging heart, it has been suggested that supplements of acetyl-l-carnitine (ALCAR) and (R)-alpha-lipoic acid can improve myocardial bioenergetics and decrease the oxidative stress associated with aging [60]. Old rats fed with ALCAR have shown a reversal of the age-related decline in carnitine levels and improved mitochondrial fatty acid β-oxidation in a number of tissues studied. However, ALCAR supplementation does not appear to reverse the age-related decline in the cardiac antioxidant status and may not improve the indices of oxidative stress. Lipoic acid, a potent thiol antioxidant and mitochondrial metabolite, appears to increase low molecular weight antioxidants decreasing the age-associated oxidative insult. Seemingly, ALCAR along with lipoic acid may be effective supplemental regimens to maintain myocardial function in aging. Moreover, the lipophilic antioxidant and mitochondrial redox coupler coenzyme $Q_{10}$ may have the potential to improve energy production in the aging heart mitochondria by bypassing defective components in the respiratory chain, as well as by reducing the effects of oxidative stress. Recent studies in rats and human suggest that coenzyme $Q_{10}$ protect the aging heart against stress [61].

Judging by the popular media, it would appear that caloric restriction and the use of antioxidants to slow/stop aging-related cardiac defects is a well-established fact. However, so far, there is a lack of meticulous and carefully done research to prove this contention. There is little doubt that mitochondria represent a desirable pharmacological target and drugs that modulate mitochondrial function (e.g., targeting oxidative stress) may be helpful in the aging heart; however, it is not clear if and how much of these antioxidant agents should be administered without jeopardizing the ROS "protector side" role in the heart signaling pathways. Recently, the antioxidant organoselenium compound ebselen, a mimic of glutathione peroxidase, has been shown to prevent the structural and functional changes occurring in mitochondria of aged red blood cells of the rainbow trout, induced by oxidative stress. However, it did not prevent swelling of the organelle [62]. Whether this compound can be of any significance in reversing the changes that occur in human cardiac aging is not known at this time. Similarly, dietary restriction, which is known to retard aging and increase the lifespan of rodents, has been shown to significantly reduce the age-related accumulation of 8-oxo-2-deoxyguanosine (oxo8dG) in nuclear DNA in all tissues of male B6D23F1 mice and in most tissues of male F344 rats [63]. Dietary restriction seems also to prevent the age-related increase in oxo8dG levels in mtDNA isolated from the liver of both rats and mice; at this time, data on heart are not yet available.

That moderate exercise has beneficial effects on cardiac physiology and metabolism is well recognized. Moderate exercise in a treadmill increased the life span of male and female mice (aged from 28 to 78 wk) by 19 and 9%, respectively [64]. Moreover, moderate exercise decreased the aging-associated accumulation of oxygen free radicals, probably by reducing the decrease in antioxidant enzymes and in complex I and IV activities in a number of tissues, including the heart. These effects however, were not significant in the very old animals.

Contrary to simple organisms, such as yeast and worms, in which aging is easily altered through external stimuli, such as caloric restriction or through genetic manipulation (e.g., SIR2 genes), manipulation of aging in mammals is more complex since it includes a close relation with programmed cell death that does not tolerate well the effects of antiaging therapy [65]. With advancing age, cells are much more susceptible to certain toxins or stresses and may not adequately respond to environmental and toxicological insults that would require increased ATP production to be successfully detoxified. Further research is needed to understand the role that mitochondrial dysfunction plays in aging, as well as to identify novel strategies to slow the progression of accumulative loss of cardiomyocytes (by apoptosis or programmed cell death) and stem the metabolic decline evident with age.

# References

1. Fannin SW, Lesnefsky EJ, Slabe TJ, Hassan MO, Hoppel CL(1999) Aging selectively decreases oxidative capacity in rat heart interfibrillar mitochondria. Arch Biochem Biophys 372:399–407
2. Ramani K, Lust WD, Whittingham TS, Lesnefsky EJ (1996) ATP catabolism and adenosine generation during ischemia in the aging heart. Mech Ageing Dev 89:113–24
3. Brunt UT, Terman A (2002) The mitochondrial-lysosomal axistheory of aging: Accumulation of damaged mitochondria as a result of imperfect autophagocytosis. Eur J Biochem 269:1996–2002
4. Rooyackers OE, Adey DB, Ades PA, Nair KS (1996) Effect of age on *in vivo* rates of mitochondrial protein synthesis in human skeletal muscle. Proc Natl Acad Sci USA 93:15364–9
5. Marín-García J, Ananthakrishnan R, Goldenthal MJ (1997) Mitochondrial gene expression in rat heart and liver during growth and development. Biochem Cell Biol 75:137–42
6. Marín-García J, Ananthakrishnan R, Agrawal N, Goldenthal MJ (1994) Mitochondrial gene expression during bovine cardiac growth and development. J Mol Cell Cardiol 26:1029–36
7. Sugiyama S,Takasawa M, Hayakawa M, Ozawa T (1993) Changes in skeletal muscle, heart and liver mitochondrial electron electron transport activities in rats and dogs of various ages. Biochem Mol Biol Int 30:937–44
8. Wanagat J, Wolff MR, Aiken JM (2002) Age-associated changes

in function, structure and mitochondrial genetic and enzymatic abnormalities in the Fischer 344 x Brown Norway F(1) hybrid rat heart. J Mol Cell Cardiol 34:17–28

9. Guerrieri F, Capozza G, Kalous M, Papa S (1992) Age-related changes of mitochondrial F0F1 ATP synthase. Ann NY Acad Sci 671:395–402

10. Lesnefsky EJ, Hoppel CL (2003) Ischemia-reperfusion injury in the aged heart: Role of mitochondria. Arch Biochem Biophys 420: 287–97

11. Lenaz G, D'Aurelio M, Merlo Pich M, Genova ML, Ventura B, Bovina C, Formiggini G, Parenti Castelli G (2000) Mitochondrial bioenergetics in aging. Biochim Biophys Acta 1459:397–404

12. Castelluccio C, Baracca A, Fato R, Pallotti F, Maranesi M, Barzanti V, Gorini A, Villa RF, Parenti Castelli G, Marchetti M (1994) Mitochondrial activities of rat heart during ageing. Mech Ageing Dev 76:73–88

13. Miro O, Casademont J, Casals E, Perea M, Urbano-Marquez A, Rustin P, Cardellach F (2000) Aging is associated with increased lipid peroxidation in human hearts, but not with mitochondrial respiratory chain enzyme defects. Cardiovasc Res 47:624–31

14. Kim JH, Shrago E, Elson CE (1988) Age-related changes in respiration coupled to phosphorylation. II. Cardiac mitochondria. Mech Ageing Dev 46:279–90

15. McMillin JB, Taffet GE, Taegtmeyer H, Hudson EK, Tate CA (1993) Mitochondrial metabolism and substrate competition in the aging Fischer rat heart. Cardiovasc Res 27:2222–8

16. Hansford RG, Tsuchiya N, Pepe S (1999) Mitochondria in heart ischemia and aging. Biochem Soc Symp 66:141–7

17. Paradies G, Ruggiero FM, Dinoi P (1992) Decreased activity of the phosphate carrier and modification of lipids in cardiac mitochondria from senescent rats. Int J Biochem 24:783–7

18. Gadaleta MN, Petruzzella V, Renis M, Fracasso F, Cantatore P (1990) Reduced transcription of mitochondrial DNA in the senescent rat. Tissue dependence and effect of L-carnitine. Eur J Biochem 187: 501–6

19. Hudson EK, Tsuchiya N, Hansford RG (1998) Age-associated changes in mitochondrial mRNA expression and translation in the Wistar rat heart. Mech Ageing Dev 103:179–93

20. Bodyak N, Kang PM, Hiromura M, Sulijoadikusumo I, Horikos-

hi N, Khrapko K, Usheva A (2002) Gene expression profiling of the aging mouse cardiac myocytes. Nucleic Acids Res 30:3788–94

21. Goyns MH, Charlton MA, Dunford JE, Lavery WL, Merry BJ, Salehi M, Simoes DC (1998) Differential display analysis of gene expression indicates that age-related changes are restricted to a small cohort of genes. Mech Ageing Dev 101:73–90

22. Barazzoni R, Short KR, Nair KS (2000) Effects of aging on mitochondrial DNA copy number and cytochrome c oxidase gene expression in rat skeletal muscle, liver, and heart. J Biol Chem 275:3343–7

23. Andreu AL, Arbos MA, Perez-Martos A, Lopez-Perez MJ, Asin J, Lopez N, Montoya J, Schwartz S (1998) Reduced mitochondrial DNA transcription in senescent rat heart. Biochem Biophys Res Commun 252:577–81

24. Hansford RG, Castro F (1982) Age-linked changes in the activity of enzymes of the tricarboxylate cycle and lipid oxidation, and of carnitine content, in muscles of the rat. Mech Ageing Dev 19:191–200

25. Craig EE, Hood DA (1997) Influence of aging on protein import into cardiac mitochondria. Am J Physiol 272: H2983–8

26. Hansford RG, Castro F (1982) Effect of senescence on Ca2+-ion transport by heart mitochondria. Mech Ageing Dev 19:5–13

27. Paradies G, Ruggiero FM, Petrosillo G, Quagliariello E (1997) Age-dependent decline in the cytochrome c oxidase activity in rat heart mitochondria: Role of cardiolipin. FEBS Lett 406:136–8

28. Hayakawa M, Hattori K, Sugiyama S, Ozawa T (1992) Age-associated oxygen damage and mutations in mitochondrial DNA in human hearts. Biochem Biophys Res Commun 189:979–85

29. Richter C (1995) Oxidative damage to mitochondrial DNA and its relationship to ageing. Int J Biochem Cell Biol 27:647–53

30. Lee HC, Pang CY, Hsu HS, Wei YH (1994) Differential accumulations of 4,977 bp deletion in mitochondrial DNA of various tissues in human ageing. Biochim Biophys Acta 1226:37–43

31. Pamplona R, Portero-Otin M, Bellmun MJ, Gredilla R, Barja G (2002) Aging increases Nepsilon-(carboxymethyl)lysine and caloric restriction decreases Nepsilon-(carboxyethyl)lysine and Nepsilon-(malondialdehyde) lysine in rat heart mitochondrial proteins. Free Radic Res 36:47–54

32. Lucas DT, Szweda LI (1998) Cardiac reperfusion injury: Aging, lipid peroxidation, and mitochondrial dysfunction. Proc Natl Acad Sci USA 95:510–4

33. Melov S (2000) Mitochondrial oxidative stress: Physiologic consequences and potential for a role in aging. Ann NY Acad Sci 908:219–25

34. Suh JH, Heath SH, Hagen T (2003) Two subpopulations of mitochondria in the aging rat heart display heterogenous levels of oxidative stress. Free Radic Biol Med 35:1064–72

35. Leichtweis S, Leeuwenburgh C, Bejma J, Ji LL (2001) Aged rat hearts are not more susceptible to ischemia-reperfusion injury in vivo: Role of glutathione. Mech Ageing Dev 122:503–18

36. Vertechy M, Cooper MB, Ghirardi O, Ramacci MT (1989) Antioxidant enzyme activities in heart and skeletal muscle of rats of different ages. Exp Gerontol 24:211–8

37. Phaneuf S, Leeuwenburgh C (2002) Cytochrome c release from mitochondria in the aging heart: A possible mechanism for apoptosis with age. Am J Physiol Integr Comp Physiol 282:R423–30

38. Simonetti I, De Tata V, Del Roso A, Gori Z, Bergamini E (1990) Changes in the transmural distribution of antioxidant enzyme activities across the left ventricle heart wall from rats fed ad libitum or food-restricted during growth and aging. Arch Gerontol Geriatr 10:163–71

39. Adler A, Messina E, Sherman B, Wang Z, Huang H, Linke A, Hintze TH (2003) NAD(P)H oxidase-generated superoxide anion accounts for reduced control of myocardial $O_2$ consumption by NO in old Fischer 344 rats. Am J Physiol Heart Circ Physiol 285:H1015–22

40. Cook SA, Sugden PH, Clerk A (1999) Regulation of Bcl-2 family proteins during development and in response to oxidative stress in cardiac myocytes: association with changes in mitochondrial membrane potential. Circ Res 85:940–9

41. Long X, Goldenthal MJ, Wu GM, Marín-García J (2004) Mitochondrial Ca2+ flux and respiratory enzyme activity decline are early events in cardiomyocyte response to $H_2O_2$. J Mol Cell Cardiol 37:63–70

42. Pollack M, Phaneuf S, Dirks A, Leeuwenburgh C (2002) The role of apoptosis in the normal aging brain, skeletal muscle, and heart. Ann N Y Acad Sci 959:93–107

43. Torella D, Rota M, Nurzynska D, Musso E, Monsen A, Shiraishi I, Zias E, Walsh K, Rosenzweig A, Sussman MA, Urbanek K, Nadal-

Ginard B, Kajstura J, Anversa P, Leri A (2004) Cardiac stem cell and myocyte aging, heart failure, and insulin-like growth factor-1 overexpression. Circ Res 94:514–24

44. Chomyn A, Attardi G (2003) MtDNA mutations in aging and apoptosis. Biochem Biophys Res Commun 304:519–29

45. Marín-García J, Zoubenko O, Goldenthal MJ (2002) Mutations in the cardiac mtDNA control region associated with cardiomyopathy and aging. J Cardiac Failure 8:93–100

46. Marín-García J, Goldenthal MJ, Pierpont ME, Ananthakrishnan R and Perez-Atayde A (1999) Is age a contributory factor of mitochondrial bioenergetic decline and DNA defects in idiopathic dilated cardiomyopathy? Cardiovascular Pathology 8:217–22

47. Nekhaeva E, Bodyak ND, Kraytsberg Y, McGrath SB, Van Orsouw NJ, Pluzhnikov A, Wei JY, Vijg J, Khrapko K (2002) Clonally expanded mtDNA point mutations are abundant in individual cells of human tissues. Proc Natl Acad Sci USA 99:5521–6

48. Diaz F, Bayona-Bafaluy MP, Rana M, Mora M, Hao H, Moraes CT (2002) Human mitochondrial DNA with large deletions repopulates organelles faster than full-length genomes under relaxed copy number control. Nucleic Acids Res 30:4626–33

49. Khrapko K, Bodyak N, Thilly WG, van Orsouw NJ, Zhang X, Coller HA, Perls TT, Upton M, Vijg J, Wei J (1999) Cell-by-cell scanning of whole mitochondrial genomes in aged human heart reveals a significant fraction of myocytes with clonally expanded deletions. Nucleic Acids Res 27:2434–41

50. Szibor M, Holtz J (2002) Mitochondrial ageing. Basic Res Cardiol 98:210–8

51. Miller FJ, Rosenfeldt FL, Zhang C, Linnane AW, Nagley P (2003) Precise determination of mitochondrial DNA copy number in human skeletal and cardiac muscle by a PCR-based assay: Lack of change of copy number with age. Nucleic Acids Res 31:e61.

52. Welle S, Bhatt K, Shah B, Needler N, Delehanty JM, Thornton (2003) Reduced amount of mitochondrial DNA in aged human muscle. J Appl Physiol 94:1479–84

53. Dinardo MM, Musicco C, Fracasso F, Milella F, Gadaleta MN, Gadaleta G, Cantatore P (2003) Acetylation and level of mitochondrial transcription factor A in several organs of young and old rats. Biochem Biophys Res Commun 301:187–91

54. Wallace DC (1992) Diseases of the mitochondrial DNA. Annu Rev Biochem 61:1175–212.

55. Trifunovic A, Wredenberg A, Falkenberg M, Spelbrink JN, Rovio AT, Bruder CE, Bohlooly-Y M, Gidlof S, Oldfors A, Wibom R, Tornell J, Jacobs HT, Larsson NG (2004) Premature ageing in mice expressing defective mitochondrial DNA polymerase. Nature 27:417–23

56. Wanrooij S, Luoma P, van Goethem G, van Broeckhoven C, Suomalainen A, Spelbrink JN (2004) Twinkle and POLG defects enhance age-dependent accumulation of mutations in the control region of mtDNA. Nucleic Acids Res 32:3053–64

57. Gadaleta MN, Rainaldi G, Lezza AM, Milella F, Fracasso F, Cantatore P (1992) Mitochondrial DNA copy number and mitochondrial DNA deletion in adult and senescent rats. Mutat Res 275:181–93

58. Yan L, Ge H, Li H, Lieber SC, Natividad F, Resuello RR, Kim SJ, Akeju S, Sun A, Loo K, Peppas AP, Rossi F, Lewandowski ED, Thomas AP, Vatner SF, Vatner DE (2004) Gender-specific proteomic alterations in glycolytic and mitochondrial pathways in aging monkey hearts. J Mol Cell Cardiol 37:921–9

59. Van Coster R, Smet J, George E, De Meirleir L, Seneca S, Van Hove J, Sebire G, Verhelst H, De Bleecker J, Van Vlem B, Verloo P, Leroy J (2001) Blue native polyacrylamide gel electrophoresis: A powerful tool in diagnosis of oxidative phosphorylation defects. Pediatr Res 50:658–65

60. Hagen TM, Moreau R, Suh JH, Visioli F (2002) Mitochondrial decay in the aging rat heart: Evidence for improvement by dietary supplementation with acetyl-L-cartinine and/or lipoic acid. Ann NY Acad Sci 959:491–507

61. Rosenfeldt FL, Pepe S, Linnane A, Nagley P, Rowland M, Ou R, Marasco S, Lyon W, Esmore D (2002) Coenzyme Q10 protects the aging heart against stress: Studies in rats, human tissues, and patients. Ann NY Acad Sci 959:355–9

62. Tiano L, Fedeli D, Santoni G, Davies I, Wakabayashi T, Falcioni (2003) Ebselen prevents mitochondrial ageing due to oxidative stress: in vitro study of fish erytrocytes. Mitochondrion 2:428–36

63. Hamilton ML, Van Remmen H, Drake JA, Yang H, Guo ZM, Kewitt K, Walter CA, Richardson A (2001) Does oxidative damage to DNA increase with age? Proc Natl Acad Sci USA 98:10469–74

64. Navarro A, Gomez C, Lopez-Cepero JM, Boveris M (2004) Beneficial effects of moderate exercise on mice aging: Survival,

behavior, oxidative stress and mitochondrial electron transfer. Am J Physiol Regul Integr Comp Physiol 286:R505–11

65. Guarente LP (2004) Forestalling the great beyond with the help of SIR2. The Scientist 18:34–5

# Chapter 10

# Heart Mitochondria Signaling Pathways

## Overview

The contribution that mitochondria make to cardiac function goes well beyond their critical bioenergetic role as a provider of ATP. The organelle performs an essential role in the regulatory and signaling events that occur in response to physiological stresses, including but not limited to myocardial ischemia and reperfusion, hypoxia, oxidative stress, hormonal, and cytokine stimuli. Research studies on both intact cardiac muscle tissue and cultured cardiomyocytes are beginning to examine the nature and the extent of mitochondrial involvement in interorganelle communication, hypertrophic growth, and cell death. In this chapter, particular aspects of the newly emerging field of mitochondrial medicine are presented, including assessment of organelle participation at the molecular and biochemical levels, in the multiple and interrelated signaling pathways, gauging the effect that mitochondria have as a receiver, integrator, and transmitter of signals on cardiac phenotype. In addition, future directions that may impact on the treatment of cardiac diseases are discussed.

## Introduction

Mitochondrial signaling can be defined as the process by which the organelle communicates with its environment as a transmitter and receiver of signals. The contribution that mitochondria make to cardiac function extends well beyond their critical bioenergetic role as ATP producer. The organelle plays an integral part in the regulatory and signaling events that occur in response to physiological stresses, including but not limited to myocardial ischemia and reperfusion, hypoxia, oxidative stress, hormonal, and cytokine stimuli. Research on both intact cardiac muscle tissue and cultured cardiomyocytes has just begun to probe the nature and extent of mitochondrial involvement in interorganelle communication, hypertrophic growth, and cell death.

In this chapter, an in-depth analysis of the multiple roles that the organelle plays as an integrator and receiver of signals in cardiac pathophysiology is presented.

## Mitochondrial abnormalities, signaling defects, and myocardial disease

As previously noted, pathogenic point mutations and large-scale deletions in cardiac mtDNA have severe consequences for the heart [1]. Specific mtDNA mutations with associated mitochondrial respiratory dysfunction have been identified in isolated cases of cardiomyopathy as well as in systemic encephalomyopathies with cardiac involvement, including Leigh disease, MELAS, and MERRF [1]. In addition, the depletion of cardiac mtDNA levels concomitant with myocardial mitochondrial respiratory dysfunction has been found in patients with both DCM and HCM and in patients and animal models treated with zidovudine [2–3]. While the dependence of cardiac homeostasis on functional mitochondria is primarily attributed to needed ATP derived from OXPHOS for maintaining myocardial contractility, the role of cardiac mitochondria in responding to a variety of intracellular and extracellular signals, metabolic substrates, and physiological stresses has recently become of increasing interest. Examination of cardiomyocytes containing specific pathogenic mtDNA point mutations and deletions or depleted mtDNA levels for their effect(s) on mitochondrial signaling may provide further information on the role of a mitochondrial cytopathy in the pathogenesis of cardiac diseases.

In addition to mtDNA defects, mutations at several different nuclear gene loci have been described in conjunction with mitochondrial OXPHOS deficiencies in cardiomyopathies associated with Leigh syndrome, COX deficiency, and FRDA [4–6]. In addition, mutations in nuclear genes that contribute to the observed cardiac disease-associated mitochondrial enzyme and mtDNA defects (including the elevated incidence of large-scale mtDNA deletions and mtDNA depletion) have been recently reported [7]. The involvement of both genomes in mitochondrial biogenesis and mitochondria-based pathogenesis serves as an important rationale for examining the crosstalk and regulatory signaling between both genomes as well as to expand the search for mutations involved in mitochondrial biogenesis.

Understanding the intergenomic signaling pathways may also prove illuminating about cardiac dysfunction involving various mitochondrial targets (including non-OXPHOS function) both in genetic syndromes/diseases and with physiological insults.

Defects in mitochondrial carnitine, fatty acid (FA) transport, and FAO have a crucial role in cardiac sudden death, bioenergetic dysfunction, cardiac arrhythmias, and cardiomyopathy [1]. In transgenic mice, the disruption of specific nuclear genes-encoding mitochondrial proteins (engaged in a broad array of functions) leads to cardiomyopathy and HF. Knockout mutations in ANT, MnSOD, mtTFA, and the frataxin gene (encoding a mitochondrial iron transporter associated with FRDA) leads to phenotypic cardiomyopathy and HF [8–11]. In FRDA, the disease phenotype is very prominent in the heart and less in striated muscle and clearly impacts mitochondrial bioenergetic function [6].These findings underscore the importance of the mitochondrial organelle in the overall maintenance of a functional cardiac phenotype. In particular, the mitochondrial role in myocardial apoptosis (i.e., ANT is an essential component of the mitochondrial PT pore, which mediates early apoptotic progression) and mitochondrial antioxidant response (e.g., MnSOD) to oxidative stress, a critical element of myocardial ischemia and mitochondrial cytoprotection, need to be emphasized.

## *Mitochondrial signaling in myocardial ischemia and cardioprotection*

When the supply of oxygen is disrupted as found with myocardial ischemia, both mitochondrial ETC flux and OXPHOS decline, the myocardial reserves of high-energy phosphates are rapidly depleted, pyruvate oxidation decreases, and ATP production is impaired. The hydrolysis of glycolytic-derived ATP and the resulting accumulation of lactate and pyruvate leads to intracellular acidosis (which has a direct effect on cardiac contractile function) and to the accumulation of myocardial sodium and calcium. Moreover, the energy deficit occurring as a result of ATP depletion is further compounded by the deployment of ATP to reestablish the disturbed myocardial ionic balance rather than to fuel contraction. AMP and other intermediates also accumulate with subsequent mitochondrial swelling and degeneration. In addition, the activity levels of respiratory complexes IV and V decrease in myocardial ischemia and may lead to increased levels of mtDNA deletions [12–14]. While ultimately, sustained myocardial ischemia leads to ATP depletion and necrotic cell death, there is ample evidence that both ischemia and hypoxia can activate cardio-myocyte mitochondrial death pathway by promoting the PT pore opening concomitant with mitochondrial membrane depolarization, eventual disruption of the mitochondrial membranes, and release of cytochrome *c* [15].

Increased mitochondrial function can also exacerbate ischemic da-mage, especially at the onset of reperfusion when FA influx increases and unbalanced FAO occurs [16]. Excess acetyl-CoA is produced, saturating the TCA cycle at the expense of glucose and pyruvate oxidation. Increased OXPHOS elevates mitochondrial ROS produc-tion and myocardial lipid peroxidation resulting in cardiolipin depletion with severe effect on both complex I and IV activities [17]. These enzyme activities can be restored to normal levels by the addition of exogenous cardiolipin or by the induction of antioxidants MnSOD and catalase.

Analysis of the events of ischemic preconditioning has revealed that its cardioprotective effect is at least partially mediated by $Ca^{++}$ over-loading in the mitochondrial matrix and by increased mitochondrial ROS generation, leading to further protein kinase activation. The cascade of cardioprotective events can be initiated by the binding of a variety of ligands (e.g. adenosine, opioids, bradykinin, acetylcholine) to sarcolemmal G-coupled receptors with the subsequent activation of calcium flux, tyrosine protein kinases, and the pI3k/Akt pathway (Figure 10.1). In addition, marked changes in mitochondrial matrix volume associated with the cardiomyocyte mitoK$_{ATP}$ channel opening may also play a contributory role in cytoprotection [18–19]. Drugs such as diazoxide and nicorandil specifically activate the mitoK$_{ATP}$ channel opening eliciting CP and can also inhibit $H_2O_2$-induced apoptotic progression in cardiomyocytes, suggesting that mitoK$_{ATP}$ channels also play a significant regulatory role in oxidative-stress signals in mitochondrial apoptosis [20]. While considerable attention has focused on the opening of the mitoK$_{ATP}$ channel as the primary regulatory event in mitochondrial cardioprotective signaling [21–23], this view has recently been challenged by recent evidence implicating the cardioprotective effects of mitoK$_{ATP}$ and associated channel openers (e.g., KCOs) with respiratory function inhibition in addition to mitoK$_{ATP}$ channel activity [24–25]. The precise temporal order of

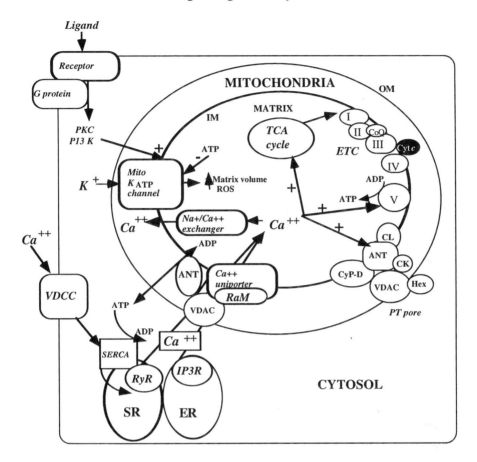

**Figure 10.1. Mitochondrial ion channels are pivotal signal transducers in myocardium.** *The cardioprotection pathway involving the mitochondrial $K^+$ channels (mitoK$_{ATP}$) is located in the inner membrane and is mediated by ROS, ligands binding to an assortment of G-coupled membrane receptors, and protein kinases (PKC/PI3K). Calcium enters the mitochondria in response to a variety of stimuli via a complex of membrane proteins, including the outer-membrane (OM) voltage-dependent anion carrier (VDAC), the inner-membrane (IM) proteins, rapid mode of $Ca^{++}$ uptake (RaM), and the $Ca^{++}$ uniporter. High $Ca^{++}$ levels can be supplied from ryanodine release (RyR) and phosphatidylinositol 3 (IP3R) receptors located in the sarcoplasmic (SR) and endoplasmic (ER) reticulum, respectively, and is coupled to the entry of calcium into the cardiomyocyte through the voltage-dependent $Ca^{++}$ channel (VDCC). Entry of high calcium levels into the mitochondria can increase activities of several enzymes of TCA cycle, electron transport chain (ETC), and complex V. Calcium also modulates the opening of the permeability transition (PT) pore shown with its accessory components, including VDAC, adenine nucleotide translocator (ANT), hexokinase (Hex), creatine kinase (CK), cyclophilin D (CyP-D), and cardiolipin (CL); calcium efflux is primarily managed by the $Na^+/Ca^{2+}$ exchanger.*

events in the mitochondrial CP cascade and the exact molecular nature of the mitoK$_{ATP}$ channel still remain to be precisely defined [21–22]

CP associated with mitochondrial signaling has also been demonstrated with brief periods of hypothermia prior to a prolonged ischemic insult [26]. The preservation of myocardial function and ATP levels are accompanied by increased expression of stress proteins (e.g., HSP70) and constitutive mitochondrial proteins (e.g., ANT and ATP synthase-β).

## *Mitochondrial signaling and myocardial hypertrophy*

The concept that cardiac cells have the ability to grow in number is controversial. Although there is general agreement that cardiomyocytes are postmitotic with limited proliferative capacity, recent studies have suggested that cardiomyocyte growth regulation may be disturbed in hearts undergoing severe remodeling (such as in late-stage HF) [27]. In normal postnatal cardiomyocyte growth, an increase in cardiac cell size and not in cell number is more commonly accepted [28]. Stimuli that provoke myocardial hypertrophy include increases in mechanical and hemodynamic loads (volume and pressure overloads/mechanical stretch), inflammatory cytokines, peptide growth factors, neuroendocrine factors (e.g., norepinephrine and angiotensin), and oxidative stress.

Molecular features of the hypertrophic response include changes in the myocardial gene expression program (fetal gene transcription) with a large array of nuclear transcription factors and activators identified, multiple signaling cascade pathways featuring an array of protein kinases [29] with resulting effects on cellular protein synthesis (including ribosomes), activated membrane ATPase pumps and calcium handlers (e.g., sarco-/endoplasmic reticulum Ca$^{++}$ ATPase), and induced protein synthesis of the sarcomeric contractile apparatus (e.g., specific myosin isoforms).

Cardiac hypertrophy resulting from primarily physiological stimuli generally does not lead to heart failure, in contrast to cardiac hypertrophy resulting from pathological stimuli (decompensation), which often does [30]. The former tends to be concentric, manifested largely by cardiac myocyte thickening, while eccentric hypertrophy is characterized by cell elongation. These growth responses are mediated by different signal transduction pathways. In addition, cardiac cells undergoing hypertrophy from pathological stimuli display both an increased sensitivity to apoptotic stimuli and an expression pattern favoring proapoptotic regulation of Fas, the Bcl-2 protein family, and caspases [31].

In cardiac hypertrophy, the effects on heart mitochondria are manifold. There is a significant down-regulation of mitochondrial pathways involving FAO/FA transport system occurring as part of a shift in cardiac bioenergetic substrate utilization from FA to glucose (glycolytic pathways) [32]. Both experimental and clinical studies of cardiac hypertrophy and HF have demonstrated reduced levels of carnitine required for mitochondrial FA import and FAO [33–34]. Moreover, the levels of MCAD, a key enzyme in FAO, have been shown to be both transcriptionally and translationally down-regulated in the rat pressure-overload model and during HF and is mediated in part by modulation of the levels of the global transcription factor PPAR-α [35]. Decline in PPAR-α in myocardial hypertrophy not only impacts the expression of genes involved in the FAO pathway but also effects the regulation of the mitochondrial carnitine shuttle by malonyl-CoA by its effect on the expression of the malonyl-CoA degrading enzyme, malonyl-CoA decarboxylase (MCD) [36].

Cardiac hypertrophy (both due to physiological and pathological stimuli) is accompanied by an increase in mitochondrial number resulting from increased mitochondrial biogenesis and protein synthesis [37]. Stimuli ranging from electrical stimulation and exercise to thyroid hormone treatment elicit cardiac hypertrophy with increased mitochondrial biogenesis and function. In addition, increased mitochondrial number has been reported in both experimental animal and transgenic models of HCM and in clinical cases of mitochondria-based cardiac disease [1, 38–39]. Aberrant mitochondrial accumulation, abnormal mitochondrial function, and myocardial hypertrophy have been widely recognized in patients with an HCM phenotype presenting either as isolated cardiomyopathy or in systemic neuropathies such as MELAS, MERRF, and Leigh disease. The increase in mitochondria is considered to be a compensatory response to mitochondrial bioenergetic dysfunction, observable in these animal models and patients, and is often discernible by increased RRF in cardiomyocytes [38]. The precise elements involved in signaling the events leading to mitochondrial biogenesis during cardiac hypertrophy and HCM remain to be identified.

Cardiac hypertrophy is also associated with shifts in mitochondrial metabolism elicited by signaling proteins (e.g., Akt/PI3K/ mammalian target of rapamycin [mTOR] pathway), which coordinate hypertrophic growth responses to a variety of physiological stimuli (e.g., glucose and serum deprivation). The critical role played by bioenergetic substrates/products (e.g., fatty acids, ATP, pyruvate, and phosphocreatine) and their regulators (e.g., AMP kinase and malonyl-CoA) in myocardial hypertrophy, and the commonality of many of the signaling elements in the hypertrophic and apoptotic pathways further support a pivotal mitochondrial role in committing the myocardial cell to growth/hypertrophy or to cell death (by apoptosis or necrosis) [29, 32, 40].

## Signaling the mitochondria: Key players

### *Nuclear gene activation*

Nuclear transcriptional modulators have been identified that govern the expression of a wide array of mitochondrial proteins in response to diverse cellular stimuli and signals. For instance, nuclear transcription factors such as nuclear respiratory factors NRF-1 and NRF-2 are implicated in the activation of mitochondrial biogenesis [41–43]. These factors exert a direct effect on the synthesis of specific nuclear-encoded subunits of the mitochondrial respiratory enzymes as well as up-regulate levels of mtTFA, involved in both mtDNA replication and transcription (Figure 10.2). In addition to the nuclear global regulatory transcription factors such as PPARs and their transcriptional coactivators (e.g., RXR-α), which play a pivotal regulatory role in the expression of mitochondrial FAO pathways integral to myocardial bioenergetic metabolism [44–46], the transcription coactivator PGC-1α, which is abundantly expressed in cardiac muscle, activates expression of transcription factors NRF-1 and NRF-2, providing an important regulatory link between mitochondrial biogenesis and FAO capacity [47]. Transcriptional control by these activators is affected by hypoxia, ischemia, and cardiac failure [48-49]. PGC-1α expression and mitochondrial bio-

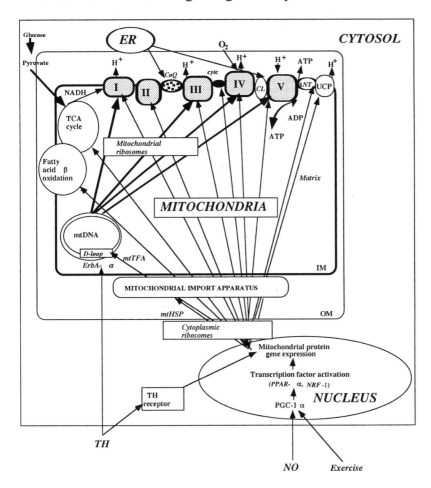

**Figure 10.2. Myocardial mitochondrial biogenesis and bioenergetic pathways are signal driven.** *Shown are the major mitochondrial bioenergetic pathways, including the matrix-localized TCA cycle, the inner-membrane (IM) associated fatty acid oxidation pathway, and the respiratory complexes (I–V) with closely associated adenine nucleotide translocator (ANT) involved in ATP/ADP mitochondria transport and uncoupling proteins (UCP) effecting proton transport. Also depicted are thyroid hormone (TH) and nitric oxide (NO) activation of transcription factors in the nucleus (e.g., PGC-1α, PPAR-α, and NRF-1) and a subset of factors (e.g., Erb-Aα and mtTFA) that activate mtDNA transcription by interaction with D-loop sequences promoting mitochondrial biogenesis. All but 13 mitochondrial proteins are encoded in the nucleus, translated on cytoplasmic ribosomes, and incorporated through the complex outer membrane by a mitochondrial import apparatus utilizing chaperones such as heat-shock proteins (HSPs) as shown. Also shown are the endoplasmic reticulum (ER) that provides important mitochondrial membrane phospholipids, (e.g., coenzyme Q [CoQ] and cardiolipin [CL]).*

genesis are modulated by the activation of a calcium/calmodulin-dependent protein kinase, indicating that the $Ca^{++}$-regulated signaling pathway plays a significant role in transcriptional activation of genes governing mitochondrial biogenesis [50]. Moreover, these nuclear activators are modulated during cardiac development [51–52]. Activation of the nuclear factor activated T-cell (NFAT) family of transcription factors has been shown to be crucial in early cardiac development and is required to maintain myocardial mitochondrial oxidative function. Targeted cardiac gene disruption of the NFATc-3 and NFATc-4 genes results in cardiomyocyte ETC dysfunction, reduced ventricular size, and aberrant cardiomyocyte structure in the mouse embryo [52].

Evidence that these nuclear transcriptional factors modulate the cardiac phenotype comes largely from studies in transgenic animals bearing either mutations in specific transcriptional factors or over-expressed genes [44–53]. Also, it has been found that specific nuclear transcription factors are essential for normal cardiac phenotype and mitochondrial function. For instance, cardiac-specific PGC-1α over-expression in transgenic mice results in uncontrolled mitochondrial proliferation and extensive loss of sarcomeric structure leading to DCM [44]. The myocardial overexpression of PPAR-α may lead to severe cardiomyopathy with both increased myocardial FA uptake and mitochondrial FAO [53]. Similarly, mutations targeting mtTFA produce inactivation of myocardial mitochondrial gene expression and ETC dysfunction resulting in DCM and atrioventricular conduction defects [11].

## *Protein kinases*

Evidence that mitochondria contain multiple phosphoprotein substrates for protein kinases and that a number of protein kinases are translocated into heart mitochondria strongly suggests that protein phosphorylation within the mitochondria is a critical component of mitochondrial signaling pathways [54]. However, it is important to note that the detection of a protein in a phosphorylated state does not directly implicate phosphorylation as playing a regulatory role. Many proteins can be phosphorylated *in vitro* by protein kinases yet show no changes in activity. Thus far, protein kinases identified in heart mitochondria include PDH kinase, branched-chain α-ketoacid dehydrogenase kinase, protein kinase A (PKA), protein kinase C (PKCδ and ε isoforms), and c-Jun N-terminal kinase kinase [55–60]. Their characterization has offered new insights into the fundamental mechanisms regulating mitochondrial responses to diverse physiological stimuli and stresses.

In cardiomyocytes, PKCε, after translocation to the mitochondria, forms a signaling module by forming complexes with specific mitogen-activated protein kinases (e.g., extracellular signal-regulated kinase, P38, and c-Jun N-terminal kinase), resulting in the phosphorylation of the proapoptotic protein Bad [59]. Also, PKCε forms physical interaction with components of the cardiac PT pore (in particular, the VDAC and ANT) [61]. This interaction may inhibit the pathological opening of the pore, including $Ca^{++}$-induced opening and subsequent mitochondrial swelling, contributing to PKCε-induced CP. While PKC activation in CP likely precedes mitoK$_{ATP}$ channel opening, its direct interaction with the mitoK$_{ATP}$ channels has not been demonstrated. Following treatment with diazoxide, PKCδ is also translocated to cardiac mitochondria [58]; however, several studies have shown that PKCδ does not play a contributory role in the CP provided by IPC [62–63].

A cAMP-dependent protein kinase (mtPKA) as well as its protein substrates have been localized to the matrix side of the inner mitochondrial membrane [57]. In cardiomyocytes, the 18-kDa subunit of complex I (NDUFS4) is phosphorylated by mtPKA, and increased levels of cAMP promote NDUFS4 phosphorylation, enhancing both complex I activity and NAD-linked mitochondrial respiration [57, 64–65]. These posttranslational changes can be reversed by dephosphorylation via a mitochondria-localized phosphatase. Phosphorylation of several subunits of COX including COXI, III, and Vb occurs at serine residues by mtPKA modulating COX activity [66] and has been considered to be a critical element of respiratory control. This cAMP-dependent phosphorylation occurs with high ATP/ADP ratios and results in the allosteric inhibition of COX activity. At the same time, this regulatory control can result in reduced mitochondrial membrane potential and more efficient energy transduction in the resting state. Conversely, increases in mitochondrial phosphatase ($Ca^{++}$-induced) activity reverse the allosteric COX inhibition/respiratory control resulting in increased membrane potential and ROS formation. Various stress stimuli leading to increased mitochondrial $Ca^{++}$

flux result in increased membrane potential and mitochondrial ROS formation.

With the development of new technologies, including improved kinase inhibitors assays and proteomic analysis, a variety of mitochondrial phosphoprotein targets for these kinases have been reported. A set of proteins has been identified in the mitochondrial phosphoprotein proteome of the bovine heart as targets of kinase-mediated phosphorylation [67]. The majority of identified phosphoproteins were involved in mitochondrial bioenergetic function either in the TCA cycle (e.g., aconitase, isocitrate, and pyruvate dehydrogenase), as respiratory complex subunits (e.g., NDUFA 10 of complex I, SDH flavoprotein subunit of complex II, core I and core III subunits of complex III, and $\alpha$ and $\beta$ subunits of complex V), or as essential players in mitochondrial bioenergetic homeostasis (e.g., creatine kinase and ANT). In addition, during myocardial ischemia, phosphorylation of the elongation factor EF-Tu, a key regulatory protein of the cardiac mitochondrial protein translation apparatus, is modulated [68].

## *Calcium signaling*

The import of $Ca^{++}$ from cytosol into cardiac mitochondria is an important regulatory event in cell signaling. Recently, mitochondrial calcium flux, particularly in cultured cardiomyocytes, has become detectable using advanced cell-imaging techniques with fluorescent dyes, confocal microscopy, and recombinantly derived $Ca^{++}$ sensitive photoprobes [69–70]. Mitochondrial $Ca^{++}$ influx is primarily provided by a $Ca^{++}$ pump uniporter located in the inner membrane driven by the mitochondrial membrane potential as well as by low matrix $Ca^{++}$ levels and can be blocked by ruthenium red [71]. Mitochondrial $Ca^{++}$ uptake is significantly and rapidly elevated in cardiomyocytes during physiological $Ca^{++}$ signaling and is often accompanied by a highly localized transient mitochondrial depolarization [70]. Efflux of $Ca^{++}$ from cardiomyocyte mitochondria is mediated by a $Na^+/Ca^{++}$ exchanger linked to ETC proton pumping, although calcium efflux also occurs with PT pore opening. Activation of the PT pore and mitochondrial $Ca^{++}$ flux also occurs in early myocardial apoptosis and ischemia/reperfusion and is involved in the generation of a calcium wave delivering system between adjacent mitochondria [72].

A major consequence of increased mitochondrial $Ca^{++}$ uptake is the up-regulation of energy metabolism and stimulation of mitochondrial OXPHOS. Elevated mitochondrial $Ca^{++}$ levels allosterically stimulate the activity of 3 TCA cycle enzymes, including pyruvate, isocitrate, and 2-oxoglutarate dehydrogenase [73–74]. Activation of these enzymes by $Ca^{++}$ results in increased $NADH/NAD^+$ ratios and ultimately leads to increased mitochondrial ATP synthesis. Recently, a thermokinetic model of cardiac bioenergetics described calcium activation of the dehydrogenases as the rate-limiting determinant of respiratory flux regulating myocardial oxygen consumption, proton efflux, NADH, and ATP synthesis [75]. In cardiomyocytes, mitochondrial ATP synthase activity can be directly modulated by increased mitochondrial $Ca^{++}$ levels [76–77].

Intracompartment $Ca^{++}$ signaling is recognized as a key mode of signal transduction and amplification in mitochondria [69–70]. Using inositol phospholipids such as inositol 1,4,5-triphosphate (IP3) as second messengers, a variety of cell-surface hormones and neurotransmitters signal the release of $Ca^{++}$ from the ER and Golgi apparatus into the cytosol. The proximity of mitochondria to ER membranes appears to be a significant factor for ER $Ca^{++}$ release and mitochondrial $Ca^{++}$ uptake [78]. This dramatic increase in mitochondrial $Ca^{++}$ is rapidly mobilized from the ER IP3-receptor channels when in close contact to mitochondria, albeit the precise molecular mechanism of this transfer has not been fully established. Similarly, the sarcoplasmic reticulum ryanodine receptors are also located near the cardiomyocyte mitochondria undergoing calcium release [79]. Proposed mechanisms for the rapid mitochondrial $Ca^{++}$ import include the involvement of diffusible cytosolic factors that stimulate the $Ca^{++}$ uniporter, the activation of an entirely different channel in the heart mitochondrial membrane (RaM), and enhanced $Ca^{++}$ uptake by mitochondrial analogues of ryanodine receptors residing in the inner membrane [80–83]. Recently, VDAC/porin has also been identified (Figure 10.1) as a component in $Ca^{++}$ transport from ER through the outer mitochondrial membrane [84].

## *Mitochondrial receptors*

Few well-characterized heart mitochondrial receptors have been detected despite the large number of receptors that have been identified in other tissues/cell types. The thyroid hormone (TH) receptor Erb-

Aα, which was identified as an "orphan" receptor [85–86] involved in interacting with mtDNA during targeted hormonal stimulation (Figure 10.2), has not yet been documented in cardiac tissue, despite the known marked effect of TH in heart mitochondria. In addition, a large number of nuclear transcription factors described and characterized in many other tissues/cell types as translocating to mitochondria, including p53, NF-κB, PPAR-α, RXR-α, and TR3 (another "orphan receptor" of the steroid-thyroid hormone-retinoid receptor superfamily of transcription factors), have also not yet been documented in heart mitochondria. No specific mitochondrial receptors have yet been found that bind TNF-α or various cytokines known to effect cardiac mitochondrial function, despite several recent studies demonstrating that TNF-α impacts cardiomyocyte mitochondria. Moreover, in contrast to other tissues, there has been limited characterization in heart mitochondria of anchoring proteins, which bind and concentrate protein kinases.

A common theme concerning signaling and activation includes the stimuli-generated translocation of specific cytosolic proteins into the mitochondria. The growing list of such translocated entities includes many of the proapoptotic proteins (e.g., Bax and Bid) as well as protein kinases. Many of these appear to target specific proteins on the outer mitochondria membrane; others are imported as preproteins, recognized by a small set of specific receptors (translocases) on the mitochondrial translocase of the outer membrane. The import of proteins into mitochondria is often mediated by heat-shock proteins (e.g., HSP60 and HSP70) that specifically interact with a complex mitochondrial protein import apparatus (including matrix proteases). A number of physiological stimuli and stresses, including temperature changes and hormone treatment (e.g., TH), can result in modulating the cardiac mitochondrial import apparatus control [87–88].

## Signals of survival and stress impact heart mitochondria

The list of extracellular influences and intracellularly generated signals that impact the mitochondrial organelle is growing, as reflected in Table 10.1. In addition to hormonal and cytokines stimuli (e.g., TH, TNF-α, and IL-1 β), there are also pro- and antiapoptotic modulators,

**Table 10.1. Stimuli signaling myocardial mitochondrial function**

| Stimuli | Signaling Pathway | Cardiomyocyte Phenotype | Mitochondrial Effect | Ref |
|---|---|---|---|---|
| IL-1 β | NO production | Cardiac dysfunction | Decreased respiration | [89] |
| TNF-α | Ceramide pathway | Cell death | Reduced activity levels of PDH, complexes I and II | [90] |
| Heat stress | Increased levels of HSP 32, 60, 72 | Improved cardiac function after I/R | Increased complex I–V activities | [91] |
| Low glucose | Myocardial apoptosis | Cell death | Cyt $c$ release | [92] |
| Low serum | Myocardial apoptosis | Cell death | Cyt $c$ release | [92] |
| Palmitate | Myocardial apoptosis; ceramide increase | Cell death | Reduced complex III and membrane potential; increased cyt $c$ release, UCP, and swollen mitochondria | [93] |
| Ceramide | Ceramide pathway | Cell death | Decreased complex III activity | [94] |
| Electrical stimulation | NRF-1 activation | Hypertrophy | Mitochondrial proliferation | [25] |
| Nitric oxide | Peroxynitrite formation | Myocardial $O_2$ uptake decline; increased $H_2O_2$ | Complex I and IV decrease; increased cyt $c$ release | [95–96] |
| Thyroid hormone (T3/T4) | Receptor-mediated nuclear and mtDNA gene activation | Hypertrophy | Mitochondrial proliferation. increased UCP and uncoupled OXPHOS | [97–98] |

*Note:* HSP, heat-shock protein; I/R, ischemia/reperfusion; IL, interleukin; NO, nitric oxide; NRF-1, nuclear respiratory factor-1; OXPHOS, oxidative phosphorylation; PDH, pyruvate dyhydrogenase; T3, triiodothyronine; T4, thyroxin; TNF-α, tumor necrosis factor-α; UCP, uncoupling protein.

nutrient, serum, growth and mitotic stimulatory factors, as well as metabolic and stress stimuli, which are described in more detail in this section.

## *Survival signals and apoptosis*

Activation of the PI3 kinase/Akt (protein kinase B) pathway promotes cell survival primarily by intervening in the mitochondrial apoptosis cascade at events before cytochrome *c* release and caspase activation occur. Akt activation inhibits changes in the inner mitochondrial membrane potential that occur in apoptosis (suppressing apoptotic progression and the cytochrome *c* release induced by several proapoptotic proteins). While Akt also contributes to the phosphorylation and inactivation of the proapoptogenic protein Bad, it remains unclear whether Bad phosphorylation is the mechanism by which Akt ensures cell survival and mitochondrial integrity, since other mitochondrial targets of Akt remain to be identified [99]. With regards to the heart, PI3K/Akt signaling also promotes glucose uptake and the growth and survival of cardiomyocytes and has been directly implicated in heart growth [100]. Growth factors are known to affect cardiomyocyte growth (e.g., type 1 insulin-like growth factor (IGF) signal through the PI3K/Akt pathway) [101]. Recently, microarray analysis of cardiomyocytes demonstrated that IGF-1 treatment results in the differential expression of genes involved in cellular signaling and mitochondrial function and confirmed that this IGF-mediated gene regulation requires extracellular-signal regulated kinase and PI3K activation [102]. In transgenic mice with cardiac-specific expression of activated Akt, IGF-binding protein is up-regulated (consistent with its growth signaling/antiapoptotic role), and both PGC-1α and PPAR-α (activating mitochondrial FAO and mitochondrial biogenesis) are down-regulated, presumably shifting cardiomyocytes toward glycolytic metabolism [103]. Deprivation of nutrients (e.g., amino acid, glucose and serum) that can lead to cardiomyocyte apoptosis [92] has been found to signal via the mitochondrial associated mTOR protein [104]. Moreover, both the Akt pathway and the downstream mTOR protein impact cardiomyocyte survival and cell size largely through increased cytoplasmic protein synthesis by mediating activation of translational initiation factors and ribosomal proteins (Figure 10.3). In addition, serotonin binding to the serotonin

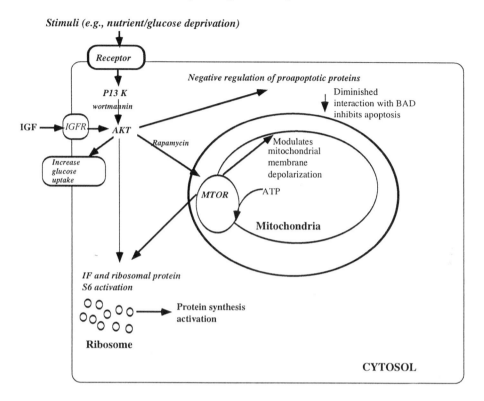

**Figure 10.3. The myocardial phosphatidylinositol 3-kinase (PI3K)/Akt signaling pathway has a mitochondrial component.** *A variety of signals, including serum and nutrients deprivation and growth factor (e.g., insulin-like growth factor, IGF) stimulation, lead to PI3K-directed phosphorylation and activation of Akt, resulting in the negative regulation of proapoptotic protein activation (e.g., Bad), apoptotic suppression, and up-regulation of glucose uptake. Mammalian target of rapamycin (MTOR; also called FRAP) located in mitochondria lies downstream of Akt and integrates the response to growth factor and nutrient deprivation, mitochondrial membrane depolarization events, and is responsive to ATP levels. Both MTOR and Akt modulate cytoplasmic protein synthesis by the activation of translation initiation factors (IF) and of ribosomal proteins (e.g., S6), which regulate cardiomyocyte size. Also shown (italics) is the response of PI3K and MTOR kinase activities, respectively, to the specific inhibitors wortmannin and rapamycin.*

2B receptor protects cardiomyocytes against serum-deprivation-induced apoptosis via the PI3K pathway impacting ANT and Bax expression. In transgenic mice harboring serotonin 2B receptor null mutations, pronounced myocardial mitochondrial defects are present in addition to altered ETC activities (i.e., complexes II and IV), ANT, and Bax expression [105].

Finally, Akt signaling also provides CP against ischemic injury in response to diverse treatments, including cardiotrophin-1, adenosine, acetylcholine, and bradykinin-mediated preconditioning [106–108], although the precise target of Akt action in mitochondria-based CP remains undetermined since Akt does not associate directly with mitoK$_{ATP}$ channels.

## Stress signals

Stresses in cardiac hypertrophy (e.g., mechanical stress) and ischemia/hypoxia (e.g., oxidative stress) elicit a variety of adaptive responses at the tissue, cellular, and molecular levels. A current model displaying a cardiac physiological response to hypoxia suggests that mitochondria function as $O_2$ sensors both by increasing ROS generation during hypoxia and via their abundant heme-containing proteins (e.g., COX), which reversibly bind oxygen [109]. Oxidant signals such as ROS act as second messengers initiating signaling cascades and are prominent features in both adaptive responses to hypoxia and mechanically stressed heart. Down-regulation of COX activity contributes to increased ROS generation and signaling observed in cardiomyocytes during hypoxia [110]. Also, hypoxia stimulates NO synthesis in cardiomyocytes [111], and NO down-regulates COX activity, with subsequent mitochondrial $H_2O_2$ production. This event has been proposed to provide a mitochondria-generated signal for further regulating redox-sensitive signaling pathways, including apoptosis, and can proceed even in the absence of marked changes in ATP levels [96]. NO synthase (NOS) has been identified in heart mitochondria although its role in regulating OXPHOS is not clear [112–113]. Mitochondrial ROS has also been shown to activate P38 kinase in hypoxic cardiomyocytes [114]. Longer-term responses to hypoxia have been shown to involve increased gene expression of hypoxia-induced factors and the activation of transcription factors such as NF-κB, which has also been implicated in the complex regulation of cardiac hypertrophy and inflammatory cytokines (e.g.,TNF-α and IL- 1). While increased ROS has been shown to be an important element in NF-κB gene activation, there is evidence that cardiomyocyte hypoxia-induced factor (HIF) gene activation can also occur in the absence of ROS [115].

## *Metabolic signals*

Mitochondria respond to changes in cellular levels of key metabolites such as adenosine, ATP, ADP, oxygen, and NADH as well as numerous substrates and coenzymes. After birth, FAO becomes the primary source of cardiac bioenergy and of electrons/NADH for the TCA cycle and ETC function [116]. Fatty acids also physically interact with mitochondria, impacting on membrane structure and function such as transport and excitability. As discussed in Chapter 7, the increased accumulation of amphiphilic long-chain fatty acids, which occurs with defective mitochondrial FAO and transport, can provide a variety of toxic effects on the electrophysiological properties of cardiac cell membranes, including disturbed ion transport and impaired gap junction activity causing cardiac arrhythmias, and contribute to cardiac failure and sudden death [36, 117]. In addition, long-chain fatty acids (e.g., palmitate) can modulate inner-membrane proton conductance (increased uncoupling) and stimulate PT pore opening, determining apoptogenic protein release into the cytosol [93].

Another major mitochondrial target of hormone signaling (TH) as well as of long-chain fatty acids (e.g., palmitate) in the myocardium is the family of uncoupling proteins (UCP1–UCP5). These inner-membrane-localized carrier proteins function to dissipate the proton gradient across the mitochondrial membrane. The myocardial expression of uncoupling proteins is up-regulated transcriptionally with either palmitate or TH treatment [118–120]. Cardiac expression of one of the uncoupling protein genes (UCP3) has also been reported to be PPAR-$\alpha$ dependent [120]. In addition, elevated expression of uncoupling proteins in cardiac muscle results in increased uncoupling of OXPHOS from respiration, decreased myocardial efficiency, and mitochondrial membrane potential [119].

## Future prospects: Therapeutic targets and directions

### *The essential role played by mitochondria in cytoprotective signaling and CP*

The recognition that mitochondria play an essential role in cytoprotective signaling and CP may stimulate further collaboration among cardiologists and others researchers in the fields of drug discovery to successfully carry out the pharmacological manipulation of mito- chondrial metabolism and signaling in cardiovascular diseases. Research in mitochondria-based CP may reveal potential target molecules (e.g., mitochondrial receptor, signaling kinase, or mem- brane channel) for highly specific pharmacological intervention, although, as a caveat, a greater understanding of the network of complex interacting pathways will be needed. For example, despite recent achievements in identifying genetic and signaling defects causing cardiac arrhythmia, the development of effective drugs (e.g., specific ion channel blockers) to substantially reduce the mortality associated with severe arrhythmias has thus far shown little success, underscoring the complex circuitry involved in evolving cardiac disease phenotypes [121]. Moreover, pharmacological agents that are cardioprotective in animal studies can have variable effects in clinical settings (e.g., diazoxide has shown negative effects, while nicorandil has proved more successful in limited clinical trials) [122].

## *Mitochondrial metabolic intermediates*

Increasing knowledge of the specific molecular and biochemical nature of mitochondrial bioenergetic defects has provided a rationale for clinical treatment using metabolic intermediates (e.g., succinate), coenzymes, and vitamins serving as electron donors, transporters, and cofactors (e.g., vitamin K, thiamine, and ascorbate) in order to bypass specific defects in OXPHOS and increase ATP production [123]. For instance, coenzyme $Q_{10}$ and its analogue idebenone have shown beneficial effects in the treatment of the cardiomyopathy associated with FRDA [124]. Shifting myocardial oxidative substrates from fatty acid to glucose has been effectively used to prevent the accumulation of long-chain acylcarnitines and in improving myocardial energy efficiency in HF [125]. In addition, dichloroacetate has shown prom- ise in stemming the lactic acidosis and declining PDH activity that accompanies myocardial ischemia and reperfusion injury [123]. Dietary therapies, including replacement of normal dietary fat by me- dium-chain triglycerides and increased carbohydrates, and carnitine supplementation have proved highly effective in treating cardiomyo- pathies due to mitochondrial long-chain FAO disorders and mitochondrial carnitine transport deficiencies and in lowering acyl-CoA accumulation [126]. Supplementation with free polyunsaturated fatty acids can provide significant cardioprotective effect against both ischemia-related ventricular fibrillation and arrhythmias [127]. A more complete description of the palliative therapies presently available to treat mitochondrial-based cardiac diseases as well as the future prospects for gene and cell transplantation therapies are presented in Chapters 11 and 12.

## Summary

At the outset, it is important to understand that the complex field of heart mitochondrial signaling is presently in its infancy. Many of the findings cited in this chapter came to light as a by-product of a large number of studies focused on understanding the mechanisms of apoptosis. Our purpose here is to direct the focus on the subject of mitochondrial signaling in its own right, knowing that a large number of potential relationships of heart mitochondria with other cellular organelles remain to be identified.

Accordingly, heart mitochondria are presented as the receiver, integrator, and transmitter of signals, involving multiple and interrelated signaling pathways at both the molecular and biochemical levels, with nuclear and cytoplasmic factors fundamentally involved in the shaping of the organelle's responses. We examine evidence that the mitochondria act as a dynamic receiver and integrator of numerous translocated signaling proteins (including protein kinases and nuclear transcription factors), regulatory $Ca^{++}$ fluxes, and membrane phospholipids as well as the transmission of mitochondria-generated oxidative stress and energy-related signaling that contribute to the overall cardiomyocyte response to myocardial ischemia and hypertrophy. While presently, there is substantial interest and information concerning the integral role of myocardial apoptosis in cardiac remodeling, myocardial mitochondrial signaling also plays fundamental roles in the cardiomyocyte proliferative pathways, nutrient and $O_2$ sensing, bioenergetic metabolite/substrate selection, interorganellar cross-talk, and the responses of cardiomyocytes to metabolic transition and physiological stresses, roles that are only recently coming to light and warrant further investigation. An increased awareness of mitochondrial signaling may lead to the delineation of the molecular mechanisms underlying different cardiovascular pathological states and enhance our understanding of the widening spectra of abnormal cardiac phenotypes known to have mitochondrial dysfunction.

# References

1.  Marín-García J, Goldenthal MJ (2002) Understanding the impact of mitochondrial defects in cardiovascular disease: A review. J Card Fail 8:347–61

2.  Marín-García J, Ananthakrishnan R, Goldenthal MJ, Pierpont ME (2000) Biochemical and molecular basis for mitochondrial cardiomyopathy in neonates and children. J Inherit Metab Dis 23:625–33

3.  Lewis W, Dalakas MC (1995) Mitochondrial toxicity of antiviral drugs. Nat Med 1:417–22

4.  Benit P, Slama A, Cartault F, Giurgea I, Chretien D, Lebon S, Marsac C, Munnich A, Rotig A, Rustin P (2004) Mutant NDUFS3 subunit of mitochondrial complex I causes Leigh syndrome. J Med Genet 41:14–17

5.  Papadopoulou LC, Sue CM, Davidson MM, Tanji K, Nishino I, Sadlock JE, Krishna S, Walker W, Selby J, Glerum DM, Coster RV, Lyon G, Scalais E, Lebel R, Kaplan P, Shanske S, De Vivo DC, Bonilla E, Hirano M, DiMauro S, Schon EA (1999) Fatal infantile cardioencephalomyopathy with COX deficiency and mutations in $SCO_2$, a COX assembly gene. Nat Genet 23:333–7

6.  Lodi R, Cooper JM, Bradley JL, Manners D, Styles P, Taylor DJ, Schapira AH (1999) Deficit of *in vivo* mitochondrial ATP production in patients with Friedreich ataxia. Proc Natl Acad Sci USA 96:11492–5

7.  Zeviani M, Spinazzola A, Carelli V (2003) Nuclear genes in mitochondrial disorders. Curr Opin Genet Dev 13:262–70

8.  Graham BH, Waymire KG, Cottrell B, Trounce IA, MacGregor GR, Wallace DC (1997) A mouse model for mitochondrial myopathy and cardiomyopathy resulting from a deficiency in the heart/muscle isoform of the adenine nucleotide translocator. Nat Genet 16:226–34

9.  Lebovitz RM, Zhang H, Vogel H, Cartwright J Jr, Dionne L, Lu N, Huang S, Matzuk MM (1996) Neurodegeneration, myocardial injury, and perinatal death in mitochondrial superoxide dismutase-deficient mice. Proc Natl Acad Sci USA 93:9782–7

10. Puccio H, Simon D, Cossee M, Criqui-Filipe P, Tiziano F, Melki J, Hindelang C, Matyas R, Rustin P, Koenig M (2001) Mouse models for Friedreich ataxia exhibit cardiomyopathy, sensory nerve defect and Fe-S enzyme deficiency followed by intramitochondrial iron deposits. Nat Genet 27:181–6

11. Wang J, Wilhelmsson H, Graff C, Li H, Oldfors A, Rustin P, Bruning JC, Kahn CR, Clayton DA, Barsh GS, Thoren P, Larsson NG (1999) Dilated cardiomyopathy and atrioventricular conduction blocks induced by heart-specific inactivation of mtDNA gene expression. Nat Genet 21:133–7

12. Corbucci GG (2000) Adaptive changes in response to acute hypoxia, ischemia and reperfusion in human cardiac cell. Minerva Anestesiol 66:523–30

13. Ylitalo K, Ala-Rami A, Vuorinen K, Peuhkurinen K, Lepojarvi M, Kaukoranta P, Kiviluoma K, Hassinen I (2001) Reversible ischemic inhibition of F(1) F(0)-ATPase in rat and human myocardium. Biochim Biophys Acta 1504:329–39

14. Corral-Debrinski M, Stepien G, Shoffner JM, Lott MT, Kanter K, Wallace DC (1991) Hypoxemia is associated with mitochondrial DNA damage and gene induction: Implications for cardiac disease. JAMA 266:1812–6

15. Regula KM, Ens K, Kirshenbaum LA (2003) Mitochondria-assisted suicide: A license to kill. J Mol Cell Cardiol 35:559–67

16. Gottleib RA, Burleson KO, Kloner RA, Babior BM, Engler RL (1994) Reperfusion injury induces apoptosis in rabbit cardiomyocytes. J Clin Invest 94:1621–8

17. Paradies G, Petrosillo G, Pistolese M, Di Venosa N, Serena D, Ruggiero FM (1999) Lipid peroxidation and alterations to oxidative metabolism in mitochondria isolated from rat heart subjected to ischemia and reperfusion. Free Radic Biol Med 27:42–50

18. Halestrap AP (1994) Regulation of mitochondrial metabolism through changes in matrix volume. Biochem Soc Trans 22:522–9

19. Garlid KD, Paucek P, Yarov-Yarovoy V, Murray HN, Darbenzio R, D'Alonzo AJ, Lodge NJ, Smith MA, Grover GJ (1997) Cardioprotective effect of diazoxide and its interaction with mitochondrial ATP-sensitive K+ channels: Possible mechanism of cardioprotection. Circ Res 81:1072–82

20. Akao M, Teshima Y, Marban E (2002) Antiapoptotic effect of nicorandil mediated by mitochondrial ATP-sensitive potassium channels in cultured cardiac myocytes. J Am Coll Cardiol 40:803–10

21. Marín-García J, Goldenthal MJ (2004) Mitochondria play a critical role in cardioprotection. J Card Fail 10:55–66

22. O'Rourke B (2004) Evidence for mitochondrial $K^+$ channels and their role in cardioprotection. Circ Res 94:420–32

23. Cohen MV, Baines CP, Downey JM (2000) Ischemic preconditioning: from adenosine receptor of KATP channel. Annu Rev Physiol 62:79–109

24. Das M, Parker JE, Halestrap AP (2003) Matrix volume measurements challenge the existence of diazoxide/glibencamide-sensitive KATP channels in rat mitochondria. J Physiol (Lond) 547: 893–902

25. Ardehali H, Chen Z, Ko Y, Mejia-Alvarez R, Marban E (2004) Multiprotein complex containing succinate dehydrogenase confers mitochondrial ATP-sensitive $K^+$ channel activity. Proc Natl Acad Sci U S A 101:11880–5

26. Ning XH, Xu CS, Song YC, Xiao Y, Hu YJ, Lupinetti FM, Portman MA (1998) Hypothermia preserves function and signaling for mitochondrial biogenesis during subsequent ischemia. Am J Physiol 274:H786–93

27. Nadal-Ginard B, Kajstura J, Leri A, Anversa P (2003) Myocyte death, growth, and regeneration in cardiac hypertrophy and failure. Circ Res 92:139–50

28. Colucci WS (1997) Molecular and cellular mechanisms of myocardial failure. Am J Cardiol 80:15L–25L

29. Hunter JJ, Chien KR (1999) Signaling pathways for cardiac hypertrophy and failure. N Engl J Med 341:1276–83

30. Katz AM (2002) Maladaptive growth in the failing heart: The cardiomyopathy of overload. Cardiovasc Drugs Ther 16:245–9

31. Kang PM, Yue P, Liu Z, Tarnavski O, Bodyak N, Izumo S (2004) Alterations in apoptosis regulatory factors during hypertrophy and heart failure. Am J Physiol Heart Circ Physiol 287:H72–80

32. Sack MN, Kelly DP (1998) The energy substrate switch during development of heart failure: Gene regulatory mechanisms. Int J Mol Med 1:17–24

33. Reibel DK, O'Rourke B, Foster KA (1987) Mechanisms for altered carnitine content in hypertrophied rat hearts. Am J Physiol 252:H561–5

34. Martin MA, Gomez MA, Guillen F, Bornstein B, Campos Y, Rubio JC, de la Calzada CS, Arenas J (2000) Myocardial carnitine

and carnitine palmitoyltransferase deficiencies in patients with severe heart failure. Biochim Biophys Acta 1502:330–6

35. Lehman JJ, Kelly DP (2002) Gene regulatory mechanisms governing energy metabolism during cardiac hypertrophic growth. Heart Fail Rev 7:175–85

36. Young ME, Goodwin GW, Ying J, Guthrie P, Wilson CR, Laws FA, Taegtmeyer H (2001) Regulation of cardiac and skeletal muscle malonyl-CoA decarboxylase by fatty acids. Am J Physiol Endocrinol Metab 280:E471–9

37. Zak R, Rabinowitz M, Rajamanickam C, Merten S, Kwiatkows-ka-Patzer B (1980) Mitochondrial proliferation in cardiac hypertrophy. Basic Res Cardiol 75:171–8

38. Lucas DT, Aryal P, Szweda LI, Koch WJ, Leinwand LA (2003) Alterations in mitochondrial function in a mouse model of hypertrophic cardiomyopathy. Am J Physiol Heart Circ Physiol 284:H575–83

39. Marín-García J, Goldenthal MJ, Moe GW (2001) Mitochondrial pathology in cardiac failure. Cardiovasc Res 49:17–26

40. Van Bilsen M, Smeets PJ, Gilde AJ, van der Vusse GJ (2004) Metabolic remodelling of the failing heart: The cardiac burn-out syndrome? Cardiovasc Res 61:218–26

41. Scarpulla RC (2002) Nuclear activators and coactivators in mammalian mitochondrial biogenesis. Biochim Biophys Acta 1576:1–14

42. Goffart S, Wiesner RJ (2003) Regulation and co-ordination of nuclear gene expression during mitochondrial biogenesis. Exp Physiol 88:33–40

43. Xia Y, Buja LM, Scarpulla RC, McMillin JB (1997) Electrical stimulation of neonatal cardiomyocytes results in sequential activation of nuclear genes governing mitochondrial proliferation and differentiation. Proc Natl Acad Sci USA 94:11399–404

44. Lehman JJ, Barger PM, Kovacs A, Saffitz JE, Medeiros DM, Kelly DP (2000) Peroxisome proliferator-activated receptor gamma coactivator-1 promotes cardiac mitochondrial biogenesis. J Clin Invest 106:847–56

45. Gilde AJ, van der Lee KA, Willemsen PH, Chinetti G, van der Leij FR, van der Vusse GJ, Staels B, van Bilsen M (2003) Peroxisome proliferator-activated receptor PPARalpha and PPARbeta/delta, but not PPARgamma, modulate the expression of genes involved in cardiac lipid metabolism. Circ Res 92:518–24

46. Barger PM, Kelly DP (2000) PPAR signaling in the control of cardiac energy metabolism. Trends Cardiovasc Med 10:238–45

47. Djouadi F, Brandt JM, Weinheimer CJ, Leone TC, Gonzalez FJ, Kelly DP (1999) The role of the peroxisome proliferator-activated receptor alpha (PPAR alfa) in the control of cardiac lipid metabolism. Prostaglandins Leukot Essent Fatty Acids 60:339–43

48. Garnier A, Fortin D, Delomenie C, Momken I, Veksler V, Ventura-Clapier R (2003) Depressed mitochondrial transcription factors and oxidative capacity in rat failing cardiac and skeletal muscles. J Physiol (Lond) 551:491–501

49. Huss JM, Levy FH, Kelly DP (2001) Hypoxia inhibits the peroxisome proliferator-activated receptor alpha/retinoid X receptor gene regulatory pathway in cardiac myocytes: A mechanism for $O_2$-dependent modulation of mitochondrial fatty acid oxidation. J Biol Chem 276:27605–12

50. Wu H, Kanatous SB, Thurmond FA, Gallardo T, Isotani E, Bassel-Duby R, Williams RS (2002) Regulation of mitochondrial biogenesis in skeletal muscle by CaMK. Science 296:349–52

51. Sack MN, Harrington LS, Jonassen AK, Mjos OD, Yellon DM (2000) Coordinate regulation of metabolic enzyme encoding genes during cardiac development and following carvedilol therapy in spontaneously hypertensive rats. Cardiovasc Drugs Ther 14:31–9

52. Bushdid PB, Osinska H, Waclaw RR, Molkentin JD, Yutzey KE (2003) NFATc3 and NFATc4 are required for cardiac development and mitochondrial function. Circ Res 92:1305–13

53. Finck BN, Lehman JJ, Leone TC, Welch MJ, Bennett MJ, Kovacs A, Han X, Gross RW, Kozak R, Lopaschuk GD, Kelly DP (2002) The cardiac phenotype induced by PPARalpha overexpression mimics that caused by diabetes mellitus. J Clin Invest 109:121–30

54. Thomson M (2002) Evidence of undiscovered cell regulatory mechanisms: Phosphoproteins and protein kinases in mitochondria. Cell Mol Life Sci 59:213–9

55. Orfali KA, Fryer LG, Holness MJ, Sugden MC (1993) Long-term regulation of pyruvate dehydrogenase kinase by high-fat feeding. Experiments in vivo and in cultured cardiomyocytes. FEBS Lett 336: 501–5

56. Doering CB, Danner DJ (2000) Amino acid deprivation induces translation of branched-chain alpha-ketoacid dehydrogenase kinase. Am J Physiol Cell Physiol 279:C1587–94

57. Technikova-Dobrova Z, Sardanelli AM, Stanca MR, Papa S (1994) cAMP-dependent protein phosphorylation in mitochondria of bovine heart. FEBS Lett 350:187–91

58. Wang Y, Hirai K, Ashraf M (1999) Activation of mitochondrial ATP-sensitive K (+) channel for cardiac protection against ischemic injury is dependent on protein kinase C activity. Circ Res 85:731–41

59. Baines CP, Zhang J, Wang GW, Zheng YT, Xiu JX, Cardwell EM, Bolli R, Ping P (2002) Mitochondrial PKCepsilon and MAPK form signaling modules in the murine heart: Enhanced mitochondrial PKCepsilon-MAPK interactions and differential MAPK activation in PKCepsilon-induced cardioprotection. Circ Res 90:390–7

60. He H, Li HL, Lin A, Gottlieb RA (1999) Activation of the JNK pathway is important for cardiomyocyte death in response to simulated ischemia. Cell Death Differ 6:987–91

61. Baines CP, Song CX, Zheng YT, Wang GW, Zhang J, Wang OL, Guo Y, Bolli R, Cardwell EM, Ping P (2003) Protein kinase Cepsilon interacts with and inhibits the permeability transition pore in cardiac mitochondria. Circ Res 92:873–80

62. Fryer RM, Schultz JE, Hsu AK, Gross GJ (1999) Importance of PKC and tyrosine kinase in single or multiple cycles of preconditioning in rat hearts. Am J Physiol Heart Circ Physiol 276:H1229–35

63. Chen L, Hahn H, Wu G, Chen CH, Liron T, Schechtman D, Cavallaro G, Banci L, Guo Y, Bolli R, Dorn GW, Mochly-Rosen D (2001) Opposing cardioprotective actions and parallel hypertrophic effects of delta PKC and epsilon PKC. Proc Natl Acad Sci USA 98: 11114–9

64. Sardanelli AM, Technikova-Dobrova Z, Scacco SC, Speranza F, Papa S (1995) Characterization of proteins phosphorylated by the cAMP-dependent protein kinase of bovine heart mitochondria. FEBS Lett 377:470–4

65. Papa S (2002) The NDUFS4 nuclear gene of complex I of mitochondria and the cAMP cascade. Biochim Biophys Acta 1555: 1447–53

66. Lee I, Bender E, Kadenbach B (2002) Control of mitochondrial membrane potential and ROS formation by reversible phosphorylation of cytochrome c oxidase. Mol Cell Biochem 234–235: 63–70

67. Schulenberg B, Aggeler R, Beechem JM, Capaldi RA, Patton WF (2003) Analysis of steady-state protein phosphorylation in mitochon-

dria using a novel fluorescent phosphosensor dye. J Biol Chem 278: 27251–5

68. He H, Chen M, Scheffler NK, Gibson BW, Spremulli LL, Gottlieb RA (2001) Phosphorylation of mitochondrial elongation factor Tu in ischemic myocardium: basis for chloramphenicol-mediated cardio-protection. Circ Res 89:461–7

69. Rutter GA, Rizzuto R (2000) Regulation of mitochondrial metabolism by ER Ca++ release: An intimate connection. Trends Biochem Sci 25:215–22

70. Duchen M (1999) Contributions of mitochondria to animal physiology: From homeostatic sensor to calcium signalling and cell death. J Physiol (Lond) 516:1–17

71. Griffiths EJ (2000) Use of ruthenium red as an inhibitor of mitochondrial Ca (2+) uptake in single rat cardiomyocytes. FEBS Lett 486:257–60

72. Pacher P, Hajnoczky G (2001) Propagation of the apoptotic signal by mitochondrial waves. EMBO J 20:4107–21

73. McCormack JG, Halestrap AP, Denton RM (1990) Role of calcium ions in regulation of mammalian intramitochondrial metabolism. Physiol Rev 70:391–425

74. Robb-Gaspers LD, Burnett P, Rutter GA, Denton RM, Rizzuto R, Thomas AP (1998) Integrating cytosolic calcium signals into mitochondrial metabolic responses. EMBO J 17:4987–5000

75. Cortassa S, Aon MA, Marban E, Winslow RL, O'Rourke B (2003) An integrated model of cardiac mitochondrial energy metabolism and calcium dynamics. Biophys J 84:2734–55

76. Das AM, Harris DA (1991) Control of mitochondrial ATP synthase in rat cardiomyocytes: Effects of thyroid hormone. Biochim Biophys Acta 1096:284–90

77. Territo PR, Mootha VK, French SA, Balaban RS (2000) Ca(2+) activation of heart mitochondrial oxidative phosphorylation: Role of the F(0)/F(1)-ATPase. Am J Physiol Cell Physiol 278:C423–35

78. Rizzuto R (1998) Close contacts with the endoplasmic reticulum as determinants of mitochondrial Ca++ responses. Science 280: 1763–6

79. Csordas G, Thomas AP, Hajnoczky G (2001) Calcium signal transmission between ryanodine receptors and mitochondria in cardiac muscle. Trends Cardiovasc Med 11:269–75

80. Gunter TE, Gunter KK (2001) Uptake of calcium by mitochondria: Transport and possible function. IUBMB Life 52:197–204

81.  Buntinas L, Gunter KK, Sparagna GC, Gunter TE (2001) The rapid mode of calcium uptake into heart mitochondria (RaM): Comparison to RaM in liver mitochondria. Biochim Biophys Acta 1504:248–61

82.  Crompton M, Costi A, Hayat L (1987) Evidence for the presence of a reversible Ca2+-dependent pore activated by oxidative stress in heart mitochondria. Biochem J 245:915–8

83.  Hajnoczky G, Csordas G, Yi M (2002) Old players in a new role: mitochondria-associated membranes, VDAC, and ryanodine receptors as contributors to calcium signal propagation from endoplasmic reticulum to the mitochondria. Cell Calcium 32:363–77

84.  Rapizzi E, Pinton P, Szabadkai G, Wieckowski MR, Vandecasteele G, Baird G, Tuft RA, Fogarty KE, Rizzuto R (2002) Recombinant expression of the voltage dependent anion channel enhances the transfer of Ca2+ microdomains to mitochondria. J Cell Biol 159:613–24

85.  Casas F, Rochard P, Rodier A, Cassar-Malek I, Marchal-Victorion S, Wiesner RJ, Cabello G, Wrutniak C (1999) A variant form of the nuclear triiodothyronine receptor c-ErbAalpha1 plays a direct role in regulation of mitochondrial RNA synthesis. Mol Cell Biol 19: 7913–24

86.  Scheller K, Seibel P, Sekeris CE (2003) Glucocorticoid and thyroid hormone receptors in mitochondria of animal cells. Int Rev Cytol 222:1–61

87.  Colavecchia M, Christie LN, Kanwar YS, Hood DA (2003) Functional consequences of thyroid hormone-induced changes in the mitochondrial protein import pathway. Am J Physiol Endocrinol Metab 284:E29–35

88.  Schneider JJ, Hood DA (2000) Effect of thyroid hormone on mtHsp70 expression, mitochondrial import and processing in cardiac muscle. J Endocrinol 165:9–17

89.  Oddis CV, Finkel MS (1995) Cytokine-stimulated nitric oxide production inhibits mitochondrial activity in cardiac myocytes. Biochem Biophys Res Commun 213:1002–9

90.  Zell R, Geck P, Werdan K, Boekstegers P (1997) TNF-alpha and IL-1 alpha inhibit both pyruvate dehydrogenase activity and mitochondrial function in cardiomyocytes: Evidence for primary impairment of mitochondrial function. Mol Cell Biochem 177:61–7

91.   Sammut IA, Harrison JC (2003) Cardiac mitochondrial complex activity is enhanced by heat shock proteins. Clin Exp Pharmacol Physiol 30:110–5

92.   Bialik S, Cryns VL, Drincic A, Miyata S, Wollowick AL, Srinivasan A, Kitsis RN (1999) The mitochondrial apoptotic pathway is activated by serum and glucose deprivation in cardiac myocytes. Circ Res 85:403–14

93.   Sparagna GC, Hickson-Bick DL, Buja LM, McMillin JB (2001) Fatty acid-induced apoptosis in neonatal cardiomyocytes: Redox signaling. Antioxid Redox Signal 3:71–9

94.   Gudz TI, Tserng KY, Hoppel CL (1997) Direct inhibition of mitochondrial respiratory chain complex III by cell-permeable ceramide. J Biol Chem 272:24154–8

95.   Riobo NA, Clementi E, Melani M, Boveris A, Cadenas E, Moncada S, Poderoso JJ (2001) Nitric oxide inhibits mitochondrial NADH: Ubiquinone reductase activity through peroxynitrite formation. Biochem J 359:139–45

96.   Poderoso JJ, Peralta JG, Lisdero CL, Carreras MC, Radisic M, Schopfer F, Cadenas E, Boveris A (1998) Nitric oxide regulates oxygen uptake and hydrogen peroxide release by the isolated beating rat heart. Am J Physiol 274:C112–9

97.   Wiesner RJ, Hornung TV, Garman JD, Clayton DA, O'Gorman E, Wallimann T (1999) Stimulation of mitochondrial gene expression and proliferation of mitochondria following impairment of cellular energy transfer by inhibition of phosphocreatine circuit in rat hearts. J Bioenerg Biomembr 31:559–567

98.   Tanaka T, Morita H, Koide H, Kawamura K, Takatsu T (1985) Biochemical and morphological study of cardiac hypertrophy: Effects of thyroxine on enzyme activities in the rat myocardium. Basic Res Cardiol 80:165–74

99.   Kennedy SG, Kandel ES, Cross TK, Hay N (1999) Akt/protein kinase B inhibits cell death by preventing release of cytochrome c from mitochondria. Mol Cell Biol 19:5800–10

100. Shioi T, McMullen JR, Kang PM, Douglas PS, Obata T, Franke TF, Cantley LC, Izumo S (2002) Akt/protein kinase B promotes organ growth in transgenic mice. Mol Cell Biol 22:2799–809

101. Condorelli G, Drusco A, Stassi G, Bellacosa A, Roncarati R, Iaccarino G, Russo MA, Gu Y, Dalton N, Chung C, Latronico MV, Napoli C, Sadoshima J, Croce CM, Ross J (2002) Akt induces en-

hanced myocardial contractility and cell size in vivo in transgenic mice. Proc Natl Acad Sci USA 17:12333–8

102. Liu Tj, Lai Hc, Wu W, Chinn S, Wang PH (2001) Developing a strategy to define the effects of insulin-like growth factor-1 on gene expression profile in cardiomyocytes. Circ Res 88:1231–8

103. Cook SA, Matsui T, Li L, Rosenzweig A (2002) Transcriptional effects of chronic Akt activation in the heart. J Biol Chem 277: 22528–33

104. Edinger AL, Thompson CB (2002) Akt maintains cell size and survival by increasing mTOR-dependent nutrient uptake. Mol Biol Cell 13:2276–88

105. Nebigil CG, Etienne N, Messaddeq N, Maroteaux L (2003) Serotonin is a novel survival factor of cardiomyocytes: Mitochondria as a target of 5-HT2B receptor signaling. FASEB J 17:1373–5

106. Matsui T, Tao J, del Monte F, Lee KH, Li L, Picard M, Force TL, Franke TF, Hajjar RJ, Rosenzweig A (2001) Akt activation preserves cardiac function and prevents injury after transient cardiac ischemia in vivo. Circulation 104:330–5

107. Krieg T, Qin Q, McIntosh EC, Cohen MV, Downey JM (2002) ACh and adenosine activate PI3-kinase in rabbit hearts through transactivation of receptor tyrosine kinases. Am J Physiol Heart Circ Physiol 283:H2322–30

108. Li Y, Sato T (2001) Dual signaling via protein kinase C and phosphatidylinositol 3'-kinase/Akt contributes to bradykinin B2 receptor-induced cardioprotection in guinea pig hearts. J Mol Cell Cardiol 33:2047–53

109. Chandel NS, Schumacker PT (2000) Cellular oxygen sensing by mitochondria: Old questions, new insight. J Appl Physiol 88:1880–9

110. Duranteau J, Chandel NS, Kulisz A, Shao Z, Schumacker PT (1998) Intracellular signaling by reactive oxygen species during hypoxia in cardiomyocytes. J Biol Chem 273:11619–24

111. Kacimi R, Long CS, Karliner JS (1997) Chronic hypoxia modulates the interleukin-1 stimulated inducible nitric oxide synthase pathway in cardiac myocytes. Circulation 96:1937–43

112. French S, Giulivi C, Balaban RS (2001) Nitric oxide synthase in porcine heart mitochondria: Evidence for low physiological activity. Am J Physiol Heart Circ Physiol 280:H2863–7

113. Kanai AJ, Pearce LL, Clemens PR, Birder LA, VanBibber MM, Choi SY, de Groat WC, Peterson J (2001) Identification of a neuronal

nitric oxide synthase in isolated cardiac mitochondria using electrochemical detection. Proc Natl Acad Sci USA 98:14126–31

114. Kulisz A, Chen N, Chandel NS, Shao Z, Schumacker PT (2002) Mitochondrial ROS initiate phosphorylation of p38 MAP kinase during hypoxia in cardiomyocytes. Am J Physiol Lung Cell Mol Physiol 282:L1324–9

115. Enomoto N, Koshikawa N, Gassmann M, Hayashi J, Takenaga K (2002) Hypoxic induction of hypoxia-inducible factor-1alpha and oxygen-regulated gene expression in mitochondrial DNA-depleted HeLa cells. Biochem Biophys Res Commun 297:346–52

116. Lopaschuk GD, Collins-Nakai RL, Itoi T (1992) Developmental changes in energy substrate use by the heart. Cardiovasc Res 26: 1172–80

117. Bonnet D, Martin D, De Lonlay P, Villain E, Jouvet P, Rabier D, Brivet M, Saudubray JM (1999) Arrhythmias and conduction defects as presenting symptoms of fatty acid oxidation disorders in children. Circulation 100:2248–53

118. Lanni A, De Felice M, Lombardi A, Moreno M, Fleury C, Ricquier D, Goglia F (1997) Induction of UCP2 mRNA by thyroid hormones in rat heart. FEBS Lett 418:171–4

119. Boehm EA, Jones BE, Radda GK, Veech RL, Clarke K (2001) Increased uncoupling proteins and decreased efficiency in palmitate-perfused hyperthyroid rat heart. Am J Physiol Heart Circ Physiol 280:H977–83

120. Young ME, Patil S, Ying J, Depre C, Ahuja HS, Shipley GL, Stepkowski SM, Davies PJ, Taegtmeyer H (2001) Uncoupling protein 3 transcription is regulated by peroxisome proliferator-activated receptor (alpha) in the adult rodent heart. FASEB J 15:833–45

121. Sanguinetti MC, Bennett PB (2003) Antiarrhythmic drug target choices and screening. Circ Res 93:491–9

122. Ito H, Taniyama Y, Iwakura K, Nishikawa N, Mauyama T, Kuzuya T, Hori M, Higashino Y, Fujii K, Minamino T (1999) Intravenous nicorandil can preserve microvascular integrity and myocardial viability in patients with reperfused anterior wall myocardial infarction. J Am Coll Cardiol 33:654–60

123. Shoffner JM, Wallace DC (1994) Oxidative phosphorylation diseases and mitochondrial DNA mutations: Diagnosis and treatment. Annu Rev Nutr 14:535–68

124. Rustin P, von Kleist-Retzow JC, Chantrel-Groussard K, Sidi D, Munnich A, Rotig A (1999) Effect of idebenone on cardiomyopathy in Friedreich's ataxia: A preliminary study. Lancet 354:477–9

125. Wallhaus TR, Taylor M, DeGrado TR, Russell DC, Stanko P, Nickles RJ (2001) Myocardial free fatty acid and glucose use after carvedilol treatment in patients with congestive heart failure. Circulation 103:2441–6

126. Pollitt RJ (1995) Disorders of mitochondrial long-chain fatty acid oxidation. J Inherit Metab Dis 18:473–90

127. Pepe S, Tsuchiya N, Lakatta EG, Hansford RG (1999) PUFA and aging modulate cardiac mitochondrial membrane lipid composition and Ca2+ activation of PDH. Am J Physiol 276:H149–58

# Chapter 11

# Treatment of Mitochondrial-Based Cardiac Diseases. Targeting the Organelle

## Overview

Mitochondrial research and its current application in cardiology have taken advantage of the remarkable fusion recently achieved by genetics and biochemistry in molecular biology. While this progress have been applied mainly to discoveries on the etiopathogenesis of neuromuscular, cardiovascular, and other diseases, more focused studies are critically needed to assess the extent that heart mitochondrial defects (either primary or secondary to other myocardial changes) contribute to the pathophysiology of cardiac diseases. In this way, this knowledge can be applied to the discovery of specific mitochondria-targeted drugs to treat the failing heart and also to reverse or to slow the abnormal changes in cardiac cells structure and function that occur with aging and other pathological clinical states.

## Introduction

Currently, there is no effective treatment for mitochondrial disorders despite recent major advances in understanding the pathogenesis of mitochondrial diseases. Various pharmacological treatments are being used, but there is no definitive evidence that these drugs are efficacious. The current and accelerated progress in mitochondrial research has brought increased interest in the pharmacological manipulation of mitochondria. A variety of pharmacological treatments are being used, usually in various combinations as a therapeutic "cocktail". While there are multiple reports and case studies citing the beneficial use of many of these compounds in treating cardiomyopapathies, there have been no large-scale rigorously controlled studies supporting their efficacy in patients with mitochondrial cardiomyopathy.

The development of delivery systems and carriers of mitochondrial specific drugs, although a very attractive methodology, is still in its infancy, and more research will be needed prior to its clinical use.

## Treatment of respiratory and metabolic defects

Despite recent advances in understanding the pathogenesis of mitochondrial-based cardiac disorders, at this time, there is no recognized "magic bullet" for their effective treatment. Various pharmacological modalities have been used, but there is no consensus about their efficacy [1]. Several compounds, including various vitamins and metabolic cofactors (e.g., riboflavin, thiamine, tocopherol [vitamin E], folic acid, succinate, ascorbate [vitamin C], menadione, L-carnitine and $CoQ_{10}$), have been employed, usually in various combinations as a therapeutic "cocktail". These compounds act on mitochondrial physiology at a variety of levels, including bypassing blocks in the respiratory chain caused by deficiencies of specific ETC complexes, providing increased scavenging of ROS, and increasing metabolites that might be reduced (due to either defective synthesis or transport) in patients with mitochondrial disease. Nevertheless, knowledge of the specific metabolic defect can be of great significance in defining the appropriate treatment. For instance, in patients with either primary carnitine or CoQ deficiency, treatment with the appropriate compound has been shown to be successful and (in the case of carnitine deficiency) can be life-saving. The efficacy of carnitine in treating children with carnitine-deficiency cardiomyopathy underscores the importance of gauging carnitine levels in children with unexplained cardiomyopathy, as well as the critical timing of such treatment [2–3]. Moreover, patients with cardiomyopathy and COX deficiency due to mutations in $SCO_2$, a COX-assembly protein implicated in the incorporation of copper into the COX holenzyme, have been shown to respond to copper supplementation [4]. Unfortunately, in many cases of mitochondrial cardiomyopathy, the precise genetic and biochemical locus of the mitochondrial defect is not known, and the use of the above generic "cocktails" may not be effective.

Severe blocks in the respiratory chain result in the accumulation of upstream metabolites including pyruvate, lactate, and the transaminated product, alanine. Levels of all 3 compounds are elevated in the blood and urine of patients with mitochondrial myopathies. Lactic acidosis has a range of neurotoxic effects and can be effectively controlled with the use of dichloroacetate (DCA), an inhibitor of PDH kinase.

Patients with MELAS treated with DCA have been reported to show clinical improvement [5]. By rapidly stimulating PDH activity and, therefore, promoting aerobic glucose oxidation in myocardial cells, DCA can significantly improve myocardial function in conditions of limited oxygen availability (e.g., ischemia/reperfusion and congestive heart failure) and stem the mitochondrial energy failure associated with these states [6]. In addition to decreasing lactic acidosis, the clinical use of DCA has also been associated with the suppression of myocardial long-chain fatty acid metabolism and increased left ventricular stroke work and cardiac output, without changes in myocardial oxygen consumption. Moreover, DCA stimulation of PDH activity, which is otherwise depressed in the diabetic heart, can be beneficial. The DCA-mediated increase in glucose metabolism rate, in combination with the use of partial FAO inhibitors, has been proposed as a potential therapeutic approach to diabetic cardiomyopathy [7].

In patients with cytochrome $c$ oxidase deficiency, DCA in combination with the use of aerobic training was found to improve exercise capacity and aerobic metabolism [8]. While the use of aerobic exercise itself has shown considerable benefits, including increasing work and oxidative capacity in patients with mitochondrial diseases, exercise tolerance and aerobic training have not yet been systematically examined in patients with mitochondrial cardiomyopathy.

## *Use of antioxidants*

As discussed in Chapter 4, mitochondria are an important source of free radicals. Increased ROS generation plays an important role in the pathogenesis of mitochondrial-based cardiac disorders, suggesting that antioxidants may be beneficial [9–10]. In the cardiac damage elicited by ischemia/reperfusion and the cardiomyopathies associated with FRDA and doxorubicin-induction, there is evidence that mitochondrial ROS and oxidative stress are implicated in the pathogenesis of the disease [11–12]. Several oxygen radical scavengers, including $CoQ_{10}$, vitamin E, dexrazoxane, and idebenone, have been used in their treatment [13–15]. In doxorubicin-induced cardiomyopathy, the free-radical scavenger dexrazoxane has been shown to protect the heart from doxorubicin-associated oxidative damage and has been recently recommended for clinical use to attenuate the myocardial damage that may occur in children treated with doxorubicin chemotherapy for acute lymphoblastic leukemia [16]. Both $CoQ_{10}$ and idebenone have been reported to markedly improve cardiac function and reduce cardiac hypertrophy in patients with FRDA [17–19]. The ataxia and other CNS symptoms occurring in FRDA are less affected by the administration of these antioxidants than is the cardiac phenotype. Idebenone has also been shown to improve cardiac function in mitochondrial cardiomyopathy [13]. In addition to its role as an antioxidant, CoQ also serves multiple cellular functions, including participation as an electron carrier in the respiratory chain and as an activating cofactor for the mitochondrial uncoupling proteins. It has been reported to have a beneficial effect in several neurological disorders with cardiac involvement, including MELAS and KSS syndromes [5]. $CoQ_{10}$ at relatively high doses ranging (60 to 150 mg/day) results in significant reduction of the cardiac conduction abnormalities seen in patients with KSS or CPEO syndromes [20].

Clinical improvement was seen in patients with congestive heart failure (CHF) after $CoQ_{10}$ supplementation to standard therapy [21]. However, since the sample size and the design used in these studies raised concerns as to the validity of systematic clinical use of $CoQ_{10}$ in treating CHF, a large double-blind multisite clinical trial is presently underway to test its efficacy [22–23].

ROS and cellular redox states regulate an extensive number of vital pathways in the myocardium, including energy metabolism, survival and stress responses, apoptosis, inflammatory response, and oxygen sensing. A detailed review of the literature reveals that the results using whole organ and animal models (more so than in isolated cell models) are often contradictory regarding their role in ischemia and reperfusion injury as it is in the role of antioxidants as a therapy, providing insight into why clinical trials of antioxidants frequently have shown mixed results.

## *Treatment of FAO disorders, arrhythmias, and CHF*

Treatment of disorders of mitochondrial long-chain FAO is based on the avoidance of fasting and the replacement of normal dietary fat by medium-chain triglyceride. Knowledge of the precise site of the biochemical or molecular defect can be of critical importance regarding the choice of the therapeutic modality used. For instance, deficiencies in CPT-II, carnitine acylcarnitine translocase, or MTP can be treated with drugs targeted to enhance glucose use and pyruvate oxidation energy, at the expense of FAO, to prevent the accumulation of long-chain acylcarnitines that can result in cardiac conduction defects and arrhythmias [3, 24]. In contrast, acute cardiomyopathy associated with VLCAD deficiency, which can be diagnosed by acylcarnitine analysis even in the neonatal period, can be treated with dietary therapy, including medium-chain triglycerides [25]. Long-chain fatty acid accumulation and their side-effects can also be effectively reversed by inhibition of CPT-I activity with perhexiline and amiodarone.

In the failing and ischemic heart, there is a plurality of changes in myocardial metabolism. Modulation of myocardial glucose and fatty acid metabolism is recognized as a target for therapeutic modification. The treatment of patients in CHF using carvedilol, a β-adrenoreceptor blocker, results in marked improvement in myocardial energy efficiency by shifting myocardial oxidative substrates from fatty acid to glucose [26]. Free fatty acids are a primary source of energy during cardiac ischemia and can also serve to uncouple OXPHOS and increase myocardial $O_2$ consumption. On the other hand, inhibitors of FAO can increase glucose oxidation and may improve cardiac efficiency. It is noteworthy that inhibitors of β-FAO can help to prevent the hyperglycemia that occurs in noninsulin-dependent diabetes. Since the inhibition of FAO is effective in controlling abnormalities in diabetes, FAO inhibitors targeting enzymes such as CPT-I may also prove useful in the treatment of diabetic cardiomyopathy. FAO inhibition can be achieved using a number of enzymatic inhibitors such as etomoxir, oxfenicine, perhexiline, aminocarnitine, trimetazidine, ranolazine, and DCA [27–28]. In animal models, etoxomir, an inhibitor of CPT-I, reversed changes in fetal gene expression, preserved cardiac function, and prevented ventricular dilatation [29]. In clinical studies of patients in heart failure, etoxomir improved systolic ventricular function, increased ejection fraction, and decreased pulmonary capillary pressure [30]. Ranolazine treatment reduces cellular acetyl-CoA content via partial inhibition of fatty acid oxidation (it is therefore termed a *pFOX inhibitor*) and activates PDH activity. Clinically, it has been used to treat both ischemia and angina [31]. This metabolic switch increases ATP production, reduces the rise in lactic acidosis, and improves myocardial function under conditions of reduced myocardial oxygen delivery. Trimetazidine treatment has been demonstrated to provide protective affects against myocardial ischemia, diabetic cardio-myopathy, and exercise-induced angina in numerous clinical and experimental investigations [27–28, 32]. While initially trimetazidine was thought to be an inhibitor of the activity of the long-chain isoform of the last enzyme involved in mitochondrial fatty acid β-oxidation, 3-ketoacyl coenzyme A thiolase [33], recent studies have cast doubt on FAO inhibition as being the primary mechanism by which trimetazidine mediates cardiac recovery [34]. Another related effect of trimetazidine, which may contribute to its antiischemic action, is its acceleration of phospholipid synthesis and turnover with significant consequences for α-adrenergic signaling [35].

Clinical studies have suggested that polyunsaturated fatty acids (e.g., N-3 PUFA) or fish oil supplementation appears to reduce mortality and sudden death associated with CHF [36]. Its effect on mortality and morbidity are currently being gauged in the GISSI heart failure project, a large-scale, randomized, double-blind study [37]. A somewhat smaller but carefully designed study has recently confirmed that N-3 PUFA treatment markedly reduces the incidence of both atrial and ventricular arrhythmias [38]. Among a large assortment of PUFA-mediated effects on cardiomyocyte membrane lipid organization and function, the incorporation of N-3 PUFA (normally associated with reduced arachidonic acid) induces a reduction of mitochondrial β-FAO and oxygen consumption in the heart. These effects on mitochondrial metabolism are manifested primarily during postischemic reperfusion as improved metabolic and ventricular function. Both aging and ischemia markedly decrease levels of N-3 PUFA and cardiolipin in myocardial membranes, effects that have been correlated to increased mitochondrial $Ca^{++}$ levels and the effects of $Ca^{++}$ on mitochondrial enzymatic activities [39].

**Table 11.1. Metabolic and antioxidant treatments for mitochondrial-based cardiac disorders**

| Treatment | Primary Mechanism | Disorder |
|---|---|---|
| Coenzyme Q | Antioxidant/ ETC carrier | Heart failure, FRDA, MELAS, KSS |
| Dichloroacetate | Increased PDH activity; decreased FAO | KSS, MELAS, lactic acidosis, diabetic cardiomyopathy |
| Idebenone | Antioxidant | Friedreich ataxia (FRDA), mitochondrial cardiomyopathy |
| Carnitine | Increased fatty acid transport | Cardiomyopathy and heart failure |
| Etomoxir | FAO inhibitor | FAO disorders |
| Trimetazidine | FAO inhibitor; increased phospholipid turnover | FAO disorders, myocardial ischemia/angina, diabetic cardiomyopathy |
| Ranolazine | Partial FAO inhibitor | FAO disorders, myocardial ischemia/angina |
| Perhexilene | FAO inhibitor; | Arrhythmia |
| N-3 PUFA | Reduced FAO | Arrhythmia |
| Copper supplement | Assist in COX subunit assembly | HCM due to $SCO_2$ mutation |
| Dexrazoxane | Antioxidant | Doxorubicin-induced cardiomyopathy |
| Carvedilol | β-adrenergic blocker; FAO shift to glucose | Congestive heart failure |
| Diltiazem | Inhibits release of mitochondrial $Ca^{++}$ | Cardiac arrhythmia Myocardial ischemia |

## *Cardioprotective agents*

As discussed in Chapter 5, CP can be a useful adjunct in the treatment of cardiovascular disease (Table 11.1). Animal studies have shown that the addition of specific drugs (e.g., protein kinase C inhibitors and adenosine receptor agonists) targeting different steps of the CP signaling pathways and applied at the immediate onset of reperfusion can significantly reduce the size of myocardial infarct and improve cardiac function [40–41]. Animal studies have also demonstrated that treatment with a particular pharmacological class of calcium antagonists (e.g., diltiazem and verapamil) can reduce a number of the harmful effects of calcium overload following myocardial ischemia and particularly prominent during early reperfusion, with recovery of myocardial contractility and restoration of the levels of critically needed myocardial high-energy phosphates [42–43]. Clinical studies have also shown that diltiazem and verapamil treatment can be beneficial to patients after myocardial infarct and with cardiac arrhythmias [44–45]. The clinical benefits of reducing the size of myocardial infarct and increasing the viability and recovery of regional function appear to be significant if diltiazem treatment is applied prior to myocardial perfusion [46]. Diltiazem inhibits sodium-induced $Ca^{++}$ release by isolated mitochondria; the increased mitochondrial $Ca^{++}$ matrix levels result in elevated $Ca^{++}$-induced dehydrogenase activities, increased respiration, and restored ATP levels [47]. Intravenous diltiazem can be cardioprotective both as an antiischemic and antiarrhthymogenic agent when infused in patients undergoing coronary artery bypass grafting [48].

As previously mentioned, a number of clinical studies have shown that mitochondrial-based CP elicited by IPC, as well as by the use of physiological stress and pharmacological stimuli (e.g., exercise and adenosine) can provide beneficial results in treating angina [49–50]. Moreover, in recent clinical trials, the chronic administration of the mitoK$_{ATP}$ opener nicorandil was shown to improve the prognosis of patients with coronary artery disease [51]. The further use of CP-based strategies in treating patients undergoing angioplasty, ischemic cardiomyopathy, heart transplant, and bypass surgery is currently under consideration.

Volatile anesthetic agents commonly used to maintain the state of general anesthesia, such as halothane, isoflurane, and sevoflurane, can provide CP in response to myocardial ischemia and reperfusion [52–54]. The cardioprotective signaling pathway of anesthetic preconditioning (APC) shares components with IPC, including protein kinase C activation, mitoK$_{ATP}$ channel activation, and mitochondrial ROS generation, despite the differences between these 2 stimuli. The direct inhibition of mitochondrial ETC enzymes and altered mitochondrial bioenergetics in hearts preconditioned by APC implicate the mitochondria as a primary target. Decreased mitochondrial ROS levels in ischemic and reperfused hearts preconditioned by APC have been proposed as contributory to their improved structure and function [54]. Clinical studies have confirmed that sevoflurane preconditioning preserves myocardial function, as assessed by biochemical markers, in patients undergoing coronary artery bypass graft surgery under cardioplegic arrest [55].

Another potential target of CP is the apoptotic pathway, which prominently features the permeabilization of mitochondrial membranes, leading to the release of protease and nuclease activators and to bioenergetic failure. As noted in Chapter 4, mitochondrial apoptosis plays a pivotal role in the progression of myocardial remodeling in HCM and DCM and can also result from myocardial ischemia/reperfusion. Attenuation of the mitochondrial apoptotic pathway by overexpression of the antiapoptotic protein Bcl-2 has been shown to provide CP in cultured cardiomyocytes and in animal models by treatment with antioxidants such as melatonin [56–57]. Modulating PT pore opening, a common early event in the mitochondrial apoptotic pathway, can be directly mediated by cyclosporin A or sanglifehrin A treatment providing cardioprotection against reperfusion injury [58]. Uncouplers of OXPHOS such as dinitrophenol and CCCP have also been shown to elicit CP [59–60]. Moreover, overexpression of the uncoupling protein (UCP2) in cultured neonatal rat cardiomyocytes suppressed markers of apoptotic cell death, prevented the loss of mitochondrial membrane potential, attenuated both mitochondrial $Ca^{++}$ overload and ROS production, protecting cardiomyocytes exposed to oxidative stress [61]. Therefore, the recent discovery that the KCOs diazoxide and pinacidil facilitate proton translocation through mitochondrial membranes acting as uncouplers of OXPHOS, activating state 4 respiration and depolarizing the mitochondria, is not surprising [62]. Since the majority of cardioprotective treatments targeting myocardial apoptosis (e.g., modulation of uncoupler or PT pore activity) can have profound impact on a variety of metabolic processes, their therapeutic application may prove to be problematic. Nevertheless, several reagents (mostly antioxidants) have shown promising results in preliminary clinical studies. In a group of patients undergoing cardiac surgery with cardioplegic arrest, increased myocardial apoptotic progression was effectively prevented in those infused with n-acetylcysteine, an antioxidant and sulfhydryl donor precursor for glutathione [63]. In addition, grape seed proanthocyanin extract (GSPE), a potent antioxidant, showed cardioprotective properties in both animal and human, improving postischemic left ventricular function and significantly reducing infarct size, myocardial ROS levels, and apoptotic markers [64]. This finding confirms previous studies documenting that the polyphenolic antioxidants present in red wine, such as resveratrol and proanthocyanidins, provide CP by their ability to function as *in vivo* antioxidants in addition to the alcoholic component, which also is cardioprotective by adapting the heart to oxidative stress [65–66]. Pyruvate also provides CP in both animal models [58, 67] and in human [68], although how this is mediated has not yet been determined.

A complementary approach to cardioprotective therapies targeting apoptosis, involves triggering antiapoptotic cell proliferation (or cell survival pathways). Various growth factors, including insulin-like growth factor (e.g., IGF-1), hepatocyte growth factor, endothelin-1, fibroblast growth factor, and transforming growth factor, have been shown to protect the heart against oxidative stress, largely by attenuating cardiac myocyte apoptosis [69]. Growth factor signaling such as occurs with IGF-1 is mediated via activation of the PI3K pathway, which has been shown to be cardioprotective and by the serine-threonine kinase, Akt. Concerns have been raised by the systemic administration of high levels of IGF-1 peptide. *In vivo* cardiac IGF-I gene transfer, performed prior to ischemia-reperfusion injury, achieved a more sustained activation of Akt and reduced hypoxia-induced apoptosis as compared to the effects of IGF-1 peptide treatment [70]. Somatic gene transfer of growth factors may be advantageous over systemic delivery by mediating cardiomyocyte protection without elevating serum levels of growth factors. Studies in transgenic animals with Akt overexpression showed a variety of cardiac phenotypes, including progressive cardiac hypertrophy and failure, suggesting that considerable caution is warranted in the therapeutic application of Akt expression and signaling since it is a critical mediator of hypertrophic growth [71–72]. However, in transgenic animals, hypertrophic remodeling resulting from Akt myocardial overexpression can be eliminated by nuclear-targeting of Akt , which enhances survival of cardiomyocytes with no loss of its cardioprotection against ischemia [73].

In a comparable way, a "metabolic cocktail" composed of glucose-insulin-potasssium, when administrated at early reperfusion, reduces infarct size in the rat heart *in vivo*. This is a relatively inexpensive approach to CP in which the insulin component primarily stimulates

Akt prosurvival signaling [74]. Since intravenous insulin therapy is associated with metabolic side-effects, the development of therapeutic agents that can target downstream cell-survival insulin-activated signaling events has been considered as an alternate approach to promote CP [75] (Table 11.2).

**Table 11.2.   Cardioprotective agents**

| Agent | Mechanism | Clinical (C) or Animal (A) Model |
|-------|-----------|-------------------|
| Ischemic preconditioning | Activates CP pathway | C, A |
| Nicorandil | MitoK$_{ATP}$ channel opener | C, A |
| Sevoflurane | Volatile anesthetic | C, A |
| N-acetylcysteine | Antioxidant; glutathione precursor | C, A |
| Pyruvate | Not determined | C, A |
| Proanthocyanin extract | Antioxidant | C, A |
| Glucose-insulin-potassium | Akt activation | C, A |
| Adenosine | Activates CP pathway | A |
| Moderate alcohol | Akt activation | A |
| Other polyphenols | Antioxidant | A |
| Diazoxide, Pinacidil | MitoK$_{ATP}$ channel opener | A |
| Bcl-2 overexpression | Apoptotic inhibitor | A |
| Cyclosporin A | PT pore modulator | A |
| Dinitrophenol, CCCP | Uncouplers | A |

## New approaches in treatment

### Gene therapy in cardiovascular diseases

Advances in the identification of genes affected in cardiovascular disease have lead to improved therapies, either by the use of gene replacement or gene-suppression (silencing) methodologies. Preclinical studies in a variety of animal models have shown that gene therapy can provide beneficial results in the treatment of HF, hypertension, hypertrophy, cardiac arrhythmias, and myocarditis as well as in disorders of the vascular wall, particularly in cases where drug therapy has proved to be of limited value. Gene therapy enables therapeutic concentrations of a gene product to be accumulated and maintained at optimally high levels and at a localized target site of action and also offers the possibility of minimizing systemic side effects by avoiding high plasma levels of the gene product [76]. While early phases of clinical gene therapy trials for cardiovascular diseases have shown promising results, in particular in regard to therapeutic angiogenesis and restenosis treatment, the development of improved vectors, methods of delivery, and the acquisition of safety and toxicity data remain to be critically improved before these therapies can be routinely used in a clinical setting.

Both viral vectors and naked plasmid DNAs have been employed in preclinical and clinical cardiovascular gene transfer studies. While plasmid DNA vectors have been shown to have good entry and expression in normal and ischemic muscle [77], their lower efficiency of transfection in myocardial gene delivery limits their use. Features of viral vectors can predetermine both the range of host cells that can be transduced as well as the efficiency, level, and duration of transgene expression. Adenoviral vectors can transduce both dividing and nondividing cells and are particularly efficient in transfecting postmitotic cells, including cardiomyocytes and to a lesser extent vascular cells, and have been the primary viral vector of choice. A limitation of the adenoviral vectors is their provision of transient rather than prolonged transgene expression. Moreover, adenoviral vectors pose additional safety concerns. These vectors produce increased inflammation, and long-term cell- and antibody-mediated immune responses have been widely reported [78]. Nevertheless, to date, no evidence of serious adverse effects have been reported in clinical trials of cardiovascular gene therapy using adenoviral vector-mediated involving over 150 subjects [79]. Other viral vectors are being considered for future use in cardiovascular therapies, including lentivirus and recombinant adeno-associated virus (AAV). AAV is taken up more slowly into myocardial cells. Compared to adenovirus, AAV transgene expression levels are lower but can be longer term, being sustained in rodent myocardium for 9 to 12 months, and AAV vectors have a lower potential to induce unwanted inflammation or immunocytotoxicity [76].

Another alternative gene transfer approach involves antisense strategies (e.g., using either antisense oligonucleotides or small interfering RNAs [siRNA]) that can regulate the transcription of targeted endogenous genes and selectively inhibit their expression). The antisense oligonucleotide approach can employ either single-strand or double-strand oligonucleotides to target specific gene expression, whereas siRNA involves the use of a specific double strand RNA construct to silence specific gene expression (RNAi). Double-strand oligonucleotides homologous to the *cis* regulatory sequences of the promoter of a gene of interest can be similarly employed. These can function as molecular decoys to bind specific transcription factors and therefore block the expression of genes requiring those transcription factors [80]. A similar strategy has been employed to block cell-cycle progression and modulate cell proliferation.

In addition to several well-characterized animal models of cardiac gene therapy aimed at treating restenosis, hypertension, and angiogenesis [81], a number of nuclear gene targets to elicit increased myocardial protection and improve cardiac function have been described.

Short-term protection of the heart from ischemia and oxidative stress can be provided by gene transfer and overexpression of genes encoding critical antioxidant enzymes such as superoxide dismutase (SOD) or heme oxygenase (HO-1). Introduction of a myocardial protective gene such as HO-1 employing a recombinant AAV vector into myocardium prior to coronary artery ligation significantly reduced infarct size in a rat model of ischemia and reperfusion [82]. In addition, gene-mediated CP against myocardial ischemia was achieved by introducing and overexpressing genes for the free radical scavenger enzyme SOD [83], heat-shock chaperone HSP70 [84], and antiapoptotic mitochondrial protein Bcl-2 [85]. It remains to be seen whether these vectors and genes can provide long-term CP against repeated, chronic forms of ischemic insult.

Experimental cardiac gene therapy has also provided useful information in treating cardiomyopathy and HF. In transgenic mice null for desmin, the muscle-specific member of the intermediate filament gene family, cardiomyopathy develops characterized by extensive cardiomyocyte death, fibrosis, and eventual HF. There is evidence that mitochondrial abnormalities are implicated in the onset of the cardiomyopathy. The overexpression of the Bcl-2 in the desmin null heart resulted in the correction of mitochondrial defects, reduction in the occurrence of myocardial fibrotic lesions, prevention of cardiac hypertrophy, restoration of cardiomyocyte ultrastructure, and significant improvement of cardiac function [86].

Nuclear-encoded gene products affecting mitochondrial metabolism have also recently proved to be an effective target for gene therapy in the rat CNS and human fibroblasts. The E1$\alpha$ subunit of the PDHC complex has been successfully transduced as an AAV construct; transduction of cultured fibroblasts from a patient with an E1$\alpha$ deficiency led to a partial restoration of PDH activity [87]. Given the pivotal role of PDHC in the regulation of aerobic metabolism, the delivery or modulation of this gene in cardiac tissues may prove useful in treating disorders in which cardiac aerobic metabolism is affected, including ischemia, hypertrophy, and HF.

## Mitochondria and gene therapy

### *Targeting mitochondria using nucleic acids*

Gene therapy to replace or repair defective mitochondrial genes could be an important adjunct in the treatment of mitochondrial-based cardiovascular disease. However, it has not yet been proven possible to introduce and replace (or repair) mtDNA genes in the mitochondria of either *in vitro* cultured cells or, more important, in the organelles of *in vivo* myocardium, posing a major hurdle for gene therapy of mtDNA-based disorders. While biolistic transformation using highly accelerated DNA-coated metal particles has shown success in the delivery of genes into bacteria, and the organelles of plants and yeast, this technique has not been proven applicable in the transformation of mammalian mitochondria. Another approach, electroporation of nucleic acids, while effective in the delivery of genes to the nucleus with subsequent expression has not been successfully applied to the gene delivery and expression in mitochondria of living cells [88]. In addition to the difficulties associated with a delivery system for mitochondrial genes, the replacement of endogenous multiple-copy defective genes (within multiple organelles) also poses a formidable challenge. Nevertheless, despite the present lack of a reliable mitochondrial transformation system, several approaches obtained primarily with isolated cells of individuals affected with mito-chondrial diseases or from cybrids have shown promising results [89–90; Marín-García and associates, unpublished data]. These include the selective destruction of mutant mtDNA by importing a restriction endonuclease enzyme into mitochondria [91], replacement of a mutant mtDNA encoded protein with a genetically engineered wildtype equivalent expressed from the nucleus (also called *allotopic expression*) [92–93], or using gene-replacement of defective mtDNA alleles with cognate genes transfected from other organisms [94] as shown in Table 11.3.

**Table 11.3.  Mitochondrial gene delivery methods**

| Method | Effectiveness with Mammalian Mitochondria |
|---|---|
| Electroporation | Not successful |
| Naked plasmid/viral transfection | Not successful |
| DQAsome | Successful transfection of plasmid DNA |
| PNAs (by itself) | Inefficient transfer of oligonucleotides |
| PNA + cationic liposomes | Improved transfer of oligonucleotides |
| PNA + cationic polyetheneimine | Improved transfer of oligonucleotides |
| Allotopic expression | Successful transfer of "reengineered" ATPase6 and ND4 genes targeted for nuclear/cytosolic expression and delivered to mitochondria |

Another promising strategy in mitochondrial gene therapy is to influence heteroplasmy, the ratio of mutant to wildtype genomes ("gene shifting"), using pharmacological, molecular, or physiological approachs. For instance, when grown in the presence of the ATPase inhibitor oligomycin, cultured cells containing a mixture of both the mutant pathogenic A8993G (responsible for Leigh syndrome) and the wildtype 8993 alleles exhibit a significant increase in the wild-type allele [95].

In patients with heteroplasmic mutations causing mitochondrial myopathies, segregation of mutant and wild-type mtDNAs has been reported in the skeletal muscle. In such patients, mutant mtDNAs predominate in mature myofibers but are rarely detectable in skeletal muscle satellite cells [96–97]. This pattern presumably reflects the loss of the mutation by random genetic drift in mitotically active tissues and the proliferation of mitochondria containing the mutant mtDNA in postmitotic cells. Satellite cells are dormant myoblasts that can be stimulated to reenter the cell cycle and form regenerated muscle by fusing with existing myofibers in response to signals for muscle growth and repair or following necrosis. The mtDNA genotype in mature myofibers from a patient with mitochondrial myopathy was examined after enhancing the incorporation of satellite cells by regenerative growth induced by resistance exercise training. A marked increase in the ratio of wild-type to mutant mtDNAs was found in muscle fibers with normal respiratory chain activity after a short period of exercise training [98]. Other studies have similarly demonstrated that by inducing localized muscle necrosis, muscle regeneration is stimulated along with the activation of endogenous satellite cell growth into myofibers, resulting in barely detectable levels of mutant mtDNA alleles, where previously they had been in excess, and restoring normal myogenic mitochondrial function [96]. It remains to be seen how this approach might be adapted in effectively treating specific cardiac mtDNA defects and mitochondrial dysfunction.

An alternative delivery system for nucleic acids into mitochondria involves the use of peptide nucleic acids (PNA) [99]. Initial experiments employed PNA as a selective antisense inhibitor to target the replication of a pathogenic mtDNA allele *in vitro* [100]. Decreased *in vitro* replication of the mutant nt 8344 allele for MERRF could be achieved using a PNA construct containing a short synthetic oligonucleotide complementary to the MERRF mutation, mimicking a shift in allele heteroplasmy observed in a MERRF patient. In this study, however, a PNA-induced gene shift in the extent of allele heteroplasmy could not be demonstrated in cultured cells. The difficulties associated with mitochondrial uptake of nucleic acids in living cells have been more recently surmounted by the addition of a mitochondrial-targeting leader peptide to the PNA-oligonucleotide molecule, and the introduction of the PNA-oligonucleotide construct in cationic liposomes [101–102] and, even more effectively, with cationic polyethylenimine (PEI) [103]. The latter approach successfully allowed the import of PNA-oligonucleotides into the mitochondrial matrix of living cultured cells or isolated mitochondria, a critical step in potential mitochondrial gene-specific therapy. An analogous mitochondrial-specific delivery system has been developed using DQAsomes, liposome-like vesicles formed in aqueous medium from a dicationic amphiphile called *dequalinium* [104]. These DQAsomes can bind DNA (as well as drugs), are able to transfect cells with a high efficiency, and selectively accumulate in mitochondria releasing their load [105–106]. Moreover, in addition to PNA-oligonucleotides, plasmid DNAs can be incorporated and condensed within the

DQAsomes and exclusively delivered to the mitochondrial compartment [105].

## *Targeting mitochondria using bioactive compounds*

The selective delivery of a variety of compounds (e.g., antiapoptotic drugs, antioxidants, and proton uncouplers) to the mitochondria can be envisaged as playing a fundamental role in the treatment of a number of mitochondrial-based disorders with cardiac involvement. The previously mentioned DQAsome has been shown to deliver drugs that trigger apoptosis to mitochondria and inhibit carcinoma growth in mice [105]. A synthetic ubiquinone analog (termed *mitoQ*) has been selectively targeted to mitochondria by the addition of a lipophilic triphenylphosphate cation [107]. These positively charged lipophilic molecules rapidly permeate the lipid bilayers and accumulate at high levels within negatively charged energized mitochondria [108]. Significant doses of these bioactive compounds can be administered safely by mouth to mice over long periods of time and accumulate within most organs, including the heart and brain. The incorporation of mitoQ within mitochondria can prevent apoptotic cell death and caspase activation induced by $H_2O_2$ (in isolated Jurkat cells) and can function as a potent antioxidant, preventing lipid peroxidation and protecting the mitochondria from oxidative damage. This procedure of targeting bioactive molecules to mitochondria can be adapted to other neutral bioactive molecules, offering a potential vehicle for testing other mitochondrial-specific therapies. For instance, synthetic peptide antioxidants containing dimethyltyrosine, which are cell-permeable and concentrate 1,000-fold in the mitochondria, can reduce intracellular ROS and cell death in a cell model. In ischemic hearts, these peptides potently improved contractile force in an *ex vivo* heart model [109].

The successful incorporation into the mitochondrial matrix of another modified antioxidant, a synthetic analog of vitamin E (MitoVitE), reduces mitochondrial lipid peroxidation and protein damage and can accumulate after oral administration at therapeutic concentrations within the cardiac tissue [108]. This methodology has been recently extended to develop of a thiol-specific indicator (containing a conjugated lipophilic cation) capable of quantitative labeling and assessment of mitochondrial cysteines and gauging the precise redox state of individual mitochondrial proteins in response to oxidative stress and cell death [110].

# References

1.  DiMauro S, Mancuso M, Naini A (2004) Mitochondrial encephalomyopathies: Therapeutic approach. Ann N Y Acad Sci 1011:232–45
2.  Pollitt RJ (1995) Disorders of mitochondrial long-chain fatty acid oxidation. J Inherit Metab Dis 18:473–90
3.  Pierpont ME, Breningstall GN, Stanley CA, Singh A (2000) Familial carnitine transporter defect: A treatable cause of cardiomyopathy in children. Am Heart J 139:S96–106
4.  Freisinger P, Horvath R, Macmillan C, Peters J, Jaksch M (2004) Reversion of hypertrophic cardiomyopathy in a patient with deficiency of the mitochondrial copper binding protein SCO$_2$: Is there a potential effect of copper? J Inherit Metab Dis 27:67–79
5.  Shoffner JM, Wallace DC (1994) Oxidative phosphorylation diseases and mitochondrial DNA mutations: Diagnosis and treatment. Annu Rev Nutr 14:535–68
6.  Bersin RM, Stacpoole PW (1997) Dichloroacetate as metabolic therapy for myocardial ischemia and failure. Am Heart J 134:841–55
7.  Fragasso G, Palloshi A, Bassanelli G, Steggerda R, Montano C, Margonato A (2004) Heart disease and diabetes: From pathophysiology to therapeutic options. Ital Heart J 5:4S–15S
8.  Taivassalo T, Matthews PM, De Stefano N, Sripathi N, Genge A, Karpati G, Arnold DL (1996) Combined aerobic training and dichloroacetate improve exercise capacity and indices of aerobic metabolism in muscle cytochrome oxidase deficiency. Neurology 47:529–34
9.  Ferrari R, Ceconi C, Curello S, Cargnoni A, Alfieri O, Pardini A, Marzollo P, Visioli O (1991) Oxygen free radicals and myocardial damage: Protective role of thiol-containing agents. Am J Med 1991: 95S–105S
10.  Ferrari R, Guardigli G, Mele D, Percoco GF, Ceconi C, Curello S (2004) Oxidative stress during myocardial ischaemia and heart failure. Curr Pharm Des 10:1699–711
11.  Cooper JM, Schapira AH (2003) Friedreich's Ataxia: Disease me-

hanisms, antioxidant and Coenzyme Q10 therapy. Biofactors 18:163–71

12. Santos DL, Moreno AJ, Leino RL, Froberg MK, Wallace KB (2002) Carvedilol protects against doxorubicin-induced mitochondrial cardiomyopathy. Toxicol Appl Pharmacol 185:218–27

13. Lerman-Sagie T, Rustin P, Lev D, Yanoov M, Leshinsky-Silver E, Sagie A, Ben-Gal T, Munnich A (2001) Dramatic improvement in mitochondrial cardiomyopathy following treatment with idebenone. J Inherit Metab Dis 24:28–34

14. Sayed-Ahmed M, Salman T, Gaballah H, Abou El-Naga SA, Nicolai R, Calvani M (2001) Propionyl-L-carnitine as protector against adriamycin-induced cardiomyopathy. Pharmacol Res 43: 513–20

15. Shite J, Qin F, Mao W, Kawai H, Stevens SY, Liang C (2001) Antioxidant vitamins attenuate oxidative stress and cardiac dysfunction in tachycardia-induced cardiomyopathy. J Am Coll Cardiol 38:1734–40

16. Lipshultz SE, Rifai N, Dalton VM, Levy DE, Silverman LB, Lipsitz SR, Colan SD, Asselin BL, Barr RD, Clavell LA, Hurwitz CA, Moghrabi A, Samson Y, Schorin M, Gelber R, Sallan SE (2004) The effect of dexrazoxane on myocardial injury in doxorubicin-treated children with acute lymphoblastic leukemia. N Engl J Med 351:145–53

17. Geromel V, Darin N, Chretien D, Benit P, DeLonlay P, Rotig A, Munnich A, Rustin P (2002) Coenzyme Q(10) and idebenone in the therapy of respiratory chain diseases: Rationale and comparative benefits. Mol Genet Metab 77:21–30

18. Hausse AO, Aggoun Y, Bonnet D, Sidi D, Munnich A, Rotig A, Rustin P (2002) Idebenone and reduced cardiac hypertrophy in Friedreich's ataxia. Heart 87:346–9

19. Rustin P, Munnich A, Rotig A (1999) Quinone analogs prevent enzymes targeted in Friedreich ataxia from iron-induced injury in vitro. Biofactors 9:247–51

20. Ogasahara S, Yorifuji S, Nishikawa Y, Takahashi M, Wada K, Hazama T, Nakamura Y, Hashimoto S, Kono N, Tarui S (1985) Improvement of abnormal pyruvate metabolism and cardiac conduction defect with coenzyme Q10 in Kearns-Sayre syndrome. Neurology 35:372–7

21. Mortensen SA, Vadhanavikit S, Baandrup U, Folkers K (1985) Long-term coenzyme Q10 therapy: A major advance in the

management of resistant myocardial failure. Drugs Exp Clin Res 11: 581–93

23. Hargreaves IP (2003) Ubiquinone: Cholesterol's reclusive cousin. Ann Clin Biochem 40:207–18

23. Mortensen SA (2003) Overview on coenzyme Q10 as adjunctive therapy in chronic heart failure: Rationale, design and end-points of "Q-symbio"—a multinational trial. Biofactors 18:79–89

24. Saudubray JM, Martin D, de Lonlay P, Touati G, Poggi-Travert F, Bonnet D, Jouvet P, Boutron M, Slama A, Vianey-Saban C, Bonnefont JP, Rabier D, Kamoun P, Brivet M (1999) Recognition and management of fatty acid oxidation defects: A series of 107 patients. J Inherit Metab Dis 22:488–502

25. Brown-Harrison MC, Nada MA, Sprecher H, Vianey-Saban C, Farquhar J Jr, Gilladoga AC, Roe CR (1996) Very long-chain acyl-CoA dehydrogenase deficiency: Successful treatment of acute cardio-myopathy. Biochem Mol Med 58:59–65

26. Wallhaus TR, Taylor M, DeGrado TR, Russell DC, Stanko P, Nickles RJ, Stone CK (2001) Myocardial free fatty acid and glucose use after carvedilol treatment in patients with congestive heart failure. Circulation 103:2441–6

27. Rupp H, Zarain-Herzberg A, Maisch B (2002) The use of partial fatty acid oxidation inhibitors for metabolic therapy of angina pectoris and heart failure. Herz 27:621–36

28. Stanley WC (2002) Partial fatty acid oxidation inhibitors for stable angina. Expert Opin Investig Drugs 11:615–29

29. Zarain-Herzberg A, Rupp H (1999) Transcriptional modulators targeted at fuel metabolism of hypertrophied heart. Am J Cardiol 83:31H–37H

30. Schmidt-Schweda S, Holubarsch C (2000) First clinical trial with etomoxir in patients with chronic congestive heart failure. Clin Sci 99:27–35

31. Pepine CJ, Wolff AA (1999) A controlled trial with a novel anti-ischemic agent, ranolazine, in chronic stable angina pectoris that is responsive to conventional antianginal agents. Am J Cardiol 84:46–50

32. Fragasso G, Piatti Md PM, Monti L, Palloshi A, Setola E, Pucceti P, Calori G, Lopaschuk GD, Margonato A (2003) Short- and long-term beneficial effects of trimetazidine in patients with diabetes and ischemic cardiomyopathy. Am Heart J 146:E18

33. Kantor PF, Lucien A, Kozak R, Lopaschuk GD (2000) The antianginal drug trimetazidine shifts cardiac energy metabolism from

fatty acid oxidation to glucose oxidation by inhibiting mitochondrial long-chain 3-ketoacyl coenzyme A thiolase. Circ Res 86:580–8

34. MacInnes A, Fairman DA, Binding P, Rhodes J, Wyatt MJ, Phelan A, Haddock PS, Karran EH (2003) The antianginal agent trimetazidine does not exert its functional benefit via inhibition of mitochondrial long-chain 3-ketoacyl coenzyme A thiolase. Circ Res 93:e26–32

35. Tabbi-Anneni I, Helies-Toussaint C, Morin D, Bescond-Jacquet A, Lucien A, Grynberg A (2003) Prevention of heart failure in rats by trimetazidine treatment: A consequence of accelerated phospholipid turnover? J Pharmacol Exp Ther 304:1003–9

36. Chung MK (2004) Vitamins, supplements, herbal medicines, and arrhythmias. Cardiol Rev 12:73–84

37. Tavazzi L, Tognoni G, Franzosi MG, Latini R, Maggioni AP, Marchioli R, Nicolosi GL, Porcu M (2004) Rationale and design of the GISSI heart failure trial: A large trial to assess the effects of n-3 polyunsaturated fatty acids and rosuvastatin in symptomatic congestive heart failure. Eur J Heart Fail 6:635–41

38. Singer P, Wirth M (2004) Can n-3 PUFA reduce cardiac arrhythmias? Results of a clinical trial. Prostaglandins Leukot Essent Fatty Acids 71:153–9

39. Pepe S, Tsuchiya N, Lakatta EG, Hansford RG (1999) PUFA and aging modulate cardiac mitochondrial membrane lipid composition and Ca2+ activation of PDH. Am J Physiol 276:H149–58

40. Xu Z, Jiao Z, Cohen MV, Downey JM (2002) Protection from AMP 579 can be added to that from either cariporide or ischemic preconditioning in ischemic rabbit heart. J Cardiovasc Pharmacol 40: 510–8

41. Inagaki K, Chen L, Ikeno F, Lee F, Imahashi K, Bouley D, Rezaee M, Yock P, Murphy E, Mochly-Rosen D (2003) Inhibition of protein kinase C protects against reperfusion injury of the ischemic heart. Circulation 108:2304–7

42. Inoue K, Ando S, Itagaki T, Shiojiri Y, Kashima T, Takaba T (2003) Intracellular calcium increasing at the beginning of reperfusion assists the early recovery of myocardial contractility after diltiazem cardioplegia. Jpn J Thorac Cardiovasc Surg 51:98–103

43. Kroner A, Seitelberger R, Schirnhofer J, Bernecker O, Mallinger R, Hallstrom S, Ploner M, Podesser BK (2002) Diltiazem during reperfusion preserves high energy phosphates by protection of mitochondrial integrity. Eur J Cardiothorac Surg 21:224–31

44. Bertolet BD (1999) Calcium antagonists in the post-myocardial infarction setting. Drugs Aging 15:461–70

45. Theroux P, Gregoire J, Chin C, Pelletier G, de Guise P, Juneau M (1998) Intravenous diltiazem in acute myocardial infarction. Diltiazem as adjunctive therapy to activase (DATA) trial. J Am Coll Cardiol 32:620–8.

46. Pizzetti G, Mailhac A, Li Volsi L, Di Marco F, Lu C, Margonato A, Chierchia SL. (2001) Beneficial effects of diltiazem during myocardial reperfusion: A randomized trial in acute myocardial infarction. Ital Heart J 2:757–65

47. Matlib MA, McFarland KL (1991) Diltiazem inhibition of sodium-induced calcium release. Am J Hypertens 4:435S–41S

48. Malhotra R, Mishra M, Kler TS, Kohli VM, Mehta Y, Trehan N (1997) Cardioprotective effects of diltiazem infusion in the perioperative period. Eur J Cardiothorac Surg 12:420–7

49. Leesar MA, Stoddard MF, Xuan YT, Tang XL, Bolli R (2003) Nonelectrocardiographic evidence that both ischemic preconditioning and adenosine preconditioning exist in humans. J Am Coll Cardiol 42:437–45

50. Crisafulli A, Melis F, Tocco F, Santoboni UM, Lai C, Angioy G, Lorrai L, Pittau G, Concu A, Pagliaro P (2004) Exercise-induced and nitroglycerin-induced myocardial preconditioning improves hemodynamics in patients with angina. Am J Physiol Heart Circ Physiol 287:H235–42

51. Argaud L, Ovize M (2004) How to use the paradigm of ischemic preconditioning to protect the heart? Med Sci 20:521–5

52. de Ruijter W, Musters RJ, Boer C, Stienen GJ, Simonides WS, de Lange JJ (2003)The cardioprotective effect of sevoflurane depends on protein kinase C activation, opening of mitochondrial K(+)(ATP) channels, and the production of reactive oxygen species. Anesth Anal 97:1370–6

53. Zaugg M, Lucchinetti E, Spahn DR, Pasch T, Schaub MC (2002) Volatile anesthetics mimic cardiac preconditioning by priming the activation of mitochondrial K(ATP) channels via multiple signaling pathways. Anesthesiology 97:4–14

54. Stowe DF, Kevin LG (2004) Cardiac preconditioning by volatile anesthetic agents: A defining role for altered mitochondrial bioenergetics. Antioxid Redox Signal 6:439–48

55. Julier K, da Silva R, Garcia C, Bestmann L, Frascarolo P, Zollinger A, Chassot PG, Schmid ER, Turina MI, von Segesser LK, Pasch

T, Spahn DR, Zaugg M (2003) Preconditioning by sevoflurane decreases biochemical markers for myocardial and renal dysfunction in coronary artery bypass graft surgery: A double-blinded, placebo-controlled, multicenter study. Anesthesiology 98:1315–27

56. Dziegiel P, Podhorska-Okolow M, Surowiak P, Ciesielska U, Rabczynski J, Zabel M (2003) Influence of exogenous melatonin on doxorubicin-evoked effects in myocardium and in transplantable Morris hepatoma in rats. In Vivo 17:325–8

57. Tanaka M, Nakae S, Terry RD, Mokhtari GK, Gunawan F, Balsam LB, Kaneda H, Kofidis T, Tsao PS, Robbins RC (2004) Cardiomyocyte-specific Bcl-2 overexpression attenuates ischemia-reperfusion injury, immune response during acute rejection, and graft coronary artery disease. Blood 104:3789–96

58. Halestrap AP, Clarke SJ, Javadov SA (2004) Mitochondrial permeability transition pore opening during myocardial reperfusion: A target for cardioprotection. Cardiovasc Res 61:372–85

59. Minners J, van den Bos EJ, Yellon DM, Schwalb H, Opie LH, Sack MN (2000) Dinitrophenol, cyclosporin A, and trimetazidine modulate preconditioning in the isolated rat heart: Support for a mitochondrial role in cardioprotection. Cardiovasc Res 47:68–73

60. Ganote CE, Armstrong SC (2003) Effects of CCCP-induced mitochondrial uncoupling and cyclosporin A on cell volume, cell injury and preconditioning protection of isolated rabbit cardiomyocytes. J Mol Cell Cardiol 35:749–59

61. Teshima Y, Akao M, Jones SP, Marban E (2003) Uncoupling protein-2 overexpression inhibits mitochondrial death pathway in cardiomyocytes. Circ Res 93:192–200

62. Holmuhamedov EL, Jahangir A, Oberlin A, Komarov A, Colombini M, Terzic A (2004) Potassium channel openers are un-coupling protonophores: Implication in cardioprotection. FEBS Lett 568:167–70

63. Fischer UM, Tossios P, Huebner A, Geissler HJ, Bloch W, Mehlhorn U (2004) Myocardial apoptosis prevention by radical scavenging in patients undergoing cardiac surgery. J Thorac Cardiovasc Surg 128:103–8

64. Bagchi D, Sen CK, Ray SD, Das DK, Bagchi M, Preuss HG, Vinson JA (2003) Molecular mechanisms of cardioprotection by a novel grape seed proanthocyanidin extract. Mutat Res 523–524:87–97

65. Brookes PS, Digerness SB, Parks DA, Darley-Usmar V (2002) Mitochondrial function in response to cardiac ischemia-reperfusion after oral treatment with quercetin. Free Radic Biol Med 32:1220–8

66. Sato M, Maulik N, Das D (2002) Cardioprotection with alcohol: role of both alcohol and polyphenolic antioxidants. Ann N Y Acad Sci 957:122–35

67. Olivencia-Yurvati AH, Blair JL, Baig M, Mallet RT (2003) Pyruvate-enhanced cardioprotection during surgery with cardio-pulmonary bypass. J Cardiothorac Vasc Anesth 17:715–20

68. Flood A, Hack BD, Headrick JP (2003) Pyruvate-dependent preconditioning and cardioprotection in murine myocardium. Clin Exp Pharmacol Physiol 30:145–52

69. Suzuki YJ (2003) Growth factor signaling for cardioprotection against oxidative stress-induced apoptosis. Antioxid Redox Signal 5: 741–9

70. Chao W, Matsui T, Novikov MS, Tao J, Li L, Liu H, Ahn Y, Rosenzweig A (2003) Strategic advantages of insulin-like growth factor-I expression for cardioprotection. J Gene Med 5:277–86

71. Matsui T, Li L, Wu JC, Cook SA, Nagoshi T, Picard MH, Liao R, Rosenzweig A (2002) Phenotypic spectrum caused by transgenic overexpression of activated Akt in the heart. J Biol Chem 277: 22896–901

72. Latronico MV, Costinean S, Lavitrano ML, Peschle C, Condorelli G (2004) Regulation of cell size and contractile function by AKT in cardiomyocytes. Ann N Y Acad Sci 1015:250–60

73. Shiraishi I, Melendez J, Ahn Y, Skavdahl M, Murphy E, Welch S, Schaefer E, Walsh K, Rosenzweig A, Torella D, Nurzynska D, Kajstura J, Leri A, Anversa P, Sussman MA (2004) Nuclear targeting of Akt enhances kinase activity and survival of cardiomyocytes. Circ Res 94:884–91

74. Jonassen AK, Sack MN, Mjos OD, Yellon DM (2001) Myocar-dial protection by insulin at reperfusion requires early administration and is mediated via Akt and p70s6 kinase cell-survival signaling. Circ Res 89:1191–8

75. Sack MN, Yellon DM (2003) Insulin therapy as an adjunct to reperfusion after acute coronary ischemia: A proposed direct myo-cardial cell survival effect independent of metabolic modulation. J Am Coll Cardiol 41:1404–7

76. Dzau VJ (2003) Predicting the future of human gene therapy for cardiovascular diseases: What will the management of coronary artery disease be like in 2005 and 2010? Am J Cardiol 92:32N–35N

77. Baumgartner I, Isner JM (2001) Somatic gene therapy in the cardiovascular system. Annu Rev Physiol 63:427–50

78. Pislau S, Janssens Sp, Gersh BJ, Simari RD (2002) Defining gene transfer before expecting gene therapy: Putting the horse before the cart. Circulation 106:631–6

79. Isner JM, Vale PR, Symes JF, Losordo DW (2001) Assessment of risks associated with cardiovascular gene therapy in human subjects. Circ Res 89:389–400

80. Morishita R, Higaki J, Tomita N, Ogihara T (1998) Application of transcription factor "decoy" strategy of gene therapy and study of gene expression in cardiovascular disease. Circ Res 82:1023–8

81. Chaudhri BB, del Monte F, Harding SE, Hajjar RJ (2004) Gene transfer in cardiac myocytes. Surg Clin North Am 84:141–59

82. Melo LG, Agrawal R, Zhang L, Rezvani M, Mangi AA, Ehsan A, Griese DP, Dell'Acqua G, Mann MJ, Oyama J, Yet SF, Layne MD, Perrella MA, Dzau VJ (2002) Gene therapy strategy for long-term myocardial protection using adeno-associated virus-mediated delivery of heme oxygenase gene. Circulation 105:602–7

83. Abunasra HJ, Smolenski RT, Morrison K, Yap J, Sheppard MN, O'Brien T, Suzuki K, Jayakumar J, Yacoub MH (2001) Efficacy of adenoviral gene transfer with manganese superoxide dismutase and endothelial nitric oxide synthase in reducing ischemia and reperfusion injury. Eur J Cardiothorac Surg 20:153–8

84. Jayakumar J, Suzuki K, Sammut IA, Smolenski RT, Khan M, Latif N, Abunasra H, Murtuza B, Amrani M, Yacoub MH (2001) Heat shock protein 70 gene transfection protects mitochondrial and ventricular function against ischemia-reperfusion injury. Circulation 104:I303–7

85. Chatterjee S, Stewart AS, Bish LT, Jayasankar V, Kim EM, Pirolli T, Burdick J, Woo YJ, Gardner TJ, Sweeney HL (2002) Viral gene transfer of the antiapoptotic factor Bcl-2 protects against chronic postischemic heart failure. Circulation 106:I212–7

86. Weisleder N, Taffet GE, Capetanaki Y (2004) Bcl-2 overexpression corrects mitochondrial defects and ameliorates inherited desmin null cardiomyopathy. Proc Natl Acad Sci USA 101:769–74

87. Stacpoole PW, Owen R, Flotte TR (2003) The pyruvate dehydrogenase complex as a target for gene therapy. Curr Gene Ther 3:239–45

88. McGregor A, Temperley R, Chrzanowska-Lightowlers ZM, Lightowlers RN (2001) Absence of expression from RNA internalised into electroporated mammalian mitochondria. Mol Genet Genomics 265:721–9

89. Turnbull DM, Lightowlers RN (2002) A roundabout route to gene therapy. Nat Genet 30:345–6

90. Chinnery PF (2004) New approaches to the treatment of mitochondrial disorders. Reprod Biomed Online 8:16–23

91. Tanaka M, Borgeld HJ, Zhang J, Muramatsu S, Gong JS, Yoneda M, Maruyama W, Naoi M, Ibi T, Sahashi K, Shamoto M, Fuku N, Kurata M, Yamada Y, Nishizawa K, Akao Y, Ohishi N, Miyabayashi S, Umemoto H, Muramatsu T, Furukawa K, Kikuchi A, Nakano I, Ozawa K, Yagi K (2002) Gene therapy for mitochondrial disease by delivering restriction endonuclease SmaI into mitochondria. J Biomed Sci 9:534–41

92. Guy J, Qi X, Pallotti F, Schon EA, Manfredi G, Carelli V, Martinuzzi A, Hauswirth WW, Lewin AS (2002) Rescue of a mitochondrial deficiency causing Leber hereditary optic neuropathy. Ann Neurol 52:534–42

93. Manfredi G, Fu J, Ojaimi J, Sadlock JE, Kwong JQ, Guy J, Schon EA (2002) Rescue of a deficiency in ATP synthesis by transfer of MTATP6, a mitochondrial DNA-encoded gene, to the nucleus. Nat Genet 30:394–9

94. Ojaimi J, Pan J, Santra S, Snell WJ, Schon E (2002) An algal nucleus-encoded subunit of mitochondrial ATP synthase rescues a defect in the analogous human mitochondrial-encoded subunit. Mol Biol Cell 13:3836–44

95. Manfredi G, Gupta N, Vazquez-Memije ME, Sadlock JE, Spinazzola A, De Vivo DC, Schon EA (1999) Oligomycin induces a decrease in the cellular content of a pathogenic mutation in the human mitochondrial ATPase 6 gene. J Biol Chem 274:9386–91

96. Fu K, Hartlen R, Johns T, Genge A, Karpati G, Shoubridge EA (1996) A novel heteroplasmic tRNAleu(CUN) mtDNA point mutation in a sporadic patient with mitochondrial encephalomyopathy segregates rapidly in skeletal muscle and suggests an approach to therapy. Hum Mol Genet 5:1835–40

97. Clark KM, Bindoff LA, Lightowlers RN, Andrews RM, Griffiths PG, Johnson MA, Brierley EJ, Turnbull DM (1997) Reversal of a mtDNA defect in human skeletal muscle. Nat Genet 16:222–4

98. Taivassalo T, Fu K, Johns T, Arnold D, Karpati G, Shoubridge EA (1999) Gene shifting: A novel therapy for mitochondrial myopathy. Hum Mol Genet 8:1047–52

99. Chinnery PF, Taylor RW, Diekert K, Lill R, Turnbull DM, Lightowlers RN (1999) Peptide nucleic acid delivery to human mitochondria. Gene Ther 6:1919–28

100. Taylor RW, Chinnery PF, Turnbull DM, Lightowlers RN (1997) Selective inhibition of mutant human mitochondrial DNA replication in vitro by peptide nucleic acids. Nat Genet 15:212–5

101. Muratovska A, Lightowlers RN, Taylor RW, Turnbull DM, Smith RA, Wilce JA, Martin SW, Murphy MP (2001) Targeting peptide nucleic acid (PNA) oligomers to mitochondria within cells by conjugation to lipophilic cations: Implications for mitochondrial DNA replication, expression and disease. Nucleic Acids Res 29:1852–63

102. Geromel V, Cao A, Briane D, Vassy J, Rotig A, Rustin P, Coudert R, Rigaut JP, Munnich A, Taillandier E (2001) Mitochondria transfection by oligonucleotides containing a signal peptide and vectorized by cationic liposomes. Antisense Nucleic Acid Drug Dev 11:175–80

103. Flierl A, Jackson C, Cottrell B, Murdock D, Seibel P, Wallace DC (2003) Targeted delivery of DNA to the mitochondrial compartment via import sequence-conjugated peptide nucleic acid. Mol Ther 7:550–7

104. Weissig V, Lasch J, Erdos G, Meyer HW, Rowe TC, Hughes J (1998) DQAsomes: A novel potential drug and gene delivery system made from Dequalinium. Pharm Res 15:334–7

105. D'Souza GG, Rammohan R, Cheng SM, Torchilin VP, Weissig V (2003) DQAsome-mediated delivery of plasmid DNA toward mitochondria in living cells. J Control Release 92:189–97

106. Weissig V, Cheng SM, D'Souza GG (2004) Mitochondrial pharmaceutics. Mitochondrion 3:229–44

107. Kelso GF, Porteous CM, Coulter CV, Hughes G, Porteous WK, Ledgerwood EC, Smith RA, Murphy MP (2001) Selective targeting of a redox-active ubiquinone to mitochondria within cells: Antioxidant and antiapoptotic properties. J Biol Chem 276:4588–96

108. Smith RA, Porteous CM, Gane AM, Murphy MP (2003) Delivery of bioactive molecules to mitochondria in vivo. Proc Natl Acad Sci USA 100:5407–12

109. Zhao K, Zhao GM, Wu D, Soong Y, Birk AV, Schiller PW, Szeto HH (2004) Cell-permeable peptide antioxidants targeted to inner mitochondrial membrane inhibit mitochondrial swelling, oxidative cell death and reperfusion injury. J Biol Chem 279: 34682–90

110. Lin TK, Hughes G, Muratovska A, Blaikie FH, Brookes PS, Darley-Usmar V, Smith RA, Murphy MP (2002) Specific modification of mitochondrial protein thiols in response to oxidative stress: A proteomics approach. J Biol Chem 277:17048–56

# Chapter 12

# Future Frontiers in Mitochondrial Cardiac Biology

## Overview

New discoveries in molecular genetic technology are beginning to be applied in cardiology arising from chromosomal mapping and identification of genes involved in both the primary etiology and as significant risk factors in the development of cardiac and vascular abnormalities. Novel technologies are being developed in animal models, while others are currently being evaluated in early clinical trials.

Genes and proteins involved in the regulation of cardiovascular physiology and in cardiac disease are being intensively studied. In this chapter, we discuss future frontiers in mitochondrial medicine, including the potential use of cell engineering (e.g., stem cell transplantation) in mitochondrial-based cardiac pathologies, the application of new technologies (e.g., pharmacogenetics and proteomics), and the critical issues that these technologies raise.

## Introduction

Despite evidence that mitochondria play a significant role in the maintenance of normal cardiac function and in cardiac pathology, fundamental questions remain unanswered regarding the underlying molecular and biochemical mechanisms involved, and ways this information can be used in improving clinical diagnosis and treatment. To address these often difficult questions, a number of emerging technologies are being recruited, some tested only in animal models and others being investigated in early clinical trials. Novel approaches using molecular genetic and cytogenetic technology to identify genes and proteins involved in cardiovascular regulation and cardiac diseases are presented in this chapter. Also, critical issues regarding data management and standardization, ethical concerns raised by using this novel technology, and the overall availability of research findings in this important field are addressed.

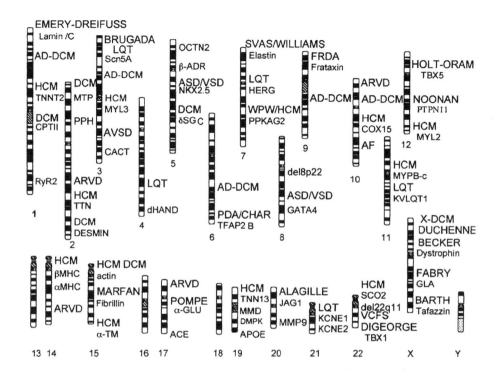

**Figure 12.1. Human chromosomal map of inherited cardiovascular disorders.**
*Disorders and affected genes are localized on ideograms of each of the human chromosomes. These include ACE, angiotensin-converting enzyme; AD-DCM, autosomal dominant dilated cardiomyopathy; AF, familial atrial fibrillation; APOE, apolipoprotein E; ARVD, arrhythmogenic right ventricular dysplasia; AVSD, atrioventricular septal defect; α-GLU, α-glucosidase; α MHC, α-myosin heavy chain; α TM, α–tropomyosin; β ADR, β adrenergic receptor; β MHC, β-myosin heavy chain; CACT, carnitine-acylcarnitine translocase; CPTII, carnitine palmitoyltransferase II; δ- SGC, δ -sarcoglycan; DCM, dilated cardiomyopathy; DMPK, myotonin protein kinase; FRDA, Friedreich's ataxia; GLA, α galactosidase; HCM, hypertrophic cardiomyopathy; HERG, human ether-a-go-go related gene; HOS, Holt-Oram syndrome; JAG1, jagged-1; KCNE1, potassium channel, voltage-gated, Isk-related subfamily member 1; KCNE2, potassium channel, voltage-gated, Isk-related subfamily member 2; KVLQT1, potassium voltage-gated long QT syndrome 1 channel; LQT, long QT syndrome; MMD, myotonic muscular dystrophy; MMP9, matrix metalloproteinase 9; MTP, mitochondrial trifunctional protein; MYBPC, myosin-binding protein C; MYL2, regulatory ventricular myosin light chain; MYL3, essential ventricular myosin light chain; NDUFS2, complex I subunit; OCTN2, organic cation carnitine transporter 2; PDA, patent ductus arteriosus/Char syndrome; PPH, primary pulmonary hypertension; PPKAγ2, AMP-activated protein kinase gamma 2; PTPN11, protein tyrosine phosphatase; RYR2, ryanodine receptor 2; SCO$_2$, synthesis of cytochrome c oxidase (COX assembly protein); SCN5A, sodium channel, voltage-gated, type V, a polypeptide; SVAS, supravalvular aortic stenosis; TBX1, T-box 1 transcription factor; TBX5, T-box 5 transcription factor;*

*TFAP2B, transcription factor of the AP-2 family; TNNT2, cardiac troponin T; TNN13, cardiac troponin I; TTN, titin; VCFS/DG, velocardiofacial syndrome/DiGeorge; WPW, Wolff-Parkinson-White syndrome; X-DCM, X-linked dilated cardiomyopathy.*

## Disease gene identification: Diagnostic application

Breakthroughs in molecular genetic technology have just begun to be applied in cardiology stemming from the use of chromosomal mapping and the identification of genes involved in the primary etiology and as significant risk factors in the development of cardiac and vascular abnormalities. Specific genetic and molecular factors have been linked to congenital heart defects (CHD) and cardiac arrhythmias allowing their identification on the human chromosome map and provide a valuable opportunity for improved genetic diagnostics and future gene therapy of cardiovascular disease (CVD) (Figure 12.1).

Many of the nuclear gene defects implicated in cardiomyopathies were originally mapped by linkage analyses in affected families, allowing the subsequent identification of candidate genes (and mutant alleles) by positional cloning and subsequent nucleotide sequence analysis. A variety of molecular techniques including polymerase chain reaction (PCR), restriction fragment length polymorphism (RFLP), and single-strand conformation polymorphism (SSCP) have been used in screening defective alleles from the proband and family members to establish inheritance patterns. In most cases, detection of novel nuclear mutations by itself is an immense undertaking involving a comprehensive analysis of large and multiple coding regions (exons) of 1, if not more, candidate genes, an undertaking less problematic with the shorter, intron-less mtDNA genes. Moreover, in the relatively well-characterized cases of familial HCM gene screening, the consensus experience has been that each specific HCM-causing mutation is rare, challenging the view of common mutations since most families have "private" or novel mutations [1]. While somewhat true of mtDNA mutations, molecular "hotspots" (e.g., tRNA$^{Leu}$ and cyt$b$ genes) appear to be more likely affected in mitochondrial cardiomyopathies [2]. The correlation of the clinical course and prognosis with specific mutations has often proved informative with nuclear gene mutations. For instance, specific ß-MHC mutations in HCM are associated with a high incidence of sudden death, whereas other mutations are associated with a better prognosis. In contrast, specific mtDNA gene mutations are more frequently associated with variable clinical phenotypes and modifying nuclear factors influencing the expression of pathogenic alleles have often been proposed as discussed below.

Recent advances in the detection of pathogenic mutations providing improved sensitivity and speed by applying high-throughput analytical techniques such as denaturing high-performance liquid chromatography (DHPLC) or capillary array electrophoresis will further advance the use of molecular genetic analysis in clinical and preclinical diagnosis [3]. Moreover, the availability of gene chip technology may allow in the near future, not only the automated and rapid screening of mtDNA and nuclear gene mutations from clinical samples but also the assessment of their impact on specific myocardial gene expression.

## Modifying Factors, Epigenetics, and SNPs

Genetic heterogeneity and intrafamilial variability have also made difficult the precise molecular elucidation of many cardiac defects, as well as the correlation of genotype with cardiac phenotype. As noted above, these difficulties may arise from the involvement of undefined multifactorial or polygenic factors that contribute to the expression of specific cardiac gene defect(s), as well as to a variety of epigenetic or acquired influences. Progress is gradually being made in defining these polygenic and epigenetic factors, a number of which have proved amenable to molecular analysis. Modifications of nuclear DNA and its nuclear environment (i.e., chromatin) may be a significant factor in the expression of cardiovascular diseases. Epigenetic alterations in chromatin (e.g., histone acetylation) have been directly implicated in the modulation of myocardial gene expression in the progression of cardiac disorders, including cardiac hypertrophy, and can play a contributory role in modulating the heart's responses to physiological insult [4–5]. Another key epigenetic mechanism involves the methylation of cytosine residues in DNA that has been implicated in genomic imprinting, gene inactivation or silencing, and changes in chromatin structure and genome stability [6]. It is well established that a major mechanism for gene expression down-regulation involves the methylation of a cytosine-

and guanosine-rich area termed the *CpG island*, often located within the promoter region of genes [7]. While there has been limited systematic study addressing the relationship of DNA methylation to the expression of cardiac genes, either during myocardial development, normal physiological transition, or during cardiac disease, a number of pivotal cardiac genes whose aberrant function can result in cardiac disorders contain CpG islands and can be regulated by methylation [8]. The stability and expression of the cardiac troponin gene associated with cardiac contractility function (and with HCM phenotype) is affected by cytosine methylation [9]. Recently, it was demonstrated that the expression of the KVLQT1 gene involved in cardiac membrane transport genes can be modulated by targeted DNA methylation [10]. Notably, defects in this gene have been definitively implicated in the etiology of long QT syndrome, cardiac arrhythmias, and sudden cardiac death [11]. Moreover, the mtTFA gene associated with mitochondrial biogenesis is also regulated by DNA methylation [12]. The promoter of human mtTFA contains 67 CpG dinucleotides localized at its NRF-1 binding site. *In vitro* methylation of the NRF-1 site by *Hha*I methylase abolished the mtTFA promoter activity up to 90%, implying that the CpG methylation of NRF-1 site inactivates mtTFA promoter-driven transcriptional activity. The role of DNA methylation in mitochondrial-based diseases awaits to be investigated.

High levels of homocysteine, an important risk factor associated with CVD, have been correlated with decreased levels of DNA methylation (or increased hypomethylation) [13]. DNA hypomethylation, associated with elevated levels of hyperacetylated and decondensed chromatin due to decreased binding of methyl-sensitive proteins (e.g., methyl CpG binding protein and histone deacetylase) may allow specific regions of DNA to be more highly susceptible to oxidative damage and DNA strand breakage. Increased homocysteine-mediated DNA hypomethylation and associated alterations in gene expression and chromatin structure may prove informative in understanding the pathogenesis of diseases related to homocysteinemia including CVD.

There is evidence that the genetic background in which deleterious mutations occur can significantly modulate their phenotypic expression. The presence of modifier genes in the genetic background that influence the phenotypic expression and severity of pathogenic HCM genes has been well established [14]. A number of maternally inherited disorders with variable penetrance, often restricted to single tissue expression, including LHON, mitochondrial nonsyndromic sensori-neural hearing loss, and a form of mitochondrial HCM, have been proposed to be caused by a primary homoplasmic mtDNA pathogenic mutation acting in concert with a nuclear modifier, which can be a common functional polymorphism in a tissue-specific protein, possibly with mitochondrial location [15]. In this disease model, the mtDNA mutation is necessary but not sufficient to induce the pathology, whereas the nuclear modifier does not induce any pathology per se but contributes to the pathogenic effect of the mito-chondrial mutation.

The identification of modifier genes, which will markedly improve the elucidation of genetic risk factors, has been assisted by large-scale genome-wide approaches to identify polymorphic variants correlated with disease severity. A list of genes with polymorphic variants associated with cardiac and mitochondrial diseases is presented in Table 12.1.

A large variety of molecular techniques are presently available for the detection of single nucleotide polymorphisms (SNPs). SNPs association studies have identified several candidate modifier genes for various cardiac disorders [16]. A number of specific genetic polymorphisms have been reported in association with myocardial infarction, coronary artery disease, and HCM. With the increased cataloging of SNPs either alone or within a larger chromosomal region (haplotypes) in available shared databases, these modifier loci can be evaluated for their effects in predisposing to specific cardiac defects and may impact on the choice of diagnostic and treatment options (e.g., pharmacogenetics). The analysis of SNPs in mtDNA has also been recently reported in Parkinson's disease, nonsyndromic hearing impairment, and LHON [17–19], but SNPS in mtDNA have not yet been assessed in association with cardiac disease.

Understanding cardiovascular disease at the genomic level may e-ventually allow for the more effective stratification of patient subclasses, opening the door to a highly targeted and optimized patient-specific therapy. The related fields of pharmacogenomics and pharmacogenetics hold the promise of improved drug development and the tailoring of drug therapy based on the individual's ability to metabolize drugs that are determined only in part by age and influenced by disease, environmental factors (e.g., diet), concurrent

**Table 12.1. Polymorphic variants associated with cardiac and mitochondrial disease**

| Site Affected (loci) | Normal Function | Associated Phenotype |
|---|---|---|
| ATP-cassette binding protein (ABC or MDR) | Lipid transport | Coronary artery disease |
| Angiotensin converting enzyme (ACE) | Renin-angiotensin regulator | Coronary artery disease |
| Apolipoprotein E (APOE) | Lipid transport | Coronary artery disease |
| β-adrenergic receptor (ADRβ 1) | Neurohormone receptor | Cardiac arrhythmia; acute myocardial infarction |
| Cholesterol ester transport protein (CETP) | Lipid transport | Coronary artery disease |
| MinK related protein (KCNE2 /MiRP1) | Potassium channel | Antibiotic-induced cardiac arrhythmia |
| Endothelin receptor A (ETA) | Vasoregulator | Idiopathic DCM |
| Plasminogen-activator inhibitor type 1 (PAI-1) | Intravascular fibrinolysis | Myocardial infarction |
| Stromelysin-1 (MMP-3) | Matrix metalloproteinase | Myocardial infarction; angina |
| *mtDNA* | | |
| T16189C in D-loop | Not known | DCM |
| tRNA$^{Leu(CUN)}$ | Protein synthesis | Cardiac conduction defects |

medications, and variable genetic factors specifying the transport, metabolism, and targets of the drug [20]. A subset of the SNPs identified in human genes (e.g., β-adrenergic receptor and angiotensin-converting enzyme) have been associated with substantial changes in the metabolism or effects of medications used in treating cardiac disease and may be informative in predicting the clinical response. Individualizing therapy may be particularly critical in establishing drug dosages and efficacy in children with cardiovascular disease, a population for which pharmacokinetics has proven to be particularly poorly defined and often unpredictable. Therefore, both immuno-logical and genetic phenotyping of patients may provide a more ef-fective therapeutic strategy, either by inhibiting or stimulating specific responses.

By utilizing a genome-wide analysis of cardiovascular disorders, a larger net can be cast for detecting associated disease-related mutations. Recent methodological advances have made it possible to simultaneously assess the entire profile of expressed genes in affected myocardium, requiring only a very limited amount of tissue usually collected by endomyocardial biopsy. Gene expression profiling, to comprehensively evaluate which genes are increased and which are decreased in expression, can be achieved by several methods, including DNA microarrays (DNA chips), serial analysis of gene expression (SAGE), differential display, and subtractive hybridization. Despite cautions regarding its use, rigorously performed DNA microarray analysis has been a highly informative tool in establishing the pathophysiological features of disease states such as myocardial hypertrophy [21], myocardial infarct [22], DCM [23], and HF [24–26]. Gene expression profiling (also termed *transcriptome analysis*) has also been examined in preconditioning models [27] in studies of early cardiac morphogenesis and development [28], and has been applied both in clinical diagnosis and in the evaluation of patients' response to therapy [29–30]. Recognition of the limitations inherent in transcriptome analysis (e.g., gene regulation occurs at levels other than transcription, and that altered transcription is not always related to phenotype changes or to altered protein synthesis) underscores the need for other complementary approaches (e.g., proteomic analysis) to gain a more complete understanding of complex cardiac disorders.

The association of defective genes with cardiac disorders uncovered by genomic analysis can be followed by proteomic analysis to establish the function and pathophysiological role played by the mutant protein and also to reveal interacting modulators. There are approximately 1,000 to 2,000 proteins constituting the human mitochondrial proteome [31]. Given the high hydrophobicity of many of its peptides, proteomic analysis of mitochondria is particularly challenging as is distinguishing mitochondrial proteins from closely related cytosolic isoforms and from contaminants present in the mitochondrial preparations.

As previously noted, most of the proteins imported into the mitochondrial organelle contain characteristic targeting sequences usually localized at the N-terminus. The alternative subcellular targeting of mitochondrial proteins can be accomplished by a variety of regulatory mechanisms to achieve differential expression of specific targeting signals of the protein isoforms, including variable transcription (using different initiation sites), mRNA splicing, and translational and post-translational modifications. In a recent survey of 31 proteins that localize to both mitochondria and other cytosolic compartments, the majority of proteins examined appear to employ a combination of regulatory mechanisms [32].

Recently, proteomic analysis of human cardiac mitochondria was carried out using sucrose-gradient centrifugation of detergent-solubi-lized mitochondria followed by 1-dimensional PAGE. Subsequent detection by mass spectrometry, tryptic peptide finger-printing, and rigorous bioinformatic analysis yielded a total of 615 distinct protein identifications, of which 20% had unknown biochemical function [33]. The human heart proteome has also been characterized using multidimensional liquid chromatography coupled with tandem mass spectrometry [34]. Other researchers have used 2-dimensional PAGE analysis of the mitochondrial proteome; however, this approach provides a limited analysis of very hydrophobic proteins due to their precipitation during first-dimension isoelectric focusing, the frequent underassessment of mitochondrial peptides with lower molecular mass, as well as the loss of functional analysis. An alternative method employs blue-native (BN) electrophoresis in the first-dimension, in which proteins are maintained in their native state and can be assessed for function, followed by denaturing SDS-PAGE coupled to tryptic peptide fingerprinting, using matrix-assisted laser desorption/ ioni-zation-time of flight mass spectrometry [35]. These techniques have also been recently adapted for the identification of a subset of mito-chondrial proteins containing posttranslational modifications (e.g., phosphorylation and thiol-reactive oxidation) [36]. Changes in the cardiac mitochondrial proteome have also recently been examined in response to oxidative stress [37] and in hearts deficient in creatine kinase [38]. A recent combined analysis of the mitochondrial pro-teome and RNA expression has also proved informative in gene identification and mitochondrial biogenesis [39].

There is also increasing interest in establishing WEB accessible resources for sharing the enormous volume of data emerging from mitochondrial proteomic studies as well as in the generation of reference and data standards, to ensure data reproducibility and validity and to assist in data interpretation [40]. These databases include a large range of relevant information about the source of the proteins, including organism, tissue, disease/physiological state, age, gender, genetic variation (transgenic or knockout), and cell type.

Once the implicated genes and their gene products have been fully identified, sequence and subsequent bioinformatic analysis can be employed to identify common structural and functional motifs and homologies with known proteins. Again, the availability of accessible searchable resources for data comparison has greatly contributed to the task of assigning function to proteins. Functional protein-protein interactions can also be further determined by the use of yeast 2-hybrid analysis. Thus far, this type of analysis has been advantageously used to delineate critical interactions between Bax and ANT proteins in the mitochondrial apoptosis pathway [41], interaction of membrane proteins (TIM50, TIM23) in the mitochondrial protein import mechanism [42], identification of mitochondrial protein kinase A anchoring proteins [43], and mitochondrial signal transducer interaction [44]. Two-hybrid analysis has also been useful in understanding the synergistic interactions of transcription factors NKX2.5 and TBX5 in early cardiac development [45]. Information derived from proteomic and functional analyses (e.g., protein-protein interaction) can be incorporated into a rational design of drugs to treat myocardium damaged by mitochondrial oxidative stress and congenital heart defects [46].

## Animal models of mitochondrial-based heart disease

One of the most exciting and successful tools to evaluate specific gene dysfunction and mitochondrial-based heart disease has been transgenic animals. The availability of animal models with mitochondrial-based cardiac disease has been extremely useful in highlighting the multiple pathways that (if perturbed) can lead to dysfunction in the human heart and in the identification of potential targets for future drug and gene therapies and can also serve as a critical substrate for directly testing novel treatment strategies [47–48]. As has been noted at several points throughout this book, null mutations in a number of nuclear-encoded genes involved in mitochondrial metabolic function can lead to cardiac dysfunction in transgenic mice (listed in Table 12.2). Unfortunately, null mutations that are easily generated in mice have not yet been generated in other rodents and animal species (e.g., rat, dog and pig). However, data from studies from a variety of organisms utilizing overexpression of specific genes have proved informative in delineating genes and pathways mediating regulation of cardiac function and onset of CVD.

**Table 12.2. Transgenic models of mitochondrial-based CVD**

| Gene Loci | Cardiac Phenotype | Ref |
|---|---|---|
| **Nuclear gene knockouts** | | |
| Adenine nucleolide translocator (ANT1) | Cardiomyopathy and defective coupled respiration | [49] |
| Mn superoxide dismutase (SOD2) | DCM and SOD deficiency | [50] |
| Heart-specific mtTFA | DCM and conduction defects; mtDNA depletion, ETC defects | [51] |
| Frataxin | HCM; ETC defect; Fe-S deposits | [52] |
| Long-chain acyl-CoA dehydrogenase (LCAD) | Cardiomyopathy and sudden death; impaired FAO | [53] |
| Mitochondrial trifunctional protein alpha subunit (MTPα) | Cardiac necrosis and sudden death; lipid accumulation with impaired FAO | [54] |
| Very long-chain acyl-CoA dehydrogenase (VLCAD) | Increased ventricular tachycardia; lipid and mitochondrial accumulation | [55] |
| RXR α | Embryonic HF with defects in ETC, and ATP levels; increased mitochondrial number | [56] |
| MEF2A | DCM and sudden death; severe mitochondrial disorganization and dysfunction | [57] |
| **Mitochondrial DNA** | | |
| Chloramphenicol resistance (CAP$^R$) | DCM and perinatal death | [58] |
| 4.7 kb deletion | Cardiomyopathy and ETC defects | [59] |

Recent studies have begun to achieve the introduction and replacement of mtDNA in animal models. Recent successes with the allotopic strategy, described in Chapter 11, in which normal mitochondrial protein is expressed by nuclear-genetic engineering, have enabled the correction of specific mitochondrial genetic and enzymatic deficiencies [60–61]. However, there are limitations in the repertoire of mitochondrial genes that can be functionally replaced in mammalian cells by allotopic expression [62].

Given the systemic nature of many mtDNA defects, a major obstacle remains in how to deliver an effective agent (e.g., functional gene or gene product) throughout the cells of a living organism for repair/therapy [63]. Strategies to address this problem include the transplant of healthy mitochondria into the germ line. This can be achieved by transfer of a nucleus from a fertilized oocyte to a healthy donor cytoplast. Several techniques have been used to successfully introduce genetically distinct mtDNA molecules into the mouse female germ line. Heteroplasmic mice have been created by the fusion of cytoplasts generated from mouse ova with single zygotes [64] by fusion of a zygote nucleus and a portion of the oocyte cytoplasm with enucleated eggs [65], and by the microinjection of somatic cell mitochondria from one species of mice into zygotes of another species generating xenocybrids [66]. The fusion of cytoplasts heteroplasmic for a 4,696-bp mtDNA deletion to pronucleus-stage zygotes has also been used to generate the first mouse model of mtDNA disease [59], including the development of cardiomyopathy. The fusion of cytoplasts to undifferentiated mouse female embryonic stem (ES) cells has also been used to introduce a well-characterized mouse mtDNA mutation, the mouse 16S rRNA mutation resulting in chloramphenicol resistance (CAP$^R$) into the mouse female germ line [58, 67]. Mice homoplasmic for the CAP$^R$ mutation exhibited myopathy, DCM, and perinatal or *in utero* lethality, validating the ES cell approach to produce transmitochondrial mice. More recently, the strategy of xenocybrid transfer of mitochondria by cytoplast fusion, combined with the use of mtDNA-depleted ES cells, enabled the generation of transmitochondrial mice with germ-line transmission of homoplasmic mitochondria containing the introduced alleles [68].

The use of transmitochondrial oocytes in human studies has a limited but controversial history. Ooplasmic transplantation has been reported in several studies in conjunction with *in vitro* fertilization clinics [69–70]. In these studies, the addition of a small amount of injected ooplasm, derived from fertile donor oocytes, into developmentally compromised oocytes from patients with recurrent preimplantation failure was reported to enhance embryo viability and led to the birth of 15 children. The mtDNA from the donor as well as the recipient cell mtDNA were found to be present in blood of the child emerging from the transplanted oocyte at 1 year of age. Excluding the numerous ethical considerations provoked by this first case of human germ-line genetic modification, several cautions have been raised by these studies, including the potential for long-term harm in chromosomal segregation and aberrant division, predicted by similar studies conducted in lower organisms, and epigenetic influences of foreign cytoplasm demonstrated in numerous studies of cytoplasmic transfer in mice [71]. In fact, 2 of the 15 pregnancies resulted in unexpected chromosomal abnormalities, including Turner syndrome. The long-term deleterious influence of heteroplasmic mtDNA has also been considered as a potential problem in this technique [72]. If we are to fully appreciate the outcomes associated with embryo manipulation, then extensive investigations with animal models that incorporate genetic, biochemical, and physiological analyses are mandated, accompanied by clinical monitoring, to demonstrate the suitability of these techniques for human use.

In patients with mitochondrial disease due to specific mtDNA defects, recommendations have been formulated regarding the use of prenatal diagnosis, including preimplantation diagnosis and chorionic villus sampling [73]. Prenatal diagnosis of defects such as Mendelian defects and syndromes caused by mutations at nt 8993 appear to be more reliable than with other maternally inherited defects, in which there is little correlation between phenotype and the amount of mutant allele (mutant load).

## Cellular engineering

Recently, there has been intense interest in the use of cell transplantation to treat myocardial damage via cardiac transplantation and cell repair. This represents a daunting challenge, since it has been estimated that millions of cardiac cells would be required to repopulate and repair a single damaged human heart.

One promising new therapeutic technique for the augmentation and regeneration of myocardium is the use of cellular cardiomyoplasty, involving transplantation of autologous skeletal myoblasts into injured myocardium. Reports from both animal and clinical investigations indicate that skeletal myoblasts grafted into infarcted myocardium survive, can generate new myocytes and improve myocardial performance [74–75]. However, studies have also shown that electromechanical coupling between grafted myogenic cells and host cells is lacking with this approach [76].

Another approach involves the introduction of undifferentiated adult stem cells of hematopoietic origin that also can successfully engraft in damaged myocardium and improve cardiac performance. This has been shown with purified mesenchymal and bone marrow cells [77–82]. A number of these studies have reported that some degree of cardiomyogenic differentiation and developmental plasticity, involving the transplanted stem cells, is present at the sites of damage, although the mechanism for the phenotypic improvement resulting from transplant of these extracardiac stem cells (whether involving transdetermination or cell fusion events) remains highly controversial [83–84]. Studies are underway to investigate and enhance the efficiency of the transplanted cell's homing to the site of injury and the differentiation process they undergo as well as to gauge the overall stability and functioning of the transplanted cells in the myocardial environment. Long-term studies of cardiac repair with transplanted hematopoietic cells have revealed that the newly formed myocytes do not fully acquire adult cardiomyocyte characteristics (e.g., size) and are subject to increased apoptosis over time, leading to concerns with their long-term efficacy in cardiac repair [84].

Stem-cell-derived cardiomyocytes can be obtained from embryonic stem (ES) cells derived from the inner cell mass of the embryonic blastocyst. These cells can still divide and can be expanded in culture and differentiate into different cardiac muscle cells (i.e., atrial, ventricular, and pacemaker) [85]. After transplantation into damaged myocardium in mice, they formed stable grafts and survived for at least 7 weeks. The selection of ES cells has to be performed with care to prevent teratoma formation, which can originate from single undifferentiated cells attached to the transferred cells. Moreover, their transfer is allogenic, making immunosuppression necessary. Also, ES cells can act as an unanticipated arrhythmogenic source after intramyocardial transplantation [86]. While the use of ES cells has also shown encouraging preliminarily results in mediating myocardial injury repair [87–88], there are significant ethical, legal, and distribution issues with their use that will have to be surmounted. The promising developmental plasticity of adult stem cells revealed by numerous studies may allow circumvention of the ethical and availability issues associated with the ES cell approach. Recently, a subpopulation of adult cardiac cells with stem-cell-like properties has been identified, recruited, and transplanted to a site of myocardial ischemic injury and shown to fully reconstitute well-differentiated myocardium, differentiating into both cardiomyocytes and new blood vessels [89–90].

A brief comparison of the advantages and limitations of the cell types presently used in cardiac transplantation is shown in Table 12.3. While no clear-cut choice has yet emerged as to the cell type to transplant in myocardial repair, there is reason to think that this will be a fruitful area of research, that may result in exciting therapies in the years to come.

## Applications of stem cells in treating mitochondrial defects and toxicology

Presently, information concerning mitochondrial structure and function in ES cells is limited, and the use of ES cell therapy has not been applied to treating cardiac diseases with extensive mitochondrial enzyme or DNA (in particular, mtDNA) abnormalities or for the testing of mitochondrial-based cardiotoxicity.

As we have previously noted, a subset of cardiac disorders, with a pronounced mitochondrial-based cytopathy and bioenergetic dysfunction, has a genetic basis due to either defects in mtDNA or nuclear DNA [2]. Recently, it has been proposed to introduce mtDNA-repaired ES cells into a patient harboring a pathogenic mtDNA mutation, thereby potentially transforming a diseased myocardium into a healthy one [91]. The mtDNA-repaired cell can be derived from the patient's own cells, whose endogenous defective mtDNA genome has been entirely eliminated by treatment with ethidium bromide and replaced by entirely wild-type mtDNA genes. In a similar vein, treatment of a patient's nuclear DNA defects would involve either specific genetic replacement (site-specific homologous recombination can be readily undertaken in ES cells), or if the precise site of the nuclear defect is not known, by replacing the entire nucleus of the patient with a wild-type nucleus. In the near future, ES cell therapy may be used in treating mitochondrial-based cardiac diseases.

**Table 12.3. Advantages and limitations of specific cell types in cell transplantation for the treatment of CVD**

| Cell Type | Advantages | Limitations |
|---|---|---|
| Skeletal myoblast | 1. Cells proliferate *in vitro* (allowing for autologous transplant)<br>2. Ischemia-resistant<br>3. Transplanted myoblasts can differentiate into slow-twitch myocytes enabling cellular cardiomyoplasty.<br>4. Reduces progressive ventricular dilatation | 1. Likely do not develop new cardiomyocytes *in vivo*<br>2. Electrical coupling to surrounding myocardial cells is poor<br>3. Long-term stability of differentiated phenotype is unknown. |
| Adult stem cells: Mesenchymal/ bone marrow | 1. Pluripotent stem cells can develop into cardiomyocytes.<br>2. Stem cells are easy to isolate and grow well in culture.<br>3. Neovascularization can also occur at site of myocardial scar, which may diminish ischemia.<br>4. Can improve myocardial contractile function<br>5. Autologous transplantation possible requiring no immune-suppression treatment | 1. New program of cell-differentiation is required.<br>2. Efficiency of differentiation into adult cardiomyocytes appears limited. |
| Cardiac stem cells | 1. Recognition of myocardial growth factors and recruitment to myocardium are likely faster and more efficient than other cell types<br>2. *In vivo* electrical coupling of transplanted cells to existing myocardium | 1. Poor cell growth *in vitro*<br>2. Transplanted cells are very sensitive to ischemic insult and apoptotic cell death. |
| Embryonic stem cells | 1. Easy propagation and well-defined cardiomyocyte differentiation process<br>2. Pluripotent | 1. Potential for tumor formation and immune rejection<br>2. Arrhythmogenic potential<br>3. Incomplete response to physiological stimuli<br>4. Difficult to isolate<br>5. Ethical objections |

Pharmacological testing and appraisal of drugs with potential cardiotoxicity can be carried out using stem cells [92–94]]. As an alternative to *in vivo* studies, a test utilizing differentiation of ES cell into cardiomyocytes (to test chemical toxicity *in vitro*) has been developed. Retinoic acid was strongly embryotoxic inhibiting cardiac cell differentiation at very low concentrations (several orders of magnitude), compared to the levels needed to exert cytotoxic effects on the viability of the ES cells [94].

# References

1.   Maron BJ, Moller JH, Seidman CE, Vincent GM, Dietz HC, Moss AJ, Sondheimer HM, Pyeritz RE, McGee G, Epstein AE (1998) Impact of laboratory molecular diagnosis on contemporary diagnostic criteria for genetically transmitted cardiovascular diseases: hypertrophic cardiomyopathy, long-QT syndrome, and Marfan syndrome. Circulation 98:1460–71

2.   Marín-García J, Goldenthal MJ (2002) Understanding the impact of mitochondrial defects in cardiovascular disease: A review. J Card Fail 8:347–61

3.   van Den Bosch BJ, de Coo RF, Scholte HR, Nijland JG, van Den Bogaard R, de Visser M, de Die-Smulders CE, Smeets HJ (2000) Mutation analysis of the entire mitochondrial genome using denaturing high performance liquid chromatography. Nucleic Acids Res 28:E89

4.   Zhang CL, McKinsey TA, Chang S, Antos CL, Hill JA, Olson EN (2002) Class II histone deacetylases act as signal-responsive repressors of cardiac hypertrophy. Cell 110:479–88

5.   Hamamori Y, Schneider MD (2003) HATs off to Hop: Recruitment of a class I histone deacetylase incriminates a novel transcriptional pathway that opposes cardiac hypertrophy. J Clin Invest 112:824–6

6.   Ferguson-Smith AC, Sasaki H, Cattanach BM, Surani MA (1993) Parental-origin-specific epigenetic modification of the mouse H19 gene. Nature 362:751–5

7.   Bird AP (1986) CpG rich islands and the function of DNA methylation. Nature 321:209–13

8. D'Cruz LG, Baboonian C, Phillimore HE, Taylor R, Elliott PM, Varnava A, Davison F, McKenna WJ, Carter ND (2000) Cytosine methylation confers instability on the cardiac troponin T gene in hypertrophic cardiomyopathy. J Med Genet 37:E18

9. Cerrato F, Vernucci M, Pedone PV, Chiariotti L, Sebastio G, Bruni CB, Riccio A (2002) The 5' end of the KCNQ1OT1 gene is hypomethylated in the Beckwith-Wiedemann syndrome. Hum Genet 111: 105–7

10. Smilinich NJ, Day CD, Fitzpatrick GV, Caldwell GM, Lossie AC, Cooper PR, Smallwood AC, Joyce JA, Schofield PN, Reik W, Nicholls RD, Weksberg R, Driscoll DJ, Maher ER, Shows TB, Higgins MJ (1999) A maternally methylated CpG island in KvLQT1 is associated with an antisense paternal transcript and loss of imprinting in Beckwith-Wiedemann syndrome. Proc Natl Acad Sci USA 196:8064-9

11. Splawski I, Shen J, Timothy KW, Lehmann MH, Prori S, Robinson JL, Moss AJ, Schwartz PJ, Towbin JA, Vincent GM, Keating MT (2000) Spectrum of mutations in long-QT syndrome genes: KVLQT1, HERG, SCN5A, KCNE1, and KCNE2. Circulation 102:1178–85

12. Choi YS, Kim S, Pak YK (2001) Mitochondrial transcription factor A (mtTFA) and diabetes. Diabetes Res Clin Pract 54:S3–9

13. James SJ, Melnyk S, Pogribna M, Pogribny IP, Caudill MA (2002) Elevation in S-adenosylhomocysteine and DNA hypomethylation: Potential epigenetic mechanism for homocysteine-related pathology. J Nutr 132:2361S–6S

14. Marian AJ (2002) Modifier genes for hypertrophic cardiomyopathy. Curr Opin Cardiol 17:242–52

15. Carelli V, Giordano C, d'Amati G (2003) Pathogenic expression of homoplasmic mtDNA mutations needs a complex nuclear-mitochondrial interaction. Trends Genet 19:257–62

16. Daley GQ, Cargill M (2001) The heart SNPs a beat: Polymorphisms in candidate genes for cardiovascular disease. Trends Cardiovasc Med 11:60–6

17. Sudoyo H, Suryadi H, Lertrit P, Pramoonjago P, Lyrawati D, Marzuki S (2002) Asian-specific mtDNA backgrounds associated with the primary G11778A mutation of Leber's hereditary optic neuropathy. J Hum Genet 47:594–604

18. Jacobs HT, Hutchin TP, Kappi T, Gillies G, Minkkinen K, Walker J, Thompson K, Rovio AT, Carella M, Melchionda S, Zelante L, Gasparini P, Pyykko I I, Shah ZH, Zeviani M, Mueller RF (2005)

Mitochondrial DNA mutations in patients with postlingual, nonsyndromic hearing impairment. Eur J Hum Genet 13:26–33

19.   van der Walt JM, Nicodemus KK, Martin ER, Scott WK, Nance MA, Watts RL, Hubble JP, Haines JL, Koller WC, Lyons K, Pahwa R, Stern MB, Colcher A, Hiner BC, Jankovic J, Ondo WG, Allen FH Jr, Goetz CG, Small GW, Mastaglia F, Stajich JM, McLaurin AC, Middleton LT, Scott BL, Schmechel DE, Pericak-Vance MA, Vance JM (2003) Mitochondrial polymorphisms significantly reduce the risk of Parkinson disease. Am J Hum Genet 72:804–11

19.   Roden DM (2003) Cardiovascular pharmacogenomics. Circulation 108:3071–4

21.   Hwang DM, Dempsey AA, Lee CY, Liew CC (2000) Identification of differentially expressed genes in cardiac hypertrophy by analysis of expressed sequence tags. Genomics 66:1–14

22.   Stanton LW, Garrard LJ, Damm D, Garrick BL, Lam A, Kapoun AM, Zheng Q, Protter AA, Schreiner GF, White RT (2000) Altered patterns of gene expression in response to myocardial infarction. Circ Res 86:939–45

23.   Barrans JD, Allen PD, Stamatiou D, Dzau VJ, Liew CC (2002) Global gene expression profiling of end-stage dilated cardiomyopathy using a human cardiovascular-based cDNA microarray. Am J Pathol 160:2035–43

24.   Ueno S, Ohki R, Hashimoto T, Takizawa T, Takeuchi K, Yamashita Y, Ota J, Choi YL, Wada T, Koinuma K, Yamamoto K, Ikeda U, Shimada K, Mano H (2003) DNA microarray analysis of *in vivo* progression mechanism of heart failure. Biochem Biophys Res Commun 307:771–7

25.   Hwang JJ, Allen PD, Tseng GC, Lam CW, Fananapazir L, Dzau VJ, Liew CC (2002) Microarray gene expression profiles in dilated and hypertrophic cardiomyopathic end-stage heart failure. Physiol Genomics 10:31–44

26.   Barrans JD, Stamatiou D, Liew C (2001) Construction of a human cardiovascular cDNA microarray: Portrait of the failing heart. Biochem Biophys Res Commun 280:964–9

27.   Sergeev P, da Silva R, Lucchinetti E, Zaugg K, Pasch T, Schaub MC, Zaugg M (2004) Trigger-dependent gene expression profiles in cardiac preconditioning: Evidence for distinct genetic programs in ischemic and anesthetic preconditioning. Anesthesiology 100:474–88

28.   Masino AM, Gallardo TD, Wilcox CA, Olson EN, Williams RS, Garry DJ (2004) Transcriptional regulation of cardiac progenitor cell populations. Circ Res 95:389–97

29.   Konstantinov IE, Coles JG, Boscarino C, Takahashi M, Gonvalves J, Ritter J, Van Arsdell GS (2004) Gene expression profiles in children undergoing cardiac surgery for right heart obstructive lesions. J Thorac Cardiovasc Surg 127:746–54

30.   Blaxall BC, Tschannen-Moran BM, Milano CA, Koch  WJ (2003) Differential gene expression and genomic patient stratification following left ventricular assist device support.  J Am Coll Cardiol 41:1096–106

31.   Lopez MF, Melov S (2002) Applied proteomics: Mitochondrial proteins and effect on function. Circ Res 90:380–9

32. Mueller JC, Andreoli C, Prokisch H, Meitinger T (2004) Mechanisms for multiple intracellular localization of human mitochondrial proteins. Mitochondrion 3:315–26

33.   Taylor SW, Fahy E, Zhang B, Glenn GM, Warnock DE, Wiley S, Murphy AN, Gaucher SP, Capaldi RA, Gibson BW, Ghosh SS (2003) Characterization of the human heart mitochondrial proteome. Nat Biotechnol 21:281–6

34.   Gaucher SP, Taylor SW, Fahy E, Zhang B, Warnock DE, Ghosh SS, Gibson BW (2004) Expanded coverage of the human heart mitochondrial proteome using multi-dimensional liquid chromatography coupled with tandem mass spectrometry. J Proteome Res 3:495–505

35.   Brookes PS, Pinner A, Ramachandran A, Coward L, Barnes S, Kim H, Darley-Usmar VM (2002) High throughput two-dimensional blue-native electrophoresis: A tool for functional proteomics of mitochondria and signaling complexes. Proteomics 2:969–77

36.   Schulenberg B, Aggeler R, Beechem JM, Capaldi RA, Patton WF (2003) Analysis of steady-state protein phosphorylation in mitochondria using a novel fluorescent phosphosensor dye. J Biol Chem 278:27251–5

37.   Taylor SW, Fahy E, Murray J, Capaldi RA, Ghosh SS (2003) Oxidative post-translational modification of tryptophan residues in cardiac mitochondrial proteins. J Biol Chem 278:19587–90

38.   Kernec F, Unlu M, Labeikovsky W, Minden JS, Koretsky AP (2001) Changes in the mitochondrial proteome from mouse hearts deficient in creatine kinase. Physiol Genomics 6:117–28

39.   Mootha VK, Bunkenborg J, Olsen JV, Hjerrild M, Wisniewski JR, Stahl E, Bolouri MS, Ray HN, Sihag S, Kamal M, Patterson N, Lander ES, Mann M (2003) Integrated analysis of protein composition, tissue diversity, and gene regulation in mouse mitochondria. Cell 115:629–40

40.   Ravichandran V, Vasquez GB, Srivatava S, Verma M, Petricoin E, Lubell J, Sriram RD, Barker PE, Gilliland GL (2004) Data standards for proteomics: Mitochondrial two-dimensional polyacrylamide gel electrophoresis data as a model system.  Mitochondrion 3:327–36

41.   Marzo I, Brenner C, Zamzami N, Jurgensmeier JM, Susin SA, Vieira HL, Prevost MC, Xie Z, Matsuyama S, Reed JC, Kroemer G (1998) Bax and adenine nucleotide translocator cooperate in the mitochondrial control of apoptosis. Science 281:2027–31

42.   Guo Y, Cheong N, Zhang Z, De Rose R, Deng Y, Farber SA, Fernandes-Alnemri T, Alnemri ES (2004) Tim50, a component of the mitochondrial translocator, regulates mitochondrial integrity and cell death. J Biol Chem 279:24813–25

43.   Wang L, Sunahara RK, Krumins A, Perkins G, Crochiere ML, Mackey M, Bell S, Ellisman MH, Taylor SS (2001) Cloning and mitochondrial localization of full-length D-AKAP2, a protein kinase A anchoring protein. Proc Natl Acad Sci USA 98:3220–5

44.   Lufei C, Ma J, Huang G, Zhang T, Novotny-Diermayr V, Ong CT, Cao X (2003) GRIM-19, a death-regulatory gene product, suppresses Stat3 activity via functional interaction. EMBO J 22: 1325–35

45.   Hiroi Y, Kudoh S, Monzen K, Ikeda Y, Yazaki Y, Nagai R, Komuro (2001) Tbx5 associates with Nkx2-5 and synergistically promotes cardiomyocyte differentiation. Nat Genet 28:276–80

46.   Gibson BW (2004) Exploiting proteomics in the discovery of drugs that target mitochondrial oxidative damage. Sci Aging Knowledge Environ 2004:pe12

47.   Larsson NG, Rustin P (2001) Animal models for respiratory chain disease. Trends Mol Med 7:578–81

48.   Schuler AM, Wood PA (2002) Mouse models for disorders of mitochondrial fatty acid beta-oxidation. ILAR J 43:57–65

49.   Graham BH, Waymire KG, Cottrell B, Trounce IA, MacGregor GR, Wallace DC (1997) A mouse model for mitochondrial myopathy and cardiomyopathy resulting from a deficiency in the heart/muscle isoform of the adenine nucleotide translocator. Nat Genet 16:226–34

50.   Lebovitz RM, Zhang H, Vogel H, Cartwright J Jr, Dionne L, Lu N, Huang S, Matzuk MM (1996) Neurodegeneration, myocardial injury, and perinatal death in mitochondrial superoxide dismutase-deficient mice. Proc Natl Acad Sci USA 93:9782–7

51.   Wang J, Wilhelmsson H, Graff C, Li H, Oldfors A, Rustin P, Bruning JC, Kahn CR, Clayton DA, Barsh GS, Thoren P, Larsson NG (1999) Dilated cardiomyopathy and atrioventricular conduction blocks induced by heart-specific inactivation of mitochondrial DNA gene expression. Nat Genet 21:133–7

52.   Puccio H, Simon D, Cossee M, Criqui-Filipe P, Tiziano F, Melki J, Hindelang C, Matyas R, Rustin P, Koenig M (2001) Mouse models for Friedreich ataxia exhibit cardiomyopathy, sensory nerve defect and Fe-S enzyme deficiency followed by intramitochondrial iron deposits. Nat Genet 27:181–6

53.   Kurtz DM, Rinaldo P, Rhead WJ, Tian L, Millington DS, Vockley J, Hamm DA, Brix AE, Lindsey JR, Pinkert CA, O'Brien WE, Wood PA (1998) Targeted disruption of mouse long-chain acyl-CoA dehydrogenase gene reveals crucial roles for fatty acid oxidation. Proc Natl Acad Sci USA 95:15592–7

54.   Ibdah JA, Paul H, Zhao Y, Binford S, Salleng K, Cline M, Matern D, Bennett MJ, Rinaldo P, Strauss AW  (2001) Lack of mitochondrial trifunctional protein in mice causes neonatal hypoglycemia and sudden death. J Clin Invest 107:1403–9

55.   Exil VJ, Roberts RL, Sims H, McLaughlin JE, Malkin RA, Gardner CD, Ni G, Rottman JN, Strauss AW (2003) Very-long-chain acyl-coenzyme a dehydrogenase deficiency in mice. Circ Res 93: 448–55

56.   Ruiz-Lozano P, Smith SM, Perkins G, Kubalak SW, Boss GR, Sucov HM, Evans RM, Chien KR (1998) Energy deprivation and a deficiency in downstream metabolic target genes during the onset of embryonic heart failure in RXRalpha-/- embryos. Development 125: 533–44

57.   Naya FJ, Black BL, Wu H, Bassel-Duby R, Richardson JA, Hill JA, Olson EN (2002) Mitochondrial deficiency and cardiac sudden death in mice lacking the MEF2A transcription factor. Nat Med 8:1303–9

58.   Sligh JE, Levy SE, Waymire KG, Allard P, Dillehay DL, Nusinowitz S, Heckenlively JR, MacGregor GR, Wallace DC (2000) Maternal germ-line transmission of mutant mtDNAs from embryonic

stem cell-derived chimeric mice. Proc Natl Acad Sci USA 97:14461–6

59.   Inoue K, Nakada K, Ogura A, Isobe K, Goto Y, Nonaka I, Hayashi JI (2000) Generation of mice with mitochondrial dysfunction by introducing mouse mtDNA carrying a deletion into zygotes. Nat Genet 26:176–81

60.   Guy J, Qi X, Pallotti F, Schon EA, Manfredi G, Carelli V, Martinuzzi A, Hauswirth WW, Lewin AS (2002) Rescue of a mitochondrial deficiency causing Leber hereditary optic neuropathy. Ann Neurol 52:534–42

61.   Manfredi G, Fu J, Ojaimi J, Sadlock JE, Kwong JQ, Guy J, Schon EA (2002) Rescue of a deficiency in ATP synthesis by transfer of MTATP6, a mitochondrial DNA-encoded gene, to the nucleus. Nat Genet 30:394–9

62.   Oca-Cossio J, Kenyon L, Hao H, Moraes CT (2003) Limitations of allotopic expression of mitochondrial genes in mammalian cells. Genetics 165:707–20

63.   Chinnery PF (2004) New approaches to the treatment of mitochondrial disorders. Reprod Biomed Online 8:16–23

64.   Jenuth JP, Peterson AC, Shoubridge EA (1997) Tissue-specific selection for different mtDNA genotypes in heteroplasmic mice. Nat Genet 16:93–5

65.   Meirelles FV, Smith LC (1997) Mitochondrial genotype segregation in a mouse heteroplasmic lineage produced by embryonic karyoplast transplantation. Genetics 145:445–51

66.   Pinkert CA, Trounce IA (2002) Production of transmitochondrial mice. Methods 26:348–57

67.   Levy SE, Waymire KG, Kim YL, MacGregor GR, Wallace DC (1999) Transfer of chloramphenicol-resistant mitochondrial DNA into the chimeric mouse. Transgenic Res 8:137–45

68.   McKenzie M, Trounce IA, Cassar CA, Pinkert CA (2004) Production of homoplasmic xenomitochondrial mice. Proc Natl Acad Sci USA 101:1685–90

69.   Barritt JA, Brenner CA, Malter HE, Cohen J (2001) Mitochondria in human offspring derived from ooplasmic transplantation. Hum Reprod 16:513–6

70.   Malter HE, Cohen J (2002) Ooplasmic transfer: Animal models assist human studies. Reprod Biomed Online 5:26–35.

71. Hawes SM, Sapienza C, Latham KE (2002) Ooplasmic donation in humans: The potential for epigenic modifications. Hum Reprod 17: 850–2

72. St John JC (2002) Ooplasm donation in humans: The need to investigate the transmission of mitochondrial DNA following cytoplasmic transfer. Hum Reprod 17:1954–8

73. Poulton J, Marchington DR (2002) Segregation of mitochondrial DNA (mtDNA) in human oocytes and in animal models of mtDNA disease: Clinical implications. Reproduction 123:751–5

74. Menasche P (2004) Skeletal myoblast transplantation for cardiac repair. Expert Rev Cardiovasc Ther 2:21–8

75. Haider HKh, Tan AC, Aziz S, Chachques JC, Sim EK (2004) Myoblast transplantation for cardiac repair: A clinical perspective. Mol Ther 9:14–23

76. Leobon B, Garcin I, Menasche P, Vilquin JT, Audinat E, Charpak S (2003) Myoblasts transplanted into rat infarcted myocard ium are functionally isolated from their host. Proc Natl Acad Sci USA 100:7808–11

77. Pittenger MF, Martin BJ (2004) Mesenchymal stem cells and their potential as cardiac therapeutics. Circ Res 95:9–20

78. Laflamme MA, Myerson D, Saffitz JE, Murry CE (2002) Evidence for cardiomyocyte repopulation by extracardiac progenitors in transplanted human hearts. Circ Res 90:634–40

79. Wollert KC, Meyer GP, Lotz J, Ringes-Lichtenberg S, Lippolt P, Breidenbach C, Fichtner S, Korte T, Hornig B, Messinger D, Arseniev L, Hertenstein B, Ganser A, Drexler H (2004) Intracoronary autologous bone-marrow cell transfer after myocardial infarction: The BOOST randomised controlled clinical trial. Lancet 364:141–8

80. Xu W, Zhang X, Qian H, Zhu W, Sun X, Hu J, Zhou H, Chen Y (2004) Mesenchymal stem cells from adult human bone marrow differentiate into a cardiomyocyte phenotype in vitro. Exp Biol Med 229:623–31

81. Orlic D, Kajstura J, Chimenti S, Limana F, Jakoniuk I, Quaini F, Nadal-Ginard B, Bodine DM, Leri A, Anversa P (2001) Mobilized bone marrow cells repair infarcted heart, improving function and survival. Proc Natl Acad Sci USA 98:10344–9

82. Orlic D, Kajstura J, Chimenti S, Jakoniuk I, Anderson SM, Li B, Pickel J, McKay R, Nadal-Ginard B, Bodine DM, Leri A, Anversa P (2001) Bone marrow cells regenerate infarcted myocardium. Nature 410:701–5

83.   Murry CE, Soonpaa MH, Reinecke H, Nakajima H, Nakajima HO, Rubart M, Pasumarthi KB, Virag JI, Bartelmez SH, Poppa V, Bradford G, Dowell JD, Williams DA, Field LJ (2004) Haematopoietic stem cells do not transdifferentiate into cardiac myocytes in myocardial infarcts. Nature 428:664–8

84.   Anversa P, Sussman MA, Bolli R (2004) Molecular genetic advances in cardiovascular medicine: Focus on the myocyte. Circulation 109:2832–8

85.   Kehat I, Kenyagin-Karsenti D, Snir M, Segev H, Amit M, Gepstein A, Livne E, Binah O, Itskovitz-Eldor J, Gepstein L (2001) Human embryonic stem cells can differentiate into myocytes with structural and functional properties of cardiomyocytes. J Clin Invest 108:407–14

86.   Zhang YM, Hartzell C, Narlow M, Dudley SC Jr. (2002) Stem cell-derived cardiomyocytes demonstrate arrhythmic potential. Circulation 106:1294–9

87.   Hodgson DM, Behfar A, Zingman LV, Kane GC, Perez-Terzic C, Alekseev AE, Puceat M, Terzic A (2004) Stable benefit of embryonic stem cell therapy in myocardial infarction. Am J Physiol Heart Circ Physiol 287:H471–9

88.   Kehat I, Gepstein L (2003) Human embryonic stem cells for myocardial regeneration. Heart Fail Rev 8:229–36

89.   Oh H, Chi X, Bradfute SB, Mishina Y, Pocius J, Michael LH, Behringer RR, Schwartz RJ, Entman ML, Schneider MD (2004) Cardiac muscle plasticity in adult and embryo by heart-derived progenitor cells. Ann N Y Acad Sci 1015:182–9

90.   Beltrami AP, Barlucchi L, Torella D, Baker M, Limana F, Chimenti S, Kasahara H, Rota M, Musso E, Urbanek K, Leri A, Kajstura J, Nadal-Ginard B, Anversa P (2003) Adult cardiac stem cells are multipotent and support myocardial regeneration. Cell 114: 763–76

91.   Zullo, SJ (2001) Gene therapy of mitochondrial DNA mutations: A brief, biased history of allotopic expression in mammalian cells. Semin Neurol 21:327–35

92.   Bremer S, Worth AP, Paparella M, Bigot K, Kolossov E, Fleischmann BK, Hescheler J, Balls M (2001) Establishment of an *in vitro* reporter gene assay for developmental cardiac toxicity. Toxicol In Vitro 15:215–23

93.   Rohwedel J, Guan K, Hegert C, Wobus AM (2001) Embryonic stem cells as an *in vitro* model for mutagenicity, cytoxicity and

embryotoxicity studies: Present state and future prospects. Toxicol In Vitro 15:741–53.

94.   Scholz G, Pohl I, Genschow E, Klemm M, Spielmann H (1999) Embryotoxicity screening using embryonic stem cells in vitro: Correlation to *in vivo* teratogenicity. Cells Tissue Organs 165:203–11

# GLOSSARY

**AAV** Adeno-associated virus. A defective human parvovirus with potential as a vector for human gene therapy of cardiovascular disorders.

**acetyl -CoA** Small water-soluble molecule that carries acetyl groups linked to coenzyme A (CoA) by a thioester bond.

**ANT** Adenine nucleotide translocator. A mitochondrial inner membrane carrier protein of ADP and ATP and part of the PT pore.

**AIF** Apoptosis-inducing factor. Released from mitochondrial intermembrane space in early apoptosis and subsequently involved in nuclear DNA fragmentation.

**ADP** Adenosine diphosphate.

**allele** One of several alternate forms of a single gene occupying a given locus on a chromosome or mtDNA.

**allotopic expression** Alternative method of mitochondrial gene therapy in which a mitochondrial gene is reengineered for expression from the nucleus and targeting its translation product to the mitochondria.

**amphipathic** Molecule with distinct hydrophobic and hydrophilic domains (e.g., phospholipids and detergents).

**amplification** Generation of many copies of a specific region of DNA.

**antimycin A** Specific inhibitor of complex III activity.

**antisense RNA** RNA complementary to a specific transcript of a gene that can hybridize to the specific RNA and block its function.

**ASO** Antisense oligonucleotides. These short, synthetic DNA molecules can reduce specific gene expression by acting either directly or as decoys of transcription factors.

**APC** Anesthetic preconditioning.

**apoptosis** Programmed cell death.

**apoptosome** Cytosolic complex involved in the activation of apoptotic caspases.

**ATP** Adenosine triphosphate.

**atractyloside** Inhibitor of the adenine nucleotide translocator.

**AZT** Zidovudine. Used to treat AIDS. An inhibitor of DNA polymerase that can cause mtDNA depletion.

**BER** Base excision repair. DNA repair in which a missing or damaged base on a single strand is recognized, excised, and replaced in the duplex by synthesizing a sequence complementary to the remaining strand.

**bilayer** Arrangement of phospholipids in biological membranes.

**biolistic transformation** Method of introducing DNA into cells using highly accelerated DNA-coated metal particles.

**bp** Base pairs.

**BMDC** Bone-marrow-derived cells.

**CAP$^R$** Resistance to the antibiotic chloramphenicol.

**cardiolipin** Anionic phospholipid located primarily in the mitochondrial inner membrane.

**carnitine** Carrier molecule involved in the transport of long-chain fatty acids into the mitochondria for β-FAO.

**caspases** Intracellular cysteine proteases activated during apoptosis that cleave substrates at their aspartic acid residues.

**CCCP** Carbonyl cyanide m-chlorophenyl hydrazone. A potent uncoupler.

**cDNA** Complementary DNA. DNA fragment that is synthesized from the mRNA strand by reverse transcriptase. This DNA copy of a mature mRNA lacks the introns that are present in the genomic DNA.

**cDNA library** Collection of cDNAs synthesized from the mRNA of an organism cloned into a vector.

**cell fusion** Fusion of two somatic cells creating a hybrid cell.

**chaperone** Protein that assists in the proper folding and assembly into larger complexes of unfolded or misfolded proteins.

**chemiosmotic coupling** Mechanism in which a gradient of hydrogen ions (pH gradient) across a membrane is used to drive an energy-requiring process such as ATP production (e.g., oxidative phosphorylation).

**chromatin** The complex of DNA and histone and nonhistone proteins found in the nucleus of a eukaryotic cell that constitutes the chromosomes.

*cis*-**acting elements** DNA sequences that affect the expression of genes only on the molecule of DNA where they reside; not protein encoding.

**CK** Creatine kinase. Both mitochondrial and cytosolic isoforms of this enzyme that catalyzes the reversible phosphorylation of creatine by ATP to form the high-energy compound phosphocreatine.

**codon** A 3-nucleotide sequence in mRNA specifying a unique amino acid.

**codon**  A 3-nucleotide sequence in mRNA specifying a unique amino acid.

**complex I**  NADH-ubiquinone oxidoreductase.

**complex II**  Succinate CoQ oxidoreductase.

**complex III**  CoQ-cytochrome *c* oxidoreductase.

**complex IV**  Cytochrome *c* oxidase.

**complex V**  Oligomycin-sensitive ATP synthase. Also termed $F_0$-$F_1$ ATPase.

**CoQ**  Coenzyme Q (also ubiquinone). Electron carrier and antioxidant.

**COX**  Cytochrome *c* oxidase (complex IV).

**CP**  Cardioprotection.

**CPEO**  Chronic progressive external ophthalmoplegia.

**CPT-I**  Carnitine palmitoyltransferase I.

**CPT-II**  Carnitine palmitoyltransferase II.

**CpG islands**: GC-rich regions of DNA often found in promoter regions.

**cristae**  Folding of inner mitochondrial membrane to enlarge the surface area.

**CsA**  Cyclosporin A. An inhibitor of PT pore opening.

**CyP-D**  Cyclophilin D. CsA-binding matrix protein component of the PT pore

**cybrid**  Hybrid cell created by the fusion of an enucleated with a nucleated cell. The enucleated cell typically contributes the mitochondria, whereas the nucleated cell may or may not have mtDNA.

**cytochrome**  A family of proteins that contain heme as a prosthetic group involved in electron transfer and identifiable by their absorption spectra.

**cytoplast**  Cell devoid of nuclei used in the generation of transmitochondrial cybrids.

**CVD**  Cardiovascular disease.

**DCCD**  Dicyclohexylcarbodiimide. An inhibitor of mitochondrial oligomycin-sensitive ATPase binding covalently to the c subunit blocking proton transfer.

**doxorubicin**  Also called *adriamycin*. Used to treat leukemia but also causes extensive mitochondrial defects and induces cardiomyopathy.

**dexrazoxane**  Antioxidant that prevents site Fe-based oxidative damage by chelating free iron; provides clinical cardioprotection against doxorubicin-induced oxidative damage.

**D loop** Noncoding regulatory region of mtDNA involved in controlling its replication and transcription.

**DQAsomes** Liposome-like vesicles formed in aqueous medium with a dicationic amphiphile dequalinium used as a mitochondrial-specific delivery system for gene therapy.

**DCM** Dilated cardiomyopathy.

**DCA** Dichloroacetate. By inhibiting PDH kinase, DCA stimulates PDH, promoting aerobic oxidation and reducing lactic acidosis.

**DNP** Dinitrophenol; uncoupling agent.

**differential display** Technique used to identify genes that are differentially expressed; RNA from the samples being compared is reverse transcribed, and the cDNA is further amplified using random primers. Genes that are differentially expressed in the chosen samples can be identified by electrophoresis.

**electroporation** Method to transfect cells with either exogenous genes or proteins using electrical field.

**epigenetic** Acquired and reversible modification of genetic material (e.g., methylation).

**ETC** Electron transport chain. A series of complexes in the mitochondrial inner membrane to conduct electrons from the oxidation of NADH and succinate to oxygen.

**ER** Endoplasmic reticulum. A membrane-bound cytosolic compartment where lipids and membrane-bound proteins are synthesized.

**ERK** Extracellular regulated kinase.

**ES** Embryonic stem cell.

**EST** Expressed sequence tags.

**exon** Segment of a gene that remains after the splicing of the primary RNA transcript and contains the coding sequences as well as 5' and 3 untranslated regions.

**expression vector** A vector that contains elements necessary for high-level and accurate transcription and translation of an inserted cDNA in a particular host or tissue.

**FAD** Flavin adenine dinucleotide. Common coenzyme of dehydrogenases; in the ETC, FAD is covalently linked to SDH.

**FADH$_2$** Flavin adenine dinucleotide (reduced form).

**FAO** Fatty acid oxidation.

**FMN** Flavin mononucleotide. A cofactor of complex I.

**Fp** Flavoprotein subunit of complex II.

**FRDA**   Friedreich ataxia. An autosomal-dominant neuromuscular disorder with frequent HCM caused by mutations in gene for frataxin, a mitochondrial-localized protein.

**glycolysis**  Cytosolic-located metabolic pathway present in all cells catalyzing the anaerobic conversion of glucose to pyruvate.

**GPx**  Glutathione peroxidase. An antioxidant enzyme with both mitochondrial and cytosolic isoforms.

**GSH**  Glutathione.

**GTP**  Guanosine triphosphate.

**G protein**   A heterotrimeric membrane-associated GTP-binding protein involved in cell-signaling pathways; activated by specific hormone or ligand binding to a 7-helix transmembrane receptor protein.

**genome**  Total genetic information carried by a cell or an organism.

**genetic code**   Correspondence between nucleotide triplets (codon) and specific amino acids in proteins.

**gene product**  The protein, tRNA, or rRNA encoded by a gene.

**genomic library**  Collection of DNA fragments (each inserted into a vector molecule) representative of the entire genome.

**genotype**  Genetic constitution of a cell or an organism.

**HCM**  Hypertrophic cardiomyopathy.

**heteroplasmy**  Presence of more than 1 genotype in a cell.

**homoplasmy**  Presence of a single genotype in a cell.

**helicase**  Enzymes that separate the strands of DNA.

**HSP**  Heat-shock protein. A family of chaperones involved in protein folding.

**hybridization**  Binding of nucleic acid sequences through complementary base pairing. The hybridization rate is influenced by temperature, G-C composition, extent of homology, and length of the sequences involved.

**hydrophobic**  Lipophilic; insoluble in water.

**ionophore**  Small hydrophobic molecule that promotes the transfer of specific ions through the membrane bilayer.

**intermembrane space**  Space between inner and outer membranes.

**intron**  A segment of a nuclear gene that is transcribed into the primary RNA transcript but is excised during RNA splicing and not present in the mature transcript.

**IPC**  Ischemic preconditioning.

**IRE**  Iron-responsive element.

**iron-sulfur center**  Nonheme iron ions complexed with cysteine chains and inorganic sulfide atoms making a protein capable of conducting electrons in electron transport or redox reactions.

**IRP**  Iron-responsive protein.

**isoforms**  Related form of the same protein generated by alternative splicing, transcriptional starts or encoded by entirely different genes.

**integral membrane protein**  Protein with at least 1 transmembrane segment requiring detergent for solubilization.

**KCOs**  Potassium channel openers (e.g., nicorandil, diazoxide, and pinacidil); can mediate cardioprotection.

**Krebs cycle**  Central metabolic pathway of aerobic respiration occurring in the mitochondrial matrix; involves oxidation of acetyl groups derived from pyruvate to $CO_2$, NADH, and $H_2O$. The NADH from this cycle is a central substrate in the OXPHOS pathway. Also termed *TCA* or *citric acid cycle*.

**KSS**  Kearns-Sayre syndrome. A mitochondrial neuropathy characterized by ptosis, ophthalmoplegia, and retinopathy with frequent cardiac conduction defects and cardiomyopathy

**knockout mutation**  A null mutation in a gene, abolishing its function (usually in mouse); allows evaluation of its phenotypic role.

**LCAD**  Long-chain acyl CoA dehydrogenase involved in FAO.

**LCHAD**  Long-chain 3-hydroxylacyl-CoA dehydrogenase.

**LHON**  Leber hereditary optical neuropathy.

**ligand**  Any molecule that binds to a specific site on a protein or a receptor molecule.

**ligase**  Enzymes that join together 2 molecules in an energy dependent process; involved in DNA replication and repair.

**MAP kinase**  Mitogen-activated protein kinases. A family of conserved serine/threonine protein kinases activated as a result of a wide range of signals involved in cell proliferation and differentiation; includes JNK and ERK.

**matrix**  Space enclosed by the mitochondrial inner membrane.

**MELAS**  Mitochondrial encephalomyopathy with lactic acidosis and strokelike episodes

**membrane potential**  Combination of proton and ion gradients across the inner membrane making the inside negative relative to the outside.

**MERRF**  Mitochondrial cytopathy including myotonus, epilepsy, and ragged-red fibers.

**MSC**  Mesenchymal stem cells.

**MCM** Mitochondrial cardiomyopathy.

**microarray** A range of oligonucleotides immobilized onto a surface (chip) that can be hybridized to determine quantitative transcript expression or mutation detection.

**mitoK$_{ATP}$ channel** Activation of the ATP-sensitive inner-membrane mitoK$_{ATP}$ channel has been implicated as a central signaling event (both as trigger and end effector) in IPC and other CP pathways.

**mitoplast** Mitochondrial preparation without outer membrane.

**mobile carrier** Small molecule shuttling electrons between complexes in the mitochondrial ETC.

**modifier gene** A gene that modifies a trait encoded by another gene.

**mRNA** Messenger RNA. Specifies the amino acid sequence of a protein; translated into protein on ribosomes.

**mtDNA polymorphism** Presence of mtDNA differing in size (due to either insertions or deletions) or in single nucleotide sequence.

**mtDNA** Mitochondrial DNA.

**mtTFA** Mitochondrial transcription factor A (also called *TFAM*).

**MT** Metallothionein. An inducible antioxidant metal-binding protein with cardioprotective properties.

**mTOR** Mammalian target of rapamycin.

**MTP** Mitochondrial trifunctional protein, part of mitochondrial FAO.

**NADH** Nicotinamide adenine dinucleotide (reduced form).

**NARP** Neuropathy, ataxia, retinitis pigmentosa.

**NO** Nitric oxide; vasodilator.

**NOS** Nitric oxide synthase.

**ND1** One of 7 ND subunits in mtDNA encoding complex I.

**NER** Nucleotide excision repair

**nonmendelian inheritance** Cytoplasmic inheritance due to genes located in mitochondria.

**northern blot** Molecular technique by which RNA separated by electrophoresis is transferred and immobilized for the detection of specific transcripts by hybridization with a labeled probe.

**NRF-1 and NRF-2** Nuclear respiratory factor.

**nt** nucleotide, the basic unit of DNA composed of a purine or pyrimidine base, a sugar, and a phosphate group.

**nucleases** Enzymes that catalyze the degradation of DNA (DNAse) or RNA (RNAse); specific nucleases have been identified that target either the 5' or 3' ends of DNA (exonuclease) or that can digest nucleic acids from internal sites (endonucleases).

**null mutation** Ablation or knockout of a gene.

$O_L$  Origin of replication for mtDNA, light strand.

$O_H$  Origin of replication for mtDNA, heavy strand.

**oligonucleotide**  Short polymer of DNA or RNA that is usually synthetic in origin.

**OXPHOS**  Oxidative phosphorylation. A process in mitochondria in which ATP formation is driven by electron transfer from NADH and $FADH_2$ to molecular oxygen and by the generation of a pH gradient and chemiosmotic coupling.

**oligomycin**  Specific inhibitor of mitochondrial ATP synthase and OXPHOS.

**PAGE**  Polyacrylamide gel electrophoresis.

**PARP**  Poly (ADP-ribose) polymerase.

**PCR**  Polymerase chain reaction. An amplification of DNA fragments using a thermostabile DNA polymerase and paired oligonucleotide primers subjected to repeated reactions with thermal cycling.

**PDH**  Pyruvate dehydrogenase.

**pharmacogenetics**  Study of the role of inheritance in interindividual variation in drug response.

**PNA**: Peptide nucleic acids; an alternative delivery system for nucleic acids to mitochondria.

**peptide**  Short polymer of amino acids that can be produced synthetically.

**peripheral membrane protein**  Protein associated with membrane via protein protein interactions; solubilized by changes in pH or salt.

**pFOX**  Partial fatty acid oxidation.

**peroxisome**  Small membrane-bounded organelle that uses oxygen to oxidize organic molecules, including fatty acids and contain enzymes that generate and degrade hydrogen peroxide ($H_2O_2$) (e.g., catalase).

**PGC-1α**  Peroxisome proliferator-activated receptor gamma co-activator. Transcriptional regulator of mitochondrial bioenergetic and biogenesis operative during physiological transitions.

**phenotype**  Observable physical characteristics of a cell or organism resulting from the interaction of its genetic constitution (genotype) with its environment.

**PKA**  Protein kinase A. Activated by cAMP.

**PKB**  Protein kinase B; also called *Akt*.

**PKC**  Protein kinase C.

**PI3K**  Phosphatidylinositol 3-kinase.

**PT pore**  Permeability transition pore. A non-specific megachannel in the mitochondrial inner membrane.

**PUFA** Polyunsaturated fatty acids.

**plasmid** DNA capable of autonomous existence in an organism; can replicate and maintain itself without integrating into the genome used as a vector.

**pleiotropic mutation** A single mutation with multiple (often unrelated) effects on an organism.

**polyadenylation** Addition of a sequence of polyadenylic acid (poly A residues) to the 3' end of RNA after its translation.

**polygenic** A large number of genes each contributing a small amount to the phenotype.

**porin** Pore-forming protein in the outer mitochondrial membrane (see VDAC).

**PPAR** Peroxisome proliferator-activated receptor.

**primer** Short nucleotide sequence that is paired with 1 strand of DNA and provides a free 3'-OH end at which a DNA polymerase starts the synthesis of a nascent chain.

**promoter** Region of DNA involved in the binding of RNA polymerase to initiate transcription.

**proteome** Entire complement of proteins contained within the eukaryotic cell.

**protein kinase** Enzyme that transfers the terminal phosphate group of ATP to a specific amino acid of a target protein.

**posttranslational modification** Postsynthetic modification of proteins by glycosylation, phosphorylation, proteolytic cleavage, or other covalent changes involving side chains or termini.

**redox reactions** Oxidation-reduction reactions in which there is a transfer of electrons from an electron donor (the reducing agent) to an electron acceptor (oxidizing agent).

**rRNA** Ribosomal RNA. A central component of the ribosome.

**ROS** Reactive oxygen species, including superoxide, hydroxyl radicals, and hydrogen peroxide.

**RFLP** Restriction fragment-length polymorphism. A variation in the length of restriction fragments due to presence or absence of a restriction site.

**RRF** Ragged red fiber.

**restriction endonucleases** Endonucleases that recognize a specific sequence in a DNA molecule (usually palindromic) and cleave the DNA at or near that site.

**rho$^0$ cells** Cells containing no mitochondrial DNA.

**rhodamine 123** A fluorescent dye used to stain mitochondria in living cells.

**Rieske Fe-S protein** A subunit and electron carrier of complex III.

**rotenone** Specific inhibitor of complex I activity.

**RXR** Retinoid X receptor. On binding 9-cis retinoic acid, RXR acts as a heterodimer and as a repressor or activator of specific gene transcription, playing a key role in cardiac development and physiological gene expression.

**SCAD** Short-chain acyl CoA dehydrogenase involved in FAO.

**SDH** Succinate dehydrogenase. A TCA cycle enzyme associated with complex II.

**SAGE** Serial analysis of gene expression. Quantitative analysis of RNA transcripts by using short sequence tags to generate a characteristic expression profile.

**signal sequence** N-terminal sequence for targeting proteins into mitochondria.

**SDS** Sodium dodecyl sulfate. An ionic detergent used for the solubilization, denaturation of proteins, and their size separation in PAGE.

**SNP** Single nucleotide polymorphism.

**SOD** Superoxide dismutase. An antioxidant ROS-scavenging enzyme with both mitochondrial and cytosolic isoforms.

**splicing** Reaction in the nucleus in which introns are removed from primary nuclear RNA and exons joined to generate mRNA.

**state 3** Respiration in coupled mitochondria in which oxygen consumption depends on the availability of ADP.

**state 4** Respiration in the absence of ADP.

**southern blot** Detection of separated restriction fragments after size separation on agarose gels, transfer to membranes and hybridization with labeled gene probes.

**SR** Sarcoplasmic reticulum. A network of internal membranes in muscle-cell cytosol that contains high $Ca^{++}$ concentration, which is released on excitation.

**TAS** Termination associated sequence. A short conserved sequence element in mtDNA that interacts with sequence-specific termination proteins involved in mtDNA replication control.

**tRNA** Transfer RNA. A small RNA molecule used in protein synthesis as an adaptor between mRNA and amino acids.

**TCA cycle** Tricarboxylic acid cycle (see Krebs cycle).

**TNF-α** Tumor necrosis factor α.

**TIM**  Protein complex in mitochondrial inner membrane required for protein import.

**TOM**  Protein complex in mitochondrial outer membrane required for protein import.

**topoisomerases**  Enzymes that change the supercoiling of DNA.

**T3** Triiodothyronine.

**transgenic animal**  Animal that has stably incorporated one or more genes from another cell or organism and can pass them on to successive generations; created by introducing new DNA sequences into the germline.

**transcript**  RNA product of DNA transcription.

**transcription factor**  Protein required for the initiation of transcription by RNA polymerase at specific sites and functioning as a regulatory factor in gene expression.

**transcriptome**  Comprehensive transcript analysis for expression profiling.

**translation**  Synthesis of protein from the mRNA template at the ribosome.

***trans*-acting elements**  Regulatory elements that mediate specific gene expression that are not located within or near the gene (e.g., proteins that bind and regulate specific promoters).

**2-dimensional electrophoresis**  Technique for separating proteins based on their size and charge differences.

**2-hybrid system**  Method to detect proteins that interact with each other using yeast gene expression.

**uncoupler**  Protein or other molecule capable of uncoupling electron transport from oxidative phosphorylation..

**UCP**  Uncoupling protein.

**VDAC**  Voltage-dependent anion channel (see porin).

**VLCAD**  Very long-chain acyl CoA-dehydrogenase; $\beta$-oxidation of fatty acids.

**western blot**  Immunochemical detection of proteins immobilized on a filter after size separation by PAGE.

**wild-type**  The common genotype or phenotype of a given organism occurring in nature.

**xenocybrid**  $Rho^{0}$ cells of 1 species repopulated with mitochondria from another species.

# INDEX

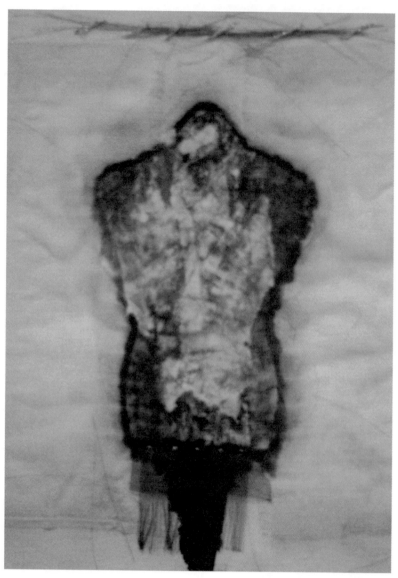

*"Aging"*                      *Danièle M. Marín*

Private Collection